Mosby's Review *for the*

PHARMACY TECHNICIAN CERTIFICATION EXAMINATION

Mosby's Review *for the*
PHARMACY TECHNICIAN CERTIFICATION EXAMINATION

SECOND EDITION

James J. Mizner Jr., MBA, RPh
Pharmacy Technician Program Director
ACT College
Arlington, Virginia

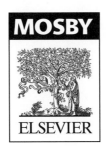

MOSBY

ELSEVIER

MOSBY
ELSEVIER

11830 Westline Industrial Drive
St. Louis, Missouri 63146

Mosby's Review for the Pharmacy Technician Certification Examination
ISBN: 978-1-4160-6204-2

Notice

Knowledge and best practice in this field are constantly changing. As new research and experience broaden our knowledge, changes in practice, treatment and drug therapy may become necessary or appropriate. Readers are advised to check the most current information provided (i) on procedures featured or (ii) by the manufacturer of each product to be administered, to verify the recommended dose or formula, the method and duration of administration, and contraindications. It is the responsibility of the practitioner, relying on their own experience and knowledge of the patient, to make diagnoses, to determine dosages and the best treatment for each individual patient, and to take all appropriate safety precautions. To the fullest extent of the law, neither the Publisher nor the Author assumes any liability for any injury and/or damage to persons or property arising out of or related to any use of the material contained in this book.

The Publisher

Library of Congress Cataloging-in-Publication Data
Mizner, James J.
    Mosby's review for the pharmacy technician certification examination / James J. Mizner Jr.—2nd ed.
        p. ; cm.
    Rev. ed. of: Mosby's review for the PTCB certification examination / James J. Mizner Jr. 2006.
    Includes bibliographical references and index.
    ISBN 978-1-4160-6204-2 (pbk. : alk. paper)
    1. Pharmacy technicians–Examinations, questions, etc. I. Mizner, James J. Mosby's review for the PTCB certification examination. II. Title. III. Title: Review for the pharmacy technician certification examination.
    [DNLM: 1. Pharmacy–Examination Questions. 2. Pharmacists' Aides–Examination Questions.   QV 18.2 M685m 2010]
    RS122.95.M59 2010
    615'.1076—dc22

                                                    2009003177

Publishing Director: Andrew Allen
Acquisitions Editor: Jennifer Janson
Developmental Editor: Kelly Brinkman
Publishing Services Manager: Patricia Tannian
Project Manager: Carrie Stetz
Designer: Paula Catalano

Last digit is the print number: 9 8 7 6 5 4 3 2

Mosby's Review for the Pharmacy Technician Certification Examination is dedicated to my wife, Mary, and son, Andrew. They have been very supportive of me throughout my life and are my source of inspiration.

Reviewers

Marcy May, Med, CPhT, PhTR
Austin Community College
Austin, Texas

Richard Nunez, CPhT
Everest College
San Francisco, California

Kathleen M. O'Malley, CPhT
Michigan Workforce Development Agency
Lansing, Michigan

Preface

Pharmacy technicians have become a major asset for both pharmacies and pharmacists in the world today. With an increasing population, longer life spans, patients taking multiple medications, and managed care playing a major role, pharmacies are seeing a major increase in processed prescriptions. A pharmacy cannot be successful in providing medications without knowledgeable pharmacy technicians assisting the pharmacists.

State boards of pharmacy realize the importance of pharmacy technicians in the drug delivery process and are committed to ensuring that pharmacy technicians possess the necessary skills to work in a pharmacy. Within the past year, Congress has been discussing the need for education and certification of **all** pharmacy technicians.

At present two organizations certify pharmacy technicians: the Pharmacy Technician Certification Board (PTCB) and the Institute for the Certification of Pharmacy Technicians (ICPT). Both organizations are accredited by the National Commission for Certifying Agencies (NCCA). The PTCB has certified more than 310,000 pharmacy technicians, and its examination is approved by 45 state boards of pharmacy. The ICPT is recognized by 32 state boards of pharmacy and has certified more than 3000 pharmacy technicians.

Mosby's Review for the Pharmacy Technician Certification Examination has been written to assist a pharmacy technician studying for the PTCB examination or the Exam for the Certification of Pharmacy Technicians (ExCPT). *Mosby's Review for the Pharmacy Technician Certification Examination* is meant to be used to augment either a formalized pharmacy technician training program or on-the-job training, not replace it. This text has been designed to review the compe-

tencies covered on the PTCB examination and material on the ExCPT. Each section of this review book is followed by multiple-choice questions similar to the type of questions seen on either of these two exams. At the end of this review book are sample tests for the student to demonstrate competency of the material expected of a pharmacy technician.

Enhancements to the second edition of *Mosby's Review for the Pharmacy Technician Certification Examination* include:

- New drug entities that have been approved by the FDA since the first edition
- An update on laws affecting the practice of pharmacy
- A discussion on USP <797>
- Six multiple-choice paper-based practice tests
- Ten multiple-choice computer-based tests
- Additional flash cards focusing on the practice of pharmacy, over-the-counter products, and herbal products

In 2008 the PTCB changed its format from a paper-based test to a computer-based test and reduced the number of questions on the examination from 140 to 100. *Mosby's Review for the Pharmacy Technician Certification Examination* is the only product currently on the market that features this format. Each question contained on either the paper or computer-based examination offers the rationale for the correct response.

The pharmacy technician should use *Mosby's Review for the Pharmacy Technician Certification Examination* as a guide to determine which topics he or she may need additional assistance in studying for either the PTCB examination or ExCPT. Good luck on the test and in your new career.

James J. Mizner Jr., MBA, RPh

Contents

Pretest

1. Which route of administration has the quickest onset of action?
   a. IM
   b. IV
   c. PO
   d. PR

2. If a physician prescribes 250 mg qid for 10 days, how many milliliters of Keflex oral suspension containing 250 mg/5 mL should be dispensed?
   a. 75 mL
   b. 100 mL
   c. 150 mL
   d. 200 mL

3. How many 250-mg capsules are needed to fill the following prescription: amoxicillin 500 mg tid for 10 days?
   a. 20
   b. 40
   c. 60
   d. 80

4. What is the percentage strength of a 1:1500 solution?
   a. 0.0006
   b. 0.0066
   c. 0.0666
   d. 0.6666

5. How should Nitrostat tablets be taken?
   a. PO
   b. PRT
   c. SC
   d. SL

6. How many grams are in 30 gr?
   a. 0.2 g
   b. 1.95 g
   c. 19.5 g
   d. 195 g

7. What is the maximum number of refills allowed on a prescription of lorazepam if authorized by a physician?
   a. None
   b. Five
   c. 12
   d. Unlimited

8. Which of the following reference books discusses the therapeutic equivalence of products?
   a. *Drug Topics Blue Book*
   b. *Drug Topics Green Book*
   c. *Drug Topics Orange Book*
   d. *Drug Topics Red Book*

9. What is the brand name for paroxetine?
   a. Effexor
   b. Paxil
   c. Prozac
   d. Zoloft

10. What is the generic name for Lodine?
    a. Diflunisal
    b. Etodolac
    c. Ibuprofen
    d. Oxaprozin

11. How many grams of hydrocortisone powder should be used to prepare 1 lb of a 0.25% hydrocortisone cream?
    a. 1.14 g
    b. 1.2 g
    c. 113.5 g
    d. 120 g

12. What is the meaning of the abbreviation of "ut dict"?
    a. As directed
    b. As needed
    c. If there is need
    d. Ointment

13. What is the meaning of the suffix *-dipsia*?
    a. Discharge
    b. Hardening
    c. Pain
    d. Thirst

14. Which organization is responsible for accrediting pharmacy education programs?
    a. ACCP
    b. ACPE
    c. APhA
    d. ASHP

15. How many tablets should be dispensed on the following prescription?

    Flagyl 250 2-week supply
    ī tab PO qid c̄ food for 2 wk for both patient and partner. No alcohol

    a. 14
    b. 28
    c. 56
    d. 112

16. What is the generic name for Augmentin?
    a. Amoxicillin-clavulanate
    b. Ampicillin-sulbactam
    c. Piperacillin-tazobactam
    d. Ticarcillin-clavulanate

17. Which of the following is not a required text in a pharmacy?
    a. A copy of the Controlled Substances Act
    b. NF
    c. PDR
    d. USP

18. Which of the following medications should be tapered off at discontinuation?
    a. Fexofenadine
    b. INH
    c. Prednisone
    d. SMZ-TMP

19. Which of the following products can be purchased as an exempt narcotic if all conditions outlined by the federal Controlled Substances Act are met?
    a. Phenobarbital
    b. Robitussin A-C
    c. Stadol NS
    d. Tussionex

20. What is the maximum weighable amount for a Class A prescription balance?
    a. 0.6 g
    b. 6 g
    c. 60 g
    d. 120 g

21. In what schedule is acetaminophen with codeine placed?
    a. II
    b. III
    c. IV
    d. V

22. In which classification of medication does acyclovir belong?
    a. Analgesic
    b. Antibiotic
    c. Antifungal
    d. Antiviral

23. How many grams of solute are in 1 L of 5% (w/v) solution?
    a. 0.5 g
    b. 5 g
    c. 50 g
    d. 5000 g

24. Which of the following products is not a combination product?
    a. Bactrim DS
    b. Dyazide
    c. Estrace
    d. Prempro

25. What is the percentage strength of an ointment if one mixes 10 g of hydrocortisone into Aquaphor to make 400 g?
    a. 0.025%
    b. 0.25%
    c. 2.5%
    d. 25%

26. What type of filter is used to prevent glass from entering the final solution when drawing from an ampule?
    a. Depth filter
    b. Filter needle
    c. Filter straw
    d. Final filter

27. In which drug classification does Singulair belong?
    a. Bronchodilator
    b. Corticosteroid
    c. Leukotriene inhibitor
    d. Xanthine derivative

28. How many grams are in 600 mL of a 1:200 (w/v) solution of a drug?
    a. 0.03 g
    b. 0.3 g
    c. 3 g
    d. 30 g

29. Why is it necessary to rotate medications on a shelf?
    a. To allocate shelf space effectively.
    b. To ensure the medication with the shortest dating is dispensed before drugs with longer dating to reduce the possibility that the medication will expire before being dispensed.
    c. To prevent dust from accumulating on the shelf.
    d. To prevent overstock from occurring.

30. Which of the following pharmacy abbreviations tells that a medication order is needed immediately?
    a. ASAP
    b. dtd
    c. NOW
    d. STAT

31. Which pharmacy legislation requires that tamper-proof pads be used for Medicaid patients?
    a. Anabolic Steroid Control Act of 2004
    b. Combat Methamphetamine Epidemic Act of 2006
    c. Isotretinoin Safety and Risk Management Act of 2004
    d. Medicaid Tamper-Resistant Prescriptions Act

32. What letter indicates a midlevel practitioner, such as a nurse practitioner or physician's assistant, who may prescribe controlled substances?
    a. A
    b. B
    c. F
    d. M

33. Which of the following medications is not a combination product?
    a. Estratest
    b. Hyzaar
    c. Lotrel
    d. Remeron

34. What is the sensitivity of a Class A prescription balance?
    a. 0.6 mg
    b. 6.0 mg
    c. 60 mg
    d. 100 mg

35. Which of the following insulin syringes is not available?
    a. One that can contain 30 units of insulin
    b. One that can contain 50 units of insulin
    c. One that can contain 100 units of insulin
    d. One that can contain 125 units of insulin

36. Which of the following are the two most common floor stock large-volume parenteral solutions?
    a. D5W and 0.45% NS
    b. D5W and 0.9% NS
    c. D5W and sterile water for injection
    d. 0.9% NS and sterile water for injection

37. What must be found on all controlled substance prescriptions?
    a. Pharmacy DEA number
    b. Physician's business license number
    c. Physician's DEA number
    d. Physician's license number

38. In which schedule does meperidine belong?
    a. II
    b. III
    c. IV
    d. V

39. Which association represents the interests of chain drugstores?
    a. APHA
    b. NABP
    c. NACDS
    d. NCPA

40. Which term refers to mistreatment of a patient based on age, gender, race, or sexual orientation?
    a. Decorum
    b. Discrimination
    c. Harassment
    d. Innuendo

41. An effervescent tablet has the following formula:

APAP	325 mg
CaCO$_3$	280 mg
Citric acid	900 mg
Potassium bicarbonate	300 mg
Sodium bicarbonate	465 mg

    How many grams would one tablet contain?
    a. 0.227 g
    b. 2.27 g
    c. 22.7 g
    d. 227 g

42. What is the generic name for Serevent?
    a. Albuterol
    b. Beclomethasone
    c. Salmeterol
    d. Triamcinolone

43. What is the weight in grams of 4 fl oz of orange peel with a specific gravity of 0.844?
    a. 84 g
    b. 101 g
    c. 112 g
    d. 142 g

44. Nitroglycerin is to nitrate as nifedipine is to:
    a. ACE inhibitor
    b. Beta-blocker
    c. Calcium channel blocker
    d. Loop diuretic

45. How many milligrams of atropine sulfate are needed to make 30 mL of a 1:200 solution?
    a. 1.5 mg
    b. 15 mg
    c. 150 mg
    d. 1500 mg

46. What is the brand name for allopurinol?
    a. Anturane
    b. Colchicine
    c. Col-Probenecid
    d. Zyloprim

47. Which of the following medications is not indicated as a smoking cessation drug?
    a. Chantix
    b. Cubucin
    c. Nicorette
    d. Zyban

48. Which of the following drugs may be used prophylactically for influenza and Parkinson's disease?
    a. Amantadine
    b. Bromocriptine
    c. Levodopa-carbidopa
    d. Selegiline

49. Which oral antidepressant is also used as a topical preparation?
    a. Amitriptyline
    b. Doxepin
    c. Imipramine
    d. Nortriptyline

50. How much time does a physician have to provide a written prescription for an "emergency prescription" for a Schedule II drug?
    a. 24 hours
    b. 48 hours
    c. 72 hours
    d. 7 days

51. The average adult dose of Tylenol is 650 mg every 6 hr. If the patient is 5 years old and weighs 54 lb and if Tylenol is available as a 160 mg/5 mL elixir, how many milliliters should be given to the patient if Clark's rule is used?
    a. 5.97 mL
    b. 7.31 mL
    c. 191 mL
    d. 234 mL

52. What is the generic name for Celexa?
    a. Citalopram
    b. Phenelzine
    c. Selegiline
    d. Tranylcypromine

53. Which of the following is not a patient's right covered under HIPAA?
    a. The right to request an amendment to his or her health record
    b. The right to obtain an accounting of any disclosures of his or her protected health information
    c. The right to obtain a copy of his or her designated record set of protected health information
    d. The right to receive compensatory and punitive damage for violations of HIPAA

54. Which form is used to inform a drug manufacturer of errors caused by commercial packaging and labeling?
    a. FDA Form 79
    b. MedWatch
    c. MERF
    d. USP-ISMP

55. You have received a medication order to prepare 500 mL of a 1:500 solution. The pharmacy has in stock a concentrate of 80%. How much of the concentrate will you need to use?
    a. 1 mL
    b. 1.25 mL
    c. 498.75 mL
    d. 499 mL

56. A physician orders KCl 40 mEq to be added to D5W 1000 mL and administered over 4 hr. The injection solution on hand is KCl 2 mEq/mL. How many milliliters of KCl should be added?
    a. 40 mL
    b. 8 mL
    c. 16 mL
    d. 20 mL

57. You have been asked to prepare 1 L of a 2% (w/v) solution. You have a 100% solution in stock. How much diluent will be needed?
    a. 2.0 mL
    b. 20 mL
    c. 200 mL
    d. 980 mL

58. If an injectable drug is labeled 0.5 mcg/2 mL and the patient is to receive 0.125 mcg, how many milliliters should the patient receive?
    a. 0.5 mL
    b. 1.0 mL
    c. 1.5 mL
    d. 2.0 mL

59. How many grams of NaCl are in 100 mL of NS solution?
    a. 0.009 g
    b. 0.09 g
    c. 0.9 g
    d. 9 g

60. Which of the following medications is approved for the treatment of diabetes?
    a. Januvia
    b. Lunesta
    c. Remeron
    d. Telithromycin

61. Which part of Medicare pays for prescriptions for senior citizens if enrolled in the prescription component of Medicare?
    a. Part A
    b. Part B
    c. Part C
    d. Part D

62. In what drug classification is quinapril?
    a. ACE inhibitor
    b. Alpha-blocker
    c. Beta-blocker
    d. Calcium channel blocker

63. Which of the following OTC medications must be recorded in a book before it is sold to the customer?
    a. Acetaminophen
    b. Pseudoephedrine
    c. Ranitidine
    d. Simethicone

64. Which of the following is an example of a drug with a sublingual dosage form?
    a. Amoxicillin
    b. Depakote
    c. Nitrostat
    d. Synthroid

65. Which of the following medications is an angiotensin II receptor antagonist?
    a. Acebutolol
    b. Clonidine
    c. Losartan
    d. Terazosin

66. Which of the following classes of antibiotics should not be taken with either fruit juices or colas?
    a. Macrolides
    b. Penicillins
    c. Quinolones
    d. Sulfas

67. If a patient is experiencing nausea and vomiting, which of the following dosage forms would be more effective?
    a. Capsule
    b. Oral solution
    c. Suppository
    d. Tablet

68. Which of the following drugs is not a bronchodilator?
    a. Albuterol
    b. Ipratropium bromide
    c. Salmeterol
    d. Theophylline

69. Which of the following medications is not a calcium channel blocker?
    a. Diovan
    b. Isoptin
    c. Plendil
    d. Tiazac

70. Drugs in which classification may cause rhinitis medicamentosa with repeated use?
    a. Antihistamines
    b. Corticosteroids
    c. Nasal decongestants
    d. Xanthine derivatives

71. How many grams of fluorouracil will a 154-lb patient receive in 5 successive days at a dose of 12 mg/kg/day?
    a. 0.42 g
    b. 0.84 g
    c. 4.2 g
    d. 8.4 g

72. Which type of syringe is used to administer an oral liquid medication to a patient?
    a. Adapt-a-Cap
    b. Hypodermic with Luer-Lok tip
    c. Hypodermic with slip tip
    d. Oral syringe

73. Which of the following medications is not a proton pump inhibitor?
    a. AcipHex
    b. Concerta
    c. Prevacid
    d. Protonix

74. How many milliliters of 95% (v/v) alcohol and 30% (v/v) alcohol should be mixed to prepare 1000 mL of a 50% (v/v) solution?
    a. 30%: 307 mL; 95%: 693 mL
    b. 30%: 444 mL; 95%: 556 mL
    c. 30%: 556 mL; 95%: 444 mL
    d. 30%: 693 mL; 95%: 307 mL

75. How many capsules each containing 250 mg of chloramphenicol are needed to provide 50 mg/kg/day for 10 days for an adult weighing 187 lb?
    a. 17
    b. 82
    c. 170
    d. 822

76. What type of drug is used to facilitate an examination or come to a conclusion regarding a condition or disease?
    a. Destructive agent
    b. Diagnostic agent
    c. Prophylactic agent
    d. Therapeutic agent

77. Which disease is characterized by glycosuria, polydipsia, and polyuria?
    a. Addison disease
    b. Cushing disease
    c. Diabetes
    d. Hypertension

78. Which of the following medications is not used to treat angina?
    a. Isosorbide dinitrate
    b. Isosorbide mononitrate
    c. Lisinopril
    d. Nitroglycerin

79. What should a pharmacy technician do if he or she observes a patient attempting to purchase Bayer aspirin while he or she is waiting for a prescription for warfarin to be filled by the pharmacy?
    a. Inform the patient of the interaction between aspirin and warfarin.
    b. Inform the pharmacist of the situation, and allow the pharmacist to counsel the patient.
    c. Point out to the patient that the "house brand" of aspirin is just as effective as Bayer aspirin.
    d. Refuse to sell the aspirin to the patient.

80. What would a message of "NDC Not Covered" indicate to the pharmacy technician?
    a. The medication has been recalled by the FDA.
    b. The patient's insurance plan does not cover the drug.
    c. The medication is a controlled substance.
    d. The medication has been backordered by the wholesaler.

81. Which of the following is the generic name for Intron?
    a. Interferon alfa-2a
    b. Interferon alfa-2b
    c. Interferon beta-1a
    d. Interferon beta-1b

82. What type of information should be collected from the patient or representative before a prescription is processed?
    a. Disease states of the patient
    b. Drug allergies
    c. Medications taken by the patient, whether prescription or OTC
    d. All the above

83. Which of the following is a prostaglandin E analog?
    a. Alginic acid
    b. Mesalamine
    c. Misoprostol
    d. Sucralfate

84. How many milligrams of epinephrine do you need to prepare 10 mL of a 1:250 epinephrine solution?
    a. 0.00004 mg
    b. 0.04 mg
    c. 40 mg
    d. 400 mg

85. How many fluid ounces of a commercially available 17% solution of benzalkonium chloride should be used to prepare 1 gallon of 1:750 solution?
    a. 0.25 fl oz
    b. 0.5 fl oz
    c. 1.0 fl oz
    d. 29.0 fl oz

86. Which of the following drugs is not used for hyperlipidemia?
    a. Folic acid
    b. Questran
    c. TriCor
    d. Zocor

87. In what drug classification does estradiol belong?
    a. Antibiotic
    b. Beta-blocker
    c. Hormone
    d. NSAID

88. Which of the following should not be mixed with Sandimmune?
    a. Carbonated beverages
    b. Chocolate milk
    c. Milk
    d. Orange juice

89. Inderal is to beta-blocker as Nasonex is to:
    a. ACE inhibitor
    b. H_2 antagonist
    c. MAOI
    d. Topical corticosteroid

90. A 143-lb patient is to receive nitroprusside 50 mg in 250 mL of an IV solution. The patient is to receive 5 mcg/kg/min. How many milligrams per hour will the patient receive?
    a. 4.29 mg/hr
    b. 19.5 mg/hr
    c. 42.9 mg/hr
    d. 19,500 mg/hr

91. Which of the following is an advantage of a parenteral drug?
    a. Difficult to reverse an overdose
    b. Rapid onset of action
    c. Possibility of injecting pathogens and pyrogens into the body
    d. Trauma to the body from the needle

92. How many grams of hydrocortisone and precipitated sulfur should be used in preparing the following compound?

    Rx: Hydrocortisone   1%
    Precipitated sulfur   20%
    Zinc oxide paste   ad 60 g

    a. Hydrocortisone 0.6 g; precipitated sulfur 12 g
    b. Hydrocortisone 2.86 g; precipitated sulfur 9.14 g
    c. Hydrocortisone 3 g; precipitated sulfur 9.60 g
    d. Hydrocortisone 6 g; precipitated sulfur 9.6 g

93. Which of the following insulins has the longest duration of action?
    a. Humalog
    b. Ultralente
    c. Regular
    d. NPH

94. Which of the following drugs is not used to treat ADHD?
    a. Amitriptyline
    b. Amphetamine-dextroamphetamine
    c. Desipramine
    d. Methylphenidate

95. Drugs in which of the following classifications are not used to treat congestive heart failure?
    a. ACE inhibitors
    b. Angiotensin II antagonists
    c. Antiarrhythmics
    d. Beta-blockers

96. How many 30-mg tablets of codeine sulfate should be used in preparing the following prescription?

    Rx: Codeine sulfate   15 mg/tsp
    Robitussin ad   120 mL

    a. 4
    b. 8
    c. 12
    d. 16

97. Which term describes the range between the minimum effective concentration and minimum toxic concentration in a blood concentration curve?
    a. Concentration at site of action
    b. Duration of action
    c. Onset of action
    d. Therapeutic window

98. What is the net profit for a prescription that has an acquisition cost of $45.00 and a dispensing cost of $3.75 and retails at $55.00?
    a. $3.75
    b. $6.25
    c. $10.00
    d. $13.75

99. Which of the following is a drug that can be used for status epilepticus?
    a. Carbamazepine
    b. Diazepam
    c. Phenytoin
    d. Primidone

100. If the dose of a drug is 150 mcg, how many doses can be prepared from 0.120 g?
    a. 8
    b. 80
    c. 800
    d. 8000

Assisting the Pharmacist in Serving Patients

FEDERAL, STATE, OR PRACTICE SITE REGULATIONS, CODES OF ETHICS, AND STANDARDS PERTAINING TO THE PRACTICE OF PHARMACY

Ethics: a philosophy of doing the correct action. Good versus evil.

CODE OF ETHICS FOR PHARMACY TECHNICIANS

Preamble

Pharmacy technicians are health care professionals who assist pharmacists in providing possible care for patients. The principles of this code, which apply to pharmacy technicians working in any and all settings, are based on the application and support of the moral obligations that guide the pharmacy profession in relationships with patients, health care professionals, and society.

Principles

- A pharmacy technician's first consideration is to ensure the health and safety of the patient and to use knowledge and skills to the best of his or her ability in serving others.
- A pharmacy technician supports and promotes honesty and integrity in the profession, which includes a duty to observe the law, maintain the highest moral and ethical conduct at all times, and uphold the ethical principles of the profession.
- A pharmacy technician assists and supports the pharmacist in the safe, efficacious, and cost-effective distribution of health services and health care resources.
- A pharmacy technician respects and values the abilities of pharmacists, colleagues, and other health care professionals.
- A pharmacy technician maintains competency in his or her practice and continually enhances his or her professional knowledge and expertise.
- A pharmacy technician respects and supports the confidentiality of a patient's records and discloses pertinent information only with proper authorization.
- A pharmacy technician never assists in the dispensing, promoting, or distribution of medications or medical devices that are not of good quality or do not meet the standards required by law.
- A pharmacy technician does not engage in any activity that will discredit the profession, and will expose, without fear or favor, illegal or unethical conduct in the profession.
- A pharmacy technician associates with and engages in the support of organizations that promote the profession of pharmacy through the use and enhancement of pharmacy technicians.

PHARMACY LAW

NOTE: This review book examines federal laws affecting the practice of pharmacy. Federal law takes precedence over state law unless the state law is stricter than the federal law, in which case the state law takes precedence. Every pharmacy technician must be aware of the state laws affecting the practice of pharmacy in his or her state.

PURE FOOD AND DRUG ACT OF 1906

Enacted in 1906 to prohibit the interstate transportation or sale of adulterated and misbranded food or drugs.

FOOD, DRUG, AND COSMETIC ACT OF 1938 (FDCA 1938)

The U.S. Food and Drug Administration (FDA) was created under FDCA 1938, which required that all new drug applications be filed with the FDA. FDCA 1938 clearly defined adulteration and misbranding of drugs and food products.

Adulteration

- Consisting "in whole or in part of any filthy, putrid, or decomposed substance"
- "[P]repared, packed, or held under unsanitary conditions"
- Prepared in containers "composed, in whole or in part, of any poisonous or deleterious substance"
- Containing unsafe color additives
- Claimed to be or represented as drugs recognized "in an official compendium" but differing in strength, quality, or purity of the drugs

Misbranding

- Labeling that is "false or misleading in any particular"
- Packaging that does not bear a label containing the name and place of business of the manufacturer, packer, or distributor or an accurate quantity of contents or is not conspicuously and clearly labeled with information required by the act
- Failure to carry a label indicating "Warning— May be habit forming" if the product is habit forming
- Failure to "bear the established name of the drug, and in case it carries more than two or more active ingredients, the quantities of the ingredients, the amount of alcohol and also including— whether active or not—the established name and quantity of certain other substances described in the act"
- Failure to label "adequate directions for use" or "adequate warnings against use in certain pathological conditions"
- Products that are "dangerous to health when used in the dosage or manner or duration prescribed, recommended or suggested in the labeling"

DURHAM-HUMPHREY ACT OF 1951

An amendment to FDCA 1938 requiring all products to have adequate directions for use unless they contain the federal legend "Caution: Federal law prohibits dispensing without a prescription."

- Separated drugs into two categories: legend and nonlegend (over the counter [OTC]). A legend drug requires a prescription, whereas an OTC drug does not require a prescription. Prescription medications require the supervision of a physician.
- Allows verbal prescriptions over the telephone.
- Allows refills to be called in from a physician's office.

KEFAUVER-HARRIS AMENDMENT OF 1962

The Kefauver-Harris Amendment requires all medications in the United States to be pure, safe, and effective.

COMPREHENSIVE DRUG ABUSE PREVENTION AND CONTROL ACT OF 1970

The Drug Enforcement Agency (DEA) was created and placed under the supervision of the Department of Justice. Controlled substances are placed in one of five schedules (classifications or categories) based on a potential for abuse and accepted medical use in the United States.

Schedules

Schedule I

No accepted medical use in the United States and possesses an extremely high potential for abuse.

Examples of Schedule I narcotics
- "Crack" cocaine
- Crystal methamphetamine
- Ecstasy
- Hashish
- Hash oil
- Heroin
- Lysergic acid diethylamide (LSD)
- Marijuana
- Mescaline
- Opium
- Phencyclidine palmitate (PCP)
- Peyote
- Psilocybin
- Rohypnol ("roofies")

Schedule II

Has a medical use but has a high abuse potential with severe psychological or physical dependency (Table 1-1).

TABLE **1-1** Examples of Schedule II Medications

BRAND NAME	GENERIC NAME
Adderall	amphetamine and dextroamphetamine
Amytal	amobarbital
Cocaine	cocaine
Codeine	codeine
Demerol	meperidine
Dexedrine	dextroamphetamine
Dilaudid	hydromorphone
Dolophine	methadone
Duragesic	fentanyl
Morphine sulfate	morphine
Numorphan	oxymorphone
OxyContin	oxycodone
Percocet	acetaminophen and oxycodone
Percodan	aspirin and oxycodone
Ritalin	methylphenidate
Seconal	secobarbital
Tylox	acetaminophen and oxycodone

Schedule III

Has accepted medical use, and the abuse potential is less than with Schedule I and II drugs (Table 1-2).

Schedule IV

Abuse potential is less than with Schedule III drugs, but administration may lead to limited physical or psychological dependence.

Schedule V

Abuse potential is less than with Schedule IV drugs; schedule includes exempt narcotics.

Drug Enforcement Agency Registration

Every facility that dispenses controlled substances must be registered with the DEA. The pharmacy registers with the DEA by submitting a DEA Form 224. The pharmacy must renew this registration every 3 years.

Ordering and Receipt

Schedule II

Schedule II medications are ordered by properly completing a DEA Form 222 (a triplicate order form). It must be signed by the individual in whose name the DEA registration is listed. A DEA Form 222 is valid for only 60 days. A DEA Form 222 must be completed with a typewriter, pen, or indelible pencil. Only one item per line, with a maximum of 10 different items per form, is permitted. The number of lines ordered must be totaled on the bottom of the form.

Unused forms must be kept in a secure location in the pharmacy. On receipt of medication, the number of packages must be recorded on a retained copy of Form 222, and the form must be dated and signed by the pharmacist (Figure 1-1). The pharmacist may not use ditto marks for the date or signature. The invoice or packing slip, in addition to the completed DEA Form 222, must be retained in a secure location of the pharmacy for a minimum of 2 years.

Schedules III to V

Drugs in Schedules III, IV, and V may be ordered by any method (written, faxed, or verbal). After receipt, the invoice or packing slip must be dated, signed, stamped with a red C, and retained in a secure location in the pharmacy for a minimum of 2 years.

Retention of Drug Enforcement Agency Records

DEA records are maintained for a minimum of 2 years, kept separately from other invoices, and kept readily retrievable. "Readily retrievable" means separated from normal business records or easily identifiable by an asterisk, a red line, or another visual identifier. A red C must be stamped on Schedule III to V records if they are filed with other invoices. They must be provided to a DEA representative within 72 hours after request.

Defective forms

A form is considered defective if it is incomplete or illegible or shows signs of alteration, erasure, or change. Defective forms must be kept for a minimum of 2 years and be readily retrievable.

Inventories

Initial inventory

The initial inventory is a complete and accurate inventory of all controlled substances before the opening of the first day of business for a pharmacy.

Biennial inventory

The biennial inventory is taken every 2 years after initial inventory is taken. An exact count for Schedule II and an estimated count for Schedule III to V drugs must be performed. Records must be kept for a minimum of 2 years.

Perpetual inventory

The perpetual inventory shows controlled substances received by the facility, supplied to other locations, returned to the pharmacy, and dispensed to patients. A perpetual inventory will show the actual number of units of a drug at a particular moment in time.

TABLE **1-2** Examples of Schedules III and IV Medications

BRAND NAME	GENERIC NAME	SCHEDULE
Ambien	zolpidem	IV
Anexsia	acetaminophen + hydrocodone	III
Ativan	lorazepam	IV
Bontril	phendimetrazine	III
Butisol	butabarbital	IV
Capital with Codeine	acetaminophen + codeine	III
Cylert	pemoline	IV
Dalmane	flurazepam	IV
Darvocet	acetaminophen + propoxyphene	IV
Darvon	propoxyphene	IV
Empirin with Codeine	aspirin + codeine	III
Equanil	meprobamate	IV
Fastin	phentermine	IV
Fioricet with Codeine	acetaminophen + butalbital + caffeine + codeine	IV
Fiorinal	aspirin + butalbital + caffeine	IV
Fiorinal with Codeine	aspirin + butalbital + caffeine + codeine	IV
Halcion	triazolam	IV
Hycodan	hydrocodone	III
Hycomine Compound	hydrocodone + chlorpheniramine + phenylephrine + acetaminophen + caffeine	III
Hycotuss	guaifenesin + hydrocodone	III
Klonopin	clonazepam	IV
Librium	chlordiazepoxide	IV
Lomotil	diphenoxylate + atropine	IV
Lorcet	acetaminophen + hydrocodone	III
Lortab	acetaminophen + hydrocodone	III
Noctec	chloral hydrate	IV
Phenobarbital	phenobarbital	IV
Restoril	temazepam	IV
Robitussin A-C	guaifenesin + codeine	IV
Soma with Codeine	carisoprodol + codeine	III
Sonata	zaleplon	IV
Stadol	butorphanol	IV
Talwin	pentazocine	IV
Talwin Nx	pentazocine + naloxone	IV
Tenuate	diethylpropion	IV
Tranxene	clorazepate	IV
Tussionex	chlorpheniramine + hydrocodone	III
Tylenol with Codeine	acetaminophen + codeine	III
Valium	diazepam	IV
Vicodin	acetaminophen + hydrocodone	III
Vicoprofen	ibuprofen + hydrocodone	III
Wygesic	acetaminophen + propoxyphene	IV
Xanax	alprazolam	IV

Return of controlled substances

Controlled substances can be returned only between DEA registrants. The DEA Form 222 is the official document for the transfer of Schedule II medications. Controlled substances cannot be returned from long-term care facilities because these facilities do not have a DEA number.

Destruction of outdated or damaged controlled substances

A DEA Form 41 must be submitted to the DEA, indicating the name, strength, and quantities of controlled substances, the date of destruction, the method of destruction, and witnesses present for the destruction. A retail pharmacy may submit one DEA Form 41 each year. Hospitals may have "blanket authorization." (Refer to Figure 1-2 for a sample DEA Form 41.)

Theft of controlled substances

After the discovery of a theft of controlled substances, the pharmacy must notify the nearest DEA diversion office, notify local police, and complete a DEA Form

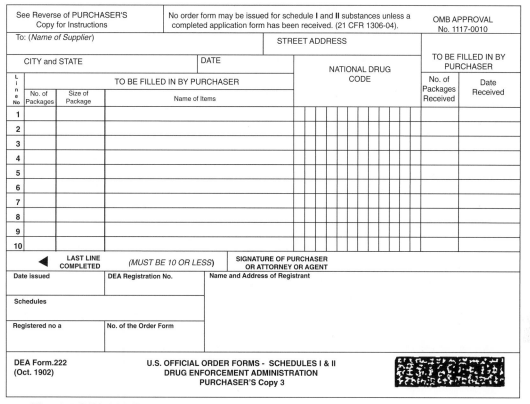

See Reverse of PURCHASER'S Copy for Instructions		No order form may be issued for schedule **I** and **II** substances unless a completed application form has been received. (21 CFR 1306-04).			OMB APPROVAL No. 1117-0010	
To: (*Name of Supplier*)			STREET ADDRESS			
CITY and STATE		DATE		NATIONAL DRUG CODE	TO BE FILLED IN BY PURCHASER	
L i n e No	TO BE FILLED IN BY PURCHASER				No. of Packages Received	Date Received
	No. of Packages	Size of Package	Name of Items			
1						
2						
3						
4						
5						
6						
7						
8						
9						
10						

◄ LAST LINE COMPLETED   *(MUST BE 10 OR LESS)*   SIGNATURE OF PURCHASER OR ATTORNEY OR AGENT

Date issued	DEA Registration No.	Name and Address of Registrant
Schedules		
Registered no a	No. of the Order Form	

DEA Form.222
(Oct. 1902)

U.S. OFFICIAL ORDER FORMS - SCHEDULES I & II
DRUG ENFORCEMENT ADMINISTRATION
PURCHASER'S Copy 3

Fig. 1-1 DEA 222 Form.

106. The pharmacy must send the original copy of the DEA Form 106 to the DEA and retain one copy for its records. Refer to Figure 1-3 for a sample DEA Form 106.

Filling of controlled substances

For Schedule II drugs, prescription can be either handwritten or computer generated but must be signed in ink by the physician with no allowable refills. A partial filling is allowed if the remaining quantity is available to the patient within 72 hours. A new prescription must be issued by the prescriber if additional quantities are to be provided after 72 hours. The pharmacist should notify the physician if the balance cannot be provided to the patient.

Emergency Filling of Schedule II Drug Prescriptions

An oral prescription can be issued to a pharmacy under the following conditions:

1. Pharmacist must make a good-faith attempt to identify the physician.
2. Prescription is limited to a quantity to treat the patient during this period.
3. Pharmacist must reduce order to writing.
4. Physician must write a prescription for this

emergency quantity, and the pharmacy must receive it within 7 days of the oral order.

Schedule II Drugs in Long-Term Care Facilities

A pharmacy may accept a faxed Schedule II drug prescription for patients in a long-term care facility as the original written prescription, and the faxed prescription must be retained as such. A partial filling of Schedule II prescriptions for residents in a long-term care facility or patients diagnosed with a terminal illness is permitted. Such prescriptions may be filled partially for up to 60 days from the date of issue of the prescription, unless the prescription is discontinued sooner. A notation must be made on the prescription such as "long-term care facility patient" or "terminally ill patient." Failure to make this notation is a violation of federal law.

Schedule III to V Drugs

A prescription may be handwritten or computer generated by a physician's office, but it must be signed by the physician in ink. The physician's office may telephone a Schedule III to V prescription in to the pharmacy or may fax one, depending on state law. A patient may receive up to five refills within 6 months

OMB Approval No. 1117 - 0007	U. S. Department of Justice / Drug Enforcement Administration **REGISTRANTS INVENTORY OF DRUGS SURRENDERED**	PACKAGE NO.

The following schedule is an inventory of controlled substances which is hereby surrendered to you for proper disposition.

FROM: *(Include Name, Street, City, State and ZIP Code in space provided below.)*

Signature of applicant or authorized agent

Registrant's DEA Number

Registrant's Telephone Number

NOTE: CERTIFIED MAIL (Return Receipt Requested) IS REQUIRED FOR SHIPMENTS OF DRUGS VIA U.S. POSTAL SERVICE. See instructions on reverse (page 2) of form.

NAME OF DRUG OR PREPARATION	Number of Con-tainers	CONTENTS *(Number of grams, tablets, ounces or other units per con-tainer)*	Con-trolled Sub-stance Con-tent, *(Each Unit)*	FOR DEA USE ONLY		
				DISPOSITION	QUANTITY	
Registrants will fill in Columns 1,2,3, and 4 ONLY.					GMS.	MGS.
1	*2*	*3*	*4*	*5*	*6*	*7*
1						
2						
3						
4						
5						
6						
7						
8						
9						
10						
11						
12						
13						
14						
15						
16						

FORM DEA-41 (9-01)   Previous edition dated **6-86** is usable.   *See instructions on reverse (page 2) of form.*

Fig. 1-2 DEA Form 41.

DEA-41 (6/1986) Pg. 2

NAME OF DRUG OR PREPARATION	Number of Con-tainers	CONTENTS *(Number of grams, tablets, ounces or other units per con-tainer)*	Con-trolled Sub-stance Con-tent, *(Each Unit)*	FOR DEA USE ONLY		
				DISPOSITION	QUANTITY	
					GMS.	MGS.
Registrants will fill in Columns 1,2,3, and 4 ONLY.						
1	*2*	*3*	*4*	*5*	*6*	*7*
17						
18						
19						
20						
21						
22						
23						
24						

The controlled substances surrendered in accordance with Title 21 of the Code of Federal Regulations, Section 1307.21, have been received in _____packages purporting to contain the drugs listed on this inventory and have been: ** (1) Forwarded tape-sealed without opening; (2) Destroyed as indicated and the remainder forwarded tape-sealed after verifying contents; (3) Forwarded tape-sealed after verifying contents.

DATE _____   DESTROYED BY: _____

** *Strike out lines not applicable.*

WITNESSED BY: _____

INSTRUCTIONS

1. List the name of the drug in column 1, the number of containers in column 2, the size of each container in column 3, and in column 4 the controlled substance content of each unit described in column 3: e.g., morphine sulfate tabs., 3 pkgs., 100 tabs., 1/4 gr. (16 mg.) or morphine sulfate tabs., 1 pkg., 83 tabs., 1/2 gr. (32mg.), etc.

2. All packages included on a single line should be identical in name, content and controlled substance strength.

3. Prepare this form in quadruplicate. Mail two (2) copies of this form to the Special Agent in Charge, under separate cover. Enclose one additional copy in the shipment with the drugs. Retain one copy for your records. One copy will be returned to you as a receipt. No further receipt will be furnished to you unless specifically requested. Any further inquiries concerning these drugs should be addressed to the DEA District Office which serves your area.

4. There is no provision for payment for drugs surrendered. This is merely a service rendered to registrants enabling them to clear their stocks and records of unwanted items.

5. Drugs should be shipped tape-sealed via prepaid express or certified mail (**return receipt requested**) to Special Agent in Charge, Drug Enforcement Administration, of the DEA District Office which serves your area.

PRIVACY ACT INFORMATION

AUTHORITY: Section 307 of the Controlled Substances Act of 1970 (PL 91-513).
PURPOSE: To document the surrender of controlled substances which have been forwarded by registrants to DEA for disposal.
ROUTINE USES: This form is required by Federal Regulations for the surrender of unwanted Controlled Substances. Disclosures of information from this system are made to the following categories of users for the purposes stated.
    A. Other Federal law enforcement and regulatory agencies for law enforcement and regulatory purposes.
    B. State and local law enforcement and regulatory agencies for law enforcement and regulatory purposes.
EFFECT: Failure to document the surrender of unwanted Controlled Substances may result in prosecution for violation of the Controlled Substances Act.

Under the Paperwork Reduction Act, a person is not required to respond to a collection of information unless it displays a currently valid OMB control number. Public reporting burden for this collection of information is estimated to average 30 minutes per response, including the time for reviewing instructions, searching existing data sources, gathering and maintaining the data needed, and completing and reviewing the collection of information. Send comments regarding this burden estimate or any other aspect of this collection of information, including suggestions for reducing this burden, to the Drug Enforcement Administration, FOI and Records Management Section, Washington, D.C. 20537; and to the Office of Management and Budget, Paperwork Reduction Project no. 1117-0007, Washington, D.C. 20503.

Fig. 1-2, Cont'd.

REPORT OF THEFT OR LOSS OF CONTROLLED SUBSTANCES

Federal Regulations require registrants to submit a detailed report of any theft or loss of Controlled Substances to the Drug Enforcement Administration. Complete the front and back of this form in triplicate. Forward the original and duplicate copies to the nearest DEA Office. Retain the triplicate copy for your records. Some states may also require a copy of this report.	OMB APPROVAL No. 1117-0001

1. Name and Address of Registrant (include ZIP Code)

ZIP CODE

2. Phone No. (Include Area Code)

3. DEA Registration Number

2 ltr. prefix   7 digit suffix

4. Date of Theft or Loss

5. Principal Business of Registrant (Check one)

1 ☐ Pharmacy   5 ☐ Distributor
2 ☐ Practitioner   6 ☐ Methadone Program
3 ☐ Manufacturer   7 ☐ Other (Specify)
4 ☐ Hospital/Clinic

6. County in which Registrant is located

7. Was Theft reported to Police?

☐ Yes   ☐ No

8. Name and Telephone Number of Police Department (Include Area Code)

9. Number of Thefts or Losses Registrant has experienced in the past 24 months

10. Type of Theft or Loss (Check one and complete items below as appropriate)

1 ☐ Night break-in   3 ☐ Employee pilferage   5 ☐ Other (Explain)
2 ☐ Armed robbery   4 ☐ Customer theft   6 ☐ Lost in transit (Complete Item 14)

11. If Armed Robbery, was anyone:

Killed? ☐ No   ☐ Yes (How many) _____
Injured? ☐ No   ☐ Yes (How many) _____

12. Purchase value to registrant of Controlled Substances taken?

$

13. Were any pharmaceuticals or merchandise taken?

☐ No   ☐ Yes (Est. Value)

$

14. IF LOST IN TRANSIT, COMPLETE THE FOLLOWING:

A. Name of Common Carrier

B. Name of Consignee

C. Consignee's DEA Registration Number

D. Was the carton received by the customer?

☐ Yes   ☐ No

E. If received, did it appear to be tampered with?

☐ Yes   ☐ No

F. Have you experienced losses in transit from this same carrier in the past?

☐ No   ☐ Yes (How Many) _____

15. What identifying marks, symbols, or price codes were on the labels of these containers that would assist in identifying the products?

16. If Official Controlled Substance Order Forms (DEA-222) were stolen, give numbers.

17. What security measures have been taken to prevent future thefts or losses?

FORM DEA - 106 (11-00) *Previous editions obsolete*   CONTINUE ON REVERSE

Fig. 1-3 DEA Form 106.

FORM DEA-106 (Nov. 2000) Pg. 2   **LIST OF CONTROLLED SUBSTANCES LOST**

Trade Name of Substance or Preparation	Name of Controlled Substance in Preparation	Dosage Strength and Form	Quantity
Examples: Desoxyn	**Methamphetamine Hydrochloride**	**5 mg Tablets**	**3 x 100**
Demerol	**Meperidine Hydrochloride**	**50 mg/ml Vial**	**5 x 30 ml**
Robitussin A-C	**Codeine Phosphate**	**2 mg/cc Liquid**	**12 Pints**
1.			
2.			
3.			
4.			
5.			
6.			
7.			
8.			
9.			
10.			
11.			
12.			
13.			
14.			
15.			
16.			
17.			
18.			
19.			
20.			
21.			
22.			
23.			
24.			
25.			
26.			
27.			
28.			
29.			
30.			
31.			
32.			
33.			
34.			
35.			
36.			
37.			
38.			
39.			
40.			
41.			
42.			
43.			
44.			
45.			
46.			
47.			
48.			
49.			
50.			

I certify that the foregoing information is correct to the best of my knowledge and belief.

Signature   Title   Date

Fig. 1-3, Cont'd.

of the date the prescription was written if authorized. Partial fillings are permitted as long as refills are indicated on the prescription; refills do not exceed the total quantity prescribed by the physician; and no partial filling occurs after 6 months of the original date of the prescription.

Exempt Narcotics

Select cough and antidiarrheal prescription items can be purchased by an individual, if permitted by state law. The quantity dispensed must be in the original manufacturer's container and must not exceed the quantity established by law. The purchaser must be at least 18 years of age and must complete the Exempt Narcotic Book with the following information: date purchased, name of purchaser, address of purchaser, name of product and quantity purchased, price of transaction, and pharmacist's signature. There is a limit of one container in a 48-hour period.

FACSIMILE PRESCRIPTIONS

A faxed prescription for a Schedule III, IV, or V drug may serve as the original prescription. The following situations are exceptions:

- A narcotic Schedule II substance that is to be compounded for direct administration to a patient by parenteral, intravenous (IV), intramuscular, subcutaneous, or intraspinal infusion.
- A Schedule II substance for a resident of a long-term care facility.
- A practitioner prescribing a Schedule II narcotic substance for a patient in hospice care, as certified by Medicare under Title XVIII or licensed by the state, may transmit a prescription to the dispensing pharmacy by fax regardless of whether the patient resides in a hospice facility or other care setting. The practitioner's agent may also transmit the prescription to the pharmacy. The practitioner will note on the prescription that it is for a hospice patient.

PRESCRIPTION MONITORING PROGRAMS

In 2005 the federal National All Schedules Prescription Electronic Reporting Act was introduced. The Act established an electronic system for practitioner monitoring of the dispensing of controlled substances in Schedules II, III, and IV. The act would have required specific information to be reported, such as a patient identifier, drug dispensed, and quantity dispensed, as well as the prescriber and the dispenser. Although the act was never enacted, the majority of states have enacted either this or similar legislation.

Transferring of Controlled Substance Prescriptions

The DEA allows transfer of the original prescription information for Schedule II, III, IV, and V controlled substances for the purpose of refill dispensing between pharmacies on a one-time basis. If pharmacies share a real-time online database, however, then the prescription may be transferred up to the maximum number of refills permitted by the law. The following are requirements:

1. The transfer is communicated directly between two licensed pharmacists, and the transferring pharmacist is responsible for the following:
   a. The word *VOID* must be written on the face of the invalidated prescription.
   b. On the reverse side of the invalidated prescription must be written the name, address, and DEA number of the pharmacy to which the prescription was transferred and the name of the pharmacist receiving the prescription information.
   c. The date of the transfer and name of the pharmacist transferring the prescription must be recorded.
2. The receiving pharmacist is responsible for the following:
   a. "Transfer" must be written on the face of the transferred prescription.
   b. The following information must be recorded:
      1. Date of issuance of the original prescription
      2. Original number of refills authorized on the original prescription
      3. Date of the original dispensing
      4. Number of valid refills remaining and dates and locations of previous refills
      5. Pharmacy's name, address, and DEA registration number and prescription number from which the prescription was transferred
      6. Name of the pharmacist who transferred the prescription
      7. Pharmacy's name, address, and DEA registration number and prescription number from which the prescription was originally filled
3. The original and transferred prescription(s) must be maintained for a period of 2 years from the date of the last refill.

POISON PREVENTION PACKAGING ACT OF 1970

The Poison Prevention Packaging Act of 1970 was enacted to reduce accidental poisoning in children. The Act requires that most OTC and legend drugs be packaged in child-resistant containers. A child-resistant container is one that cannot be opened by 80% of children younger than 5 years but can be opened by 90% of adults.

Exceptions for Child-Resistant Containers

- Single-time dispensing of product in noncompliant container as ordered by the prescriber
- Single-time or blanket dispensing of product in noncompliant container as requested by patient or customer in a signed statement
- One noncompliant size of the OTC product for elderly or handicapped patients provided that the package contains the warning "This Package for Households Without Young Children" or "Package Not Child Resistant"
- Drugs dispensed to institutionalized patients, provided that these drugs are to be administered by an employee of an institution
- Medications not requiring child-resistant containers:
  - Betamethasone with no more than 12.6 mg per package
  - Erythromycin ethylsuccinate tablets in packages containing no more than 16 g
  - Inhalation aerosols
  - Mebendazole tablets with no more than 600 mg per package
  - Methylprednisolone tablets with no more than 85 mg per package
  - Oral contraceptives taken cyclically in the manufacturer's dispensing package
  - Pancrelipase preparations
  - Powdered anhydrous cholestyramine
  - Powdered colestipol up to 5 g per packet
  - Prednisone tablets with no more than 105 mg per package
  - Sodium fluoride tablets with no more than 264 mg of sodium fluoride per package
  - Sublingual and chewable isosorbide dinitrate in doses of 10 mg or less
  - Sublingual nitroglycerin tablets

OCCUPATIONAL SAFETY AND HEALTH ACT (OSHA) OF 1970

The Occupational Safety and Health Act created the Occupational Safety and Health Administration (OSHA), which ensures a safe and healthful workplace for all employees. The law was developed to ensure job safety and health standards for employees, maintain a reporting system for job-related injuries and illness, reduce hazards in the workplace, and conduct audits to ensure compliance with the Act. Its impact on pharmacy is to address air contaminants, flammable and combustible liquids, eye and skin protection, and hazard communication standards. OSHA requires use of Material Safety Data Sheets (MSDSs), which are to be provided by the seller of a particular product to the purchaser. OSHA issues *Guidelines for Cytotoxic (Antineoplastic) Drugs.*

DRUG LISTING ACT OF 1972

Each drug is assigned a specific 11-digit number to identify it. This number is known as an NDC (National Drug Code) number. The first five digits identify the manufacturer, the next four digits identify the drug product, and the final two digits represent the package size and packaging.

ORPHAN DRUG ACT OF 1983

Orphan drugs are medications for treatment of diseases or conditions of which there are fewer than 200,000 cases in the world. The law provides tax incentives and exclusive licensing of products for manufacturers to develop and market orphan medications.

DRUG PRICE COMPETITION AND PATENT TERM RESTORATION ACT OF 1984

The Drug Price Competition and Patent Term Restoration Act of 1984 encouraged the creation of both generic and new medications by streamlining the process for generic drug approval and by extending patent licenses.

PRESCRIPTION DRUG MARKETING ACT OF 1987

- The Prescription Drug Marketing Act prohibits the reimportation of a drug into the United States by anyone except the manufacturer. The Act prohibits the sale or distribution of samples to anyone other than those licensed to prescribe them. This Act is currently being reconsidered by Congress.
- The Act requires the following label to appear on all medications to be administered to animals: "Caution: Federal law restricts this drug to use by or on an order of a licensed veterinarian."

OMNIBUS BUDGET RECONCILIATION ACT OF 1987 (OBRA-87)

The Omnibus Budget Reconciliation Act of 1987 established extensive revisions to Medicare and Medicaid Conditions of Participation regarding long-term care facilities and pharmacy. These include the following:

- Resident's drug regimen must be free of unnecessary medications.
- Antipsychotic drugs are not to be used unless the patient has a specific condition.

- Patients requiring antipsychotic medication must be documented as having been diagnosed with a condition that warrants its use.
- Patients receiving antipsychotic medication must receive gradual dose tapering.
- Behavioral modification and drug holidays are used to see if the medication may be discontinued.
- Residents are to be free of any significant medication errors.
- Routine and emergency drugs must be provided to patients.
- Long-term care facilities must have the services of a consultant pharmacist.
- Medications must be labeled according to accepted professional principles.
- Medications must be stored in locked compartments at the proper temperature according to both federal and state laws.

ANABOLIC STEROID CONTROL ACT OF 1990

The Anabolic Steroid Control Act resulted in harsher penalties for the abuse of anabolic steroids and their misuse by athletes.

OMNIBUS BUDGET RECONCILIATION ACT OF 1990 (OBRA-90)

- Requires that manufacturers provide the lowest prices to any customer or Medicaid patient by rebating each state Medicaid agency the difference between its average price and the lowest price
- Requires that an "offer to counsel" is made to every patient and drug utilization review is performed for every patient; failure to do so may result in the loss of Medicaid funds
- Authorizes government-sponsored demonstration projects relating to the provision of pharmaceutical care; patient profiles are to be maintained for all patients

FDA SAFE MEDICAL DEVICES ACT OF 1990

The Safe Medical Devices Act requires that all medical devices be tracked and records be maintained for durable medical equipment, such as infusion pumps.

AMERICANS WITH DISABILITIES ACT (ADA) OF 1990

The Americans with Disabilities Act prevents discrimination against potential employees who may possess a disability. The business must make "a reasonable accommodation" for the potential employee.

RESOURCE CONSERVATION AND RECOVERY ACT

The Environmental Protection Agency (EPA) produced federal guidelines regarding the disposal of hazardous waste. Hazardous waste includes controlled substances. Flushing is no longer an acceptable method of destruction in many states.

FDA MODERNIZATION ACT

Federal drug legend ("Federal law prohibits the dispensing of this medication without a prescription") is now represented by the abbreviation "RX" on the container.

DIETARY SUPPLEMENT HEALTH AND EDUCATION ACT (DSHEA) OF 1994

Herbal products are dietary supplements rather than drugs. The manufacturers of supplements are allowed to make claims with regard to general health promotion, but not disease claims. According to the Dietary Supplement Health and Education Act, herbal products must meet the following requirements:

- Be labeled as a dietary supplement
- Have labeling that identifies all ingredients by name
- Have labeling that lists the quantity of each ingredient
- Have packaging that identifies the plant and plant part from which the ingredient is derived
- Comply with any standards set by an official compendium
- Meet the quality, purity, and compositional specification

Guidelines are set to prevent adulteration, and manufacturers must follow good manufacturing practices.

HEALTH INSURANCE PORTABILITY AND ACCOUNTABILITY ACT (HIPAA) OF 1996

The purpose of the Health Insurance Portability and Accountability Act (HIPAA) was to improve portability and continuity of health coverage in the group and individual markets; combat waste, fraud, and abuse in health insurance and health care delivery; promote the use of medical savings accounts; improve access to long-term care services and coverage; and simplify the administration of health insurance.

HIPAA requires that health care providers ensure that patient confidentiality be maintained. HIPAA set boundaries on the use and the disclosure of protected health information and requires that patients be informed of how their protected information will be used. The information protected through HIPAA includes the following:

- Any information related to past, present, or future physical and mental health
- Past, present, or future payments for health services received
- Specific care the patient received, is receiving, or is willing to receive
- Any information that can identify the patient as the individual receiving the care
- Any information that someone could reasonably use to identify a patient as receiving care

There are two parts of HIPAA:

- Title I—Insurance Reform. Protects health insurance coverage for workers and families when they change or lose their jobs.
- Title II—Administrative Simplification. Established electronic transaction and Code Set Standards; required Health Information Privacy.

ISOTRETINOIN SAFETY AND RISK MANAGEMENT ACT OF 2004

Isotretinoin (Accutane) is a very powerful medication used to treat acne. Unfortunately, the medication has been found to cause severe birth defects; induce spontaneous abortions; and produce adverse psychiatric effects, including depression, psychosis, suicidal ideation, suicide attempts, and suicide. Because of the Isotretinoin Safety and Risk Management Act, the following are now in place:

- Mandatory registry of all patients, practitioners, and pharmacists.
- Education of all practitioners and pharmacists regarding the risks associated with the drug, including birth defects and mental health risks.
- A requirement that Accutane and its generic form are prescribed only for severe recalcitrant nodular acne, the medical condition for which Accutane was approved, that is unresponsive to conventional therapy, including antibiotics. Accutane and its generic are often prescribed for mild acne or without other medications being tried first.
- Monthly education of patients, both male and female, regarding the need to avoid pregnancy, as well as completion of a survey to warn the patient of the adverse side effects. Patient visits will include one-on-one counseling, and patients or parents must sign an informed consent form.
- Certification of medical offices and clinics as treatment centers. No Internet, phone, or mail order prescriptions may be filled.
- Thirty-day prescription allotments.
- A requirement that female patients have monthly pregnancy testing and receive a negative result before a prescription is renewed.

- Appropriate blood testing must be performed during treatment and 30 days after treatment.
- Yearly evaluation of treatment centers to ensure compliance with program.
- Mandatory quarterly reporting of all adverse reactions and mandatory reporting within 15 days of all patient deaths associated with the drug.

ANABOLIC STEROID CONTROL ACT OF 2004

On January 20, 2004, the Anabolic Steroid Control Act amended the Controlled Substances Act and replaced the existing definition of anabolic steroid with a new definition. The new definition altered the basis for all future administrative scheduling actions relating to the control of anabolic steroids as Schedule III medications by eliminating the requirement to prove muscle growth. This act increased the number of anabolic steroids to 59 substances. This amendment provided the requirements for handling substances defined as anabolic steroids to include registration, security, labeling and packaging, inventory, record maintenance, prescriptions, disposal, importation and exportation, and criminal liability.

ANY WILLING PROVIDER LAW

Any willing provider laws allow any pharmacy to participate in a prescription drug benefit plan as long as the pharmacy agrees to the terms and conditions of the plan.

FREEDOM OF CHOICE LAW

Freedom of choice laws allow a member of a prescription drug plan to select any pharmacy for his or her pharmacy benefit as long as the pharmacy agrees to the terms and conditions of the plan.

FREEDOM OF CHOICE WITH REGARD TO LONG-TERM CARE

Long-term care residents may choose an outside pharmacy for their medications if the pharmaceutical service is not provided under their contract. A long-term care facility may refuse admission to a resident if the resident refuses to use the drug distribution system already in place. Long-term care facilities may establish policies to protect patients and may require outside pharmacies to agree to policies.

PRESCRIPTION DRUG EQUITY LAW

Prescription drug equity laws prohibit a prescription drug plan from requiring mail order prescription drug coverage without also providing non–mail order coverage.

MEDICARE DRUG, IMPROVEMENT, AND MODERNIZATION ACT (MPDIMA) OF 2003

- Provides for a voluntary prescription drug benefit to Medicare beneficiaries.
- Adds preventive medical benefits to senior citizens.
- Lowers the reimbursement rates for Medicare payment for durable medical equipment.
- Created a national competitive bidding program for durable medical equipment in 2007.
- Changed the way Medicare pays for outpatient Part B drugs.
- Allowed for a voluntary Medicare-approved discount card program, begun in June 2004.
- Medicare Part D prescription plan allows beneficiaries to enroll in either regional- or national-based insurance plans.

COMBAT METHAMPHETAMINE EPIDEMIC ACT OF 2005

The Combat Methamphetamine Epidemic Act is a federal law that placed ephedrine, pseudoephedrine, and phenylpropanolamine in the Controlled Substances Act category "scheduled listed chemical products." Products containing ephedrine, pseudoephedrine, and phenylpropanolamine are subject to sales restrictions, storage requirements, and record-keeping requirements. The Act specifies a 3.6 g/day base product sales limit, a 9 g/30-day base product purchase limit, a blister package requirement, and mail order restrictions. Logbook (written or electronic) requirements have been implemented and require the following: products by name, quantity sold, names and addresses of purchasers, and date and time of sales.

MEDICAID TAMPER-RESISTANT PRESCRIPTION ACT

On April 1, 2008, physicians were required to adhere to the requirements of the Medicaid Tamper-Resistant Prescription Act. This piece of legislation applies to all handwritten prescriptions for covered outpatient drugs; drugs that are transmitted from the prescriber to the pharmacy verbally, by fax, or through e-prescribing are not affected by this legislation. The law applies whenever Medicaid pays any portion of the cost of a prescription.

As of April 1, 2008, a tamper-resistant prescription pad must include at least one of the following three characteristics:

- One or more industry-recognized features designed to prevent unauthorized copying of a completed or blank prescription form
- One or more industry-recognized features designed to prevent the erasure or modification of information written on the prescription pad by the prescriber
- One or more industry-recognized features designed to prevent the use of counterfeit prescription forms

As of October 1, 2008, a prescription pad must include all three of these characteristics to be considered tamper-resistant. These regulations do not apply to any prescriptions presented to the pharmacy before April 1, 2008. If a pharmacy receives a prescription and there are questions regarding whether the prescription meets the requirements of the Act, the pharmacy staff may contact the prescriber's office for verification. The pharmacy may accept a faxed prescription from the physician's office until it has obtained tamper-resistant prescription pads. A pharmacy may fill the prescription as an emergency prescription as long as the pharmacy receives documentation from the prescriber's office within 72 hours. A prescription may be transferred from the original pharmacy to another pharmacy by fax or telephone. The second pharmacy does not need to have direct confirmation of the original prescription from the physician.

USP <797>

USP <797> is designed to cut down on infections transmitted to patients through pharmaceutical products and to better protect staff working in pharmacies in the course of their exposure to pharmaceuticals. USP <797> contains many procedural training and quality assurance requirements for preparing sterile products. USP <797> affects all health care institutions, pharmacies, physicians' practices, and other facilities in which compounded sterile preparations are prepared, stored, and dispensed.

Facilities affected by USP <797> include those facilities in which sterile products are prepared according to manufacturer's labeling and where manipulations are performed during the compounding of sterile products that increase the potential for microbial contamination of the end product. It affects facilities where products are compounded using devices or ingredients that are not sterile to prepare compounds that must be sterilized. These products may be biologics, diagnostic agents, drugs, nutrients, or radiopharmaceuticals that include but are not limited to baths and soaks for live organs and tissues, implants, inhalations, injections, irrigations, metered sprays, and ophthalmic and otic preparations.

USP <797> addresses the following areas:

- Microbial contamination risk levels, which are defined as low-, medium-, and high-risk conditions

- Personnel training and evaluation in aseptic manipulation skills
- Clean rooms to include anterooms, air classification, physical characteristics of the construction, and gowning procedures
- Barrier isolators
- Formalized quality assurance program
- Minimum requirements for validation
- Cleaning and sanitizing workspaces
- Environmental monitoring
- Verification of automated compounding devices for nutrition compounding

REGULATORY AGENCIES

BUREAU OF ALCOHOL, TOBACCO, AND FIREARMS (ATF)

Sets regulations regarding the purchase of tax-free alcohol. Tax-free alcohol may be used in hospitals and clinics.

CENTERS FOR MEDICARE AND MEDICAID SERVICES (CMS)

Oversees Medicare and Medicaid; establishes conditions for a facility to be reimbursed for services rendered.

DRUG ENFORCEMENT AGENCY (DEA)

Enforces compliance with the Controlled Substances Act. This includes placing medications into the appropriate schedule, monitoring records and reports of controlled substances, registering pharmacies, issuing DEA Forms 222 and 41, and monitoring the destruction of controlled substances. The DEA is overseen by the Department of Justice.

ENVIRONMENTAL PROTECTION AGENCY (EPA)

Sets guidelines for the disposal of hazardous waste (includes disposal of controlled substances).

FOOD AND DRUG ADMINISTRATION (FDA)

Ensures that all pharmaceutical products are pure, safe, and effective. Reviews information supplied on MedWatch Forms. Can issue drug recalls if product is adulterated or misbranded (will perform postrecall audits to verify that manufacturers, wholesalers, pharmacists, and customers have been notified and appropriate action has occurred). Regulates the distribution of patient package inserts and the repackaging of medications. Reviews new drug applications and investigational new drug applications.

INSTITUTIONAL REVIEW BOARD

A board, committee, or other group designated by an institution to approve biomedical research in accordance with the FDA.

THE JOINT COMMISSION (TJC)

The Joint Commission (TJC), formerly known as the Joint Commission on Accreditation of Healthcare Organizations, addresses quality of patient care and patient safety. Establishes standards and accredits the following health care providers: hospitals, home health care agencies, home infusion providers, long-term care pharmacies, ambulatory infusion pharmacies, home medical equipment and home oxygen providers, ambulatory surgical centers, community health centers, college and prison health care centers, nursing homes and subacute facilities, assisted living facilities, clinical laboratories, behavioral health organizations, alcohol and chemical dependency centers, health care networks, and preferred provider organizations. Accreditation is voluntary. TJC has been granted "deemed status" for participation in Medicare. This status states that the institution has met the Medicare Conditions of Participation and can receive Medicare funding. The institution does not need to meet requirements for annual Medicare surveys by state inspectors.

NATIONAL ASSOCIATION OF THE BOARDS OF PHARMACY (NABP)

Composed of all State Boards of Pharmacy. Has no regulatory authority but meets to discuss current trends and issues in pharmacy that affect the practice of pharmacy.

STATE BOARDS OF PHARMACY (BOP)

Regulatory state agency that oversees the practice of pharmacy in a given state. Clearly defines regulations affecting pharmacy and the roles, duties, and expectations of pharmacists and pharmacy technicians in that state. Has the ability to discipline pharmacies, pharmacists, and possibly pharmacy technicians for improper behavior.

UNITED STATES PHARMACOPEIA (USP)

The United States Pharmacopeia (USP) is an official public standards–setting authority for all prescription and OTC medicines and other health care products manufactured or sold in the United States. USP also sets widely recognized standards for food ingredients and dietary supplements. USP sets standards for the quality, purity, strength, and consistency of these products—critical to public health. USP's standards are recognized and used in more than 130 countries around the globe.

PHARMACEUTICAL, MEDICAL, AND LEGAL DEVELOPMENTS THAT AFFECT THE PRACTICE OF PHARMACY

- American Society of Health System Pharmacists' *White Paper on Pharmacy Technicians*
- Computerization: method of processing, storing, and transferring prescriptions
- Online adjudication: method of billing insurance companies and ensuring payment for services
- Faxes: method of transmitting prescriptions and medication orders from a physician's office to a pharmacy
- Personal digital assistants: method of transmitting prescriptions to a pharmacy
- Medicare Prescription Drug, Improvement, and Modernization Act of 2003
- Drug Reimportation Reform: currently being examined
- Orphan Drug Act: promotes development of pharmaceutical products with small markets
- Reducing the amount of time a drug is covered by a patent, resulting in generic drugs becoming available earlier
- Revising the protocol for the development of acquired immunodeficiency syndrome (AIDS) medications
- Process for converting prescription medications to OTC status

- Allowing pharmacists to prescribe in specific situations
- Third-party health care providers
- Automation

STATE-SPECIFIC PRESCRIPTION TRANSFER REGULATIONS

Technicians must be familiar with their state laws regarding the transfer of prescriptions between pharmacies. Federal law states that controlled substance prescriptions can be transferred only one time between pharmacies. Pharmacy technicians may assist the pharmacist in the transfer of prescriptions between pharmacies. A pharmacy technician may fax a copy of a prescription to another pharmacy under the supervision of a pharmacist.

THERAPEUTIC EQUIVALENCE

According to the *Orange Book,* two drugs are therapeutically equivalent if they contain the same active ingredients and have the same strength or concentration, the same dosage form, and the same route of administration. They must have the same clinical effect and safety profile.

THERAPEUTIC INTERCHANGE

Therapeutic interchange is a substitution of one medication for another medication that is not generically equivalent but would provide the same therapeutic effect (e.g., substituting one macrolide antibiotic for another macrolide because of price) (Table 1-3).

TABLE **1-3** Therapeutic Equivalence Codes

FDA CODE	DESCRIPTION
A	Drug products that are considered to be therapeutically equivalent to other pharmaceutically equivalent products
AA	Products not presenting bioequivalence problems in conventional dosage forms
AB	Products meeting necessary bioequivalence requirements
AO	Injectable oil solutions that are considered therapeutically equivalent to other pharmaceutically equivalent products
AP	Injectable aqueous solutions
AT	Topical products that are considered therapeutically equivalent to other pharmaceutically equivalent products
B Codes	Drug products that the FDA does not consider at this time to be therapeutically equivalent to other pharmaceutically equivalent products
BC	Controlled-release tablets, controlled capsules, and controlled-release injectables (controlled-release products for which such bioequivalence data are available have been coded AB)
BD	Active ingredients and dosage forms with documented bioequivalence problems
BE	Enteric coated oral dosage forms (enteric coated oral dosage forms for which bioequivalence data are available are coded AB)
BP	Active ingredients and dosage forms with potential bioequivalence problems
BR	Suppositories or enemas for systemic use
BS	Products having standard deficiencies
BT	Topical products
BX	Insufficient data: these products are presumed to be therapeutically not equivalent until adequate information becomes available for full evaluation for therapeutic equivalence

EPIDEMIOLOGY

Epidemiology is defined as a medical science that deals with the incidence, distribution, and control of a disease in a population. It includes the factors that may control the presence or absence of a disease.

RISK FACTORS FOR DISEASE

Age
- **Pediatric patients:** Organ systems may not be fully developed, and immune system may not be fully in place.
- **Elderly:** Physiologic changes occur as one ages. These changes include auditory, gastrointestinal (GI), pulmonary, cardiovascular, urinary, hormonal, and body composition changes. Absorption, distribution, metabolism, and elimination processes are affected by age. The elderly can be subdivided into three categories:
  1. Young old: 65-74 years of age
  2. Middle old: 75-84 years of age
  3. Old old: 85 years of age and older

Gender

An individual's gender may make him or her more prone to a disease condition or may affect how a drug may work. Hormone changes have been shown to have an effect on the development of a disease.

Genetic Factors

A definitive link between heredity and disease has been shown. Many of the affective disorders may be passed from one generation to another generation. The possibility of developing either hypertension or diabetes is greatly increased in families with a history of the disease. Hemophilia is another disease that is transmitted genetically.

Immune System

An impaired immune system may make an individual more susceptible to bacterial or fungal infections. Human immunodeficiency virus (HIV) and AIDS are examples of diseases that result from an impaired immune system.

Race

Sickle cell anemia is a disease that targets individuals of African-American descent. African-American males have a higher predisposition toward hypertension, and attention deficit disorder (ADD), attention deficit–hyperactivity disorder (ADHD), and type 1 diabetes target Caucasians.

SIGNS AND SYMPTOMS OF DISEASE STATES

Angina

Chest pain is experienced because of an imbalance between oxygen supply and demand.

Anxiety

A state of uneasiness characterized by apprehension and worrying about possible events.

Asthma

Characterized by reversible small airway obstruction, progressive airway inflammation, and increased airway responsiveness from both endogenous and exogenous stimuli. Symptoms include wheezing, dyspnea, and coughing.

Bacterial Infections

Occur when the body's immune system is unable to resist bacteria. Symptoms of a bacterial infection include a fever greater than 101° F and an increase in white blood cells (>12,000).

Benign Prostatic Hypertrophy

An enlargement of the prostate of a male as he ages.

Bipolar Disease

Depressive psychosis, alternating between excessive phases of mania and depression. Mania may be characterized by exhibiting three of the following symptoms: increased need for sleep, distractibility, elevated or irritable mood, excessive involvement in pleasurable activities with a potential for painful consequences, grandiose ideas, increase in activity, pressure to keep talking, and racing thoughts.

Bronchitis

Condition in which the lungs' defense mechanisms have been destroyed by cigarette smoke, occupational dusts, fumes, environmental pollution, or bacterial infection. Characterized by a cough that produces a purulent, green, or blood-soaked sputum.

Congestive Heart Failure

Condition in which the heart is unable to meet the metabolic needs of the tissues. Congestive heart failure results in the heart pumping less blood than it receives.

Constipation

The result of low-fiber diets—decreased colon content, increased colon pressure, and decreased propulsive motility.

Depression

A psychiatric disorder that may be caused by changes in neurotransmitters (such as dopamine, norepinephrine, or serotonin) in the brain. Symptoms include a loss of interest in normal activities, low self-esteem, pessimism, self-pity, weight loss or gain, insomnia, loss of energy, feelings of worthlessness, feelings of guilt, or recurrent thoughts of death or suicide.

Diabetes

Gestational diabetes

Occurs during the second and third trimester of pregnancy. Can be treated with exercise, diet, and insulin.

Type 1 diabetes

An individual's body is unable to produce insulin, and therefore he or she becomes insulin-dependent.

Type 2 diabetes (adult onset)

Condition that occurs in individuals who have an impaired insulin secretion and are often insulin-resistant. Treatment includes weight reduction through diet and exercise.

Secondary diabetes

Diabetes with onset caused by taking various medications, such as oral contraceptives, beta-blockers, diuretics, calcium channel blockers, glucocorticoids, and phenytoin.

Drug-Induced Ulcers

Ulcers caused by medication such as aspirin, antiinflammatory agents, corticosteroids, potassium chloride, methotrexate, and iron.

Emphysema

The destruction of alveoli, walls, or air sacs of the lungs, resulting in an obstruction of the airflow on expiration. May be caused by cigarette smoke, air pollution, occupational exposure, or genetic factors.

Epilepsy

Abnormal electrical discharges in the cerebral cortex that may result in recurring, paroxysmal seizures.

Fungal Infections

Infections caused by single-cell organisms that do not have chlorophyll, possess a cell wall, and reproduce by spores. Develop in individuals whose immune system has been compromised by disease, drug therapy, or poor nutrition.

Gastroesophageal Reflux Disease (GERD)

Characterized by radiating burning or chest pain and the presence of an acid taste.

Hyperlipidemia

An elevation of one or more lipoprotein levels. May be genetically determined.

Hypertension

Systolic pressure (cardiac output) greater than 140 mm Hg and diastolic pressure (total peripheral resistance) greater than 90 mm Hg. Disease does not have symptoms.

Hyperthyroidism (Graves' Disease)

An excessive secretion of thyroid hormone characterized by decreased menses, diarrhea, exophthalmos, flushing of the skin, heat intolerance, nervousness, perspiration, tachycardia, and possible weight loss.

Hypothyroidism

A deficiency of thyroid hormone being secreted by the body, which may be attributed to an iodine deficiency, inflammation of the thyroid gland, or autoimmune destruction of the thyroid gland. Symptoms may include apathy; constipation; decreased heart rate; dry skin, nails, or scalp; fatigue; enlarged thyroid; lowered voice pitch; myxedema; puffy face; reduced mental acuity; swelling of the eyelids; enlarged and thickened tongue; and possible weight gain.

Insomnia

Characterized by the inability to sleep or remain asleep, which may be caused by situations, medications, or psychiatric or medical conditions.

Mania

Mood of extreme excitement, excessive elation, hyperactivity, agitation, and increased psychomotor activity.

Myocardial Infarction

Condition in which the heart muscle is deprived of oxygen because of a reduced oxygen supply, and muscle cells die. Myocardial infarction (MI) may be caused by angina, excessive alcohol consumption, dyspnea on exertion, reduced pulmonary vital capacity, cigarette smoking, or atherosclerosis. Symptoms are described as burning tightness or squeezing of the chest, choking, and substernal pain radiating to the neck, throat, jaw, shoulders, and arms.

Obesity

Condition in which an individual's total body weight consists of greater fat than is considered normal. For males, obesity is body weight 25% above the ideal body weight; for females, it is 35%.

Panic Disorders

Intense anxiety characterized by a sense of fear, apprehension, or a premonition of serious illness or a life-threatening attack.

Schizophrenia

Chronic psychotic disorder characterized by a retreat from reality, delusions, hallucinations, ambivalence, withdrawal, or regressive behavior.

Stroke

An interruption of the oxygen supply to a specific area of the brain caused by a rupture or obstruction (clot) of the blood vessel, resulting in a loss of consciousness. Complications may include retinopathy, neuropathy, vascular problems, or kidney damage.

Tuberculosis

A disease affecting the lungs; caused by *Mycobacterium tuberculosis* and spread by leukocytes and the lymph in the body. Tuberculosis is spread by respiratory droplets inhaled into the lungs of a person.

Ulcers

Disorders of the upper GI tract caused by excessive acid secretion. Ulcers may be categorized as gastric ulcers, which are local excavations of the gastric mucosa occurring more often in men from the Western hemisphere. Duodenal ulcers occur in the duodenum of the intestine and are usually caused by hypersecretion of acid. Stress ulcers develop from the breakdown of the natural mucosal resistance from severe physiologic stress caused by an illness.

Urinary Tract Infections

Presence of bacteria in the urinary tract with localized symptoms. Symptoms include blood in the urine, fever, and burning sensation.

Viral Infections

Diseases caused by agents smaller than bacteria, which are normally spread by direct contact, ingestion of contaminated food and water, or inhalation of airborne particles. May be acute, chronic, or slow in nature, and the infection may be local or generalized. Symptoms are more severe than in bacterial infections and include malaise, myalgia, headaches, chills, or fever.

DRUG INTERACTIONS

DRUG-DRUG INTERACTIONS

One drug alters the action of another drug; interactions include addition, antagonism, potentiation, and synergism.

- **Addition:** The combined effect of two drugs. It is equal to the sum of the effects of each drug taken alone.
- **Antagonism:** One drug works against the action of another drug.
- **Potentiation:** One drug increases or prolongs the effect of another drug. The total effect is greater than the sum of the effects of each drug alone (e.g., Vistaril and Demerol).
- **Synergism:** The joint action of drugs in which their combined effect is more intense or longer in duration than the sum of the effects of two drugs.

DRUG-DISEASE INTERACTIONS

Various diseases may inhibit the absorption, metabolism, and elimination of different drugs. An example would be taking decongestants if the patient is either hypertensive or diabetic.

DRUG-NUTRIENT INTERACTIONS

Poor nutrition may affect the metabolism of various drugs. An example of a drug-nutrient interaction occurs when warfarin and vitamin K are taken simultaneously.

DRUG-FOOD INTERACTIONS

- Improved absorption occurs if the following drugs are taken with a fatty meal: ketoconazole, nitrofurantoin, and griseofulvin.
- Decreased absorption occurs if the following drugs are taken with food: tetracycline, ciprofloxacin, etidronate, phenytoin, norfloxacin, zidovudine, levothyroxine, and didanosine.
- Grapefruit juice affects the following drugs metabolized by cytochrome P450: calcium channel blockers, estrogens, cyclosporine, midazolam, and triazolam.
- Warfarin interacts with foods high in vitamin K, such as romaine lettuce and spinach. Warfarin users should consult a cardiologist or internist for a list of these foods.

DRUG-RELATED PROBLEMS

An event or situation involving drug therapy that actually or potentially interferes with the optimum outcome. These drug-related problems include an untreated indication, improper drug selection, subtherapeutic dosage, failure to receive a drug, overdosage, and drug use without an indication.

EFFECTS OF PATIENT'S AGE ON DRUG AND NONDRUG THERAPY

Neonates

A child's organs are not fully developed until the age of 1 year. Other factors affecting the amount of drug to be given to a child depend on the child's weight, height, and body surface area (BSA).

Geriatric Patients

Physiologic changes occur and include optic, auditory, GI, pulmonary, cardiovascular, urinary, hormonal, and body composition changes. As an individual ages, the absorption, distribution, metabolism, and elimination of drugs change, affecting the amount of drug and frequency of the dose. Other age-related factors include multiple health issues, lower body weight, and an increase in adverse drug reactions.

DRUG INFORMATION SOURCES

- **Primary literature:** The original reports of scientific, clinical, technical, and administrative research projects.
- **Secondary literature:** General reference books based on primary literature. Includes abstracting services, bibliographic services, and specialized microfiche systems.
- **Tertiary literature:** Condensed works based on primary literature. Includes monographs and textbooks.

Books

- **American Hospital Formulary Service Drug Information:** Provides information on uses, interactions, pharmacokinetics, and dosage and administration of drugs, both commercial and experimental.
- **Drug Topics Red Book:** A source of information concerning prices. Sections on emergency information, clinical reference guide, practice management and professional development, pharmacy and health care organizations, drug reimbursement information, manufacturer and wholesaler information, product identification, Rx product listing, OTC and nondrug products listing, and

complementary and herbal product referencing. Drug Topics Red Book contains pricing information necessary for third-party reimbursement.

- **Goodman and Gilman's the Pharmacological Basis of Therapeutics:** The book examines the principles of pharmacokinetics as they relate to medications.
- **FDA: Approved Drug Products with Therapeutic Equivalence Evaluations (Orange Book):** Approved drugs for use in the United States.
- **Drug Facts and Comparisons:** Provides information with regard to brand and generic names, orphan and investigational drugs, drug monographs, drug identification, and dosage calculations. Updated monthly.
- **Handbook on Injectable Drugs:** References the compatibility of various parenteral drugs.
- **Handbook of Nonprescription Drugs:** OTC reference book.
- **Martindale: The Complete Drug Reference:** International reference book on medications.
- **Merck Index:** A source of chemical substance data.
- **Pharmaceutical Dosage Forms and Drug Delivery Systems:** Discusses dosage forms and delivery systems.
- **Physicians' Desk Reference:** Compilation of product inserts from the pharmaceutical manufacturers. Contains indexes of manufacturers and product category; generic and trade names; product identification guide; product information; diagnostic product information; and miscellaneous information.
- **Remington's Pharmaceutical Sciences:** Detailed book of the practice of pharmacy.
- **U.S. Pharmacopeia and National Formulary:** Official compendium of drug monographs setting official standards for pharmaceuticals.
- **USP Dictionary of USAN and International Drug Names**
- **USP Drug Information Vol. I—Drug Information for the Health Care Professional:** Describes medically accepted uses of medications, which include labeled and unlabeled uses of medications.
- **USP Drug Information Vol. II—Advice for the Patient:** This book assists the pharmacist in advising and counseling patients about their medication.
- **USP Drug Information Vol. III—Approved Drug Products and Legal Requirements:** Volume III discusses both state and federal requirements of a medication, which may include storage and dispensing information.

Pharmacy Journals of Specific Pharmacy Organizations

- AACP: *American Journal of Pharmaceutical Education*
- AAPS: *Pharmaceutical Research*
- AMCP: *Journal of Managed Care Pharmacy*
- AJHP: *American Journal of Health System Pharmacists*
- APhA: *Journal of American Pharmacists Association; Pharmacy Today*
- ASCP: *The Consultant Pharmacist*
- ASHP: *American Society of Health System Pharmacists*
- CRS: *Journal of Controlled Release*
- ISMP: *ISMP Medication Safety Alerts Newsletter*
- NCPA: *America's Pharmacist*
- NPTA: *Today's Technician*

Pharmacy Magazines

- *Chain Drug Store News*
- *Drug Topics*
- *Hospital Pharmacy*
- *Journal of Managed Care Pharmacy*
- *Pharmacy Times*
- *The Script*
- *U.S. Pharmacist*

PHARMACOLOGY

DRUG NOMENCLATURE

Prefix + root word + suffix

ANTIBIOTICS

Sulfonamides: Bacteriostatic

Mechanism of action (MOA): Interfere with para-amino-benzoic acid and folic acid formation and thus destroy bacteria.

Common indications: Urinary tract infections (UTIs), otitis media, ulcerative colitis, lower respiratory infections.

Adverse reactions: Photosensitivity resulting in rashes or sunburns, nausea and vomiting, jaundice, blood complications, kidney damage.

Special considerations: Avoid direct sunlight or use sunscreens when exposed. Drink plenty of water to prevent crystallization in the urine. Sulfamethoxazole-trimethoprim infusion fluids need to be stored at room temperature.

EXAMPLES OF SULFONAMIDES

GENERIC NAME	BRAND NAME	DOSAGE FORMS
sulfamethoxazole-trimethoprim	Bactrim, Septra	Oral suspension, tablet, IV
sulfadiazine	Silvadene	Cream
sulfasalazine	Azulfidine	Tablet, enteric coated tablet, oral suspension
sulfisoxazole	Gantrisin	Tablet, oral suspension, ophthalmic ointment

Penicillins

MOA: Prevent bacteria from forming a cell wall.

Common indications: Abscesses, meningitis, otitis media, pneumonia, respiratory infections, prophylaxis.

Adverse reactions: Diarrhea, hives, rash, wheezing, anaphylaxis.

Special considerations: Take on an empty stomach with water; avoid taking with colas or juices.

Reconstitution concerns: Amoxicillin can be stored at room temperature but will last 14 days if refrigerated. Augmentin should be refrigerated and will last 10 days. Ampicillin will last 7 days if not refrigerated but 14 days when refrigerated.

EXAMPLES OF PENICILLINS

GENERIC NAME	BRAND NAME	DOSAGE FORMS
amoxicillin	Amoxil, Polymox	Capsule, oral suspension
ampicillin	Omnipen	Capsule, oral suspension
cloxacillin	None	Capsule, powder for oral suspension, powder for injection
dicloxacillin	Dynapen	Oral suspension, oral tablet, chewable tablet
piperacillin	None	Powder for injection
piperacillin + tazobactam	Zosyn	Powder for injection, solution for injection
penicillin	Veetids	Tablet, oral suspension
ticarcillin-clavulanate	Timentin	IV

Cephalosporins

MOA: Prevent bacteria from forming a cell wall.

Indications: Dental work, heart and pacemaker procedures, orthopedic surgery, pneumonia, upper respiratory infections (URIs), and sinus infections.

Adverse reactions: Share the same side effects as penicillins.

Special considerations: Ten percent of population may have a cross-sensitivity to penicillin.

Reconstitution concerns: Reconstituted cefaclor, cephalexin, and cefadroxil should be refrigerated and will last for 14 days. Cefuroxime suspension can be stored either at room temperature or refrigerated; will expire in 10 days. Loracarbef can be stored for 14 days at room temperature on reconstitution.

EXAMPLES OF CEPHALOSPORINS

GENERIC NAME	BRAND NAME	DOSAGE FORMS
cefaclor	Ceclor	Capsule, oral suspension, extended-release tablet
cefdinir	Omnicef	Capsule, oral liquid
cefixime	Suprax	Oral suspension, tablet
cefepime	Maxipime	Injection (IV)
cefpodoxime	Vantin	Oral suspension
cefadroxil	Duricef	Capsule, oral suspension, tablet
ceftibuten	Cedax	Oral suspension, capsule
cefuroxime	Ceftin, Zinacef	Intramuscular, IV, oral suspension, tablet
cephalexin	Keflex, Keftab	Capsule, oral suspension, tablet
cephradine	Velosef	Capsule
cefprozil	Cefzil	Oral liquid, capsule

Carbapenems, Carbacephems, and Monobactams

Indications: Gram-positive and gram-negative bacteria.

Adverse reactions: Same as penicillin and cephalosporin, but there is an increased possibility of seizures.

EXAMPLES OF CARBAPENEMS

GENERIC NAME	BRAND NAME	DOSAGE FORMS
ertapenem	Invanz	Injection (IV)
imipenem-cilastatin	Primaxin	Injection (IV)

EXAMPLE OF A CARBACEPHEM

GENERIC NAME	BRAND NAME	DOSAGE FORMS
loracarbef	Lorabid	Capsule, oral liquid

EXAMPLE OF A MONOBACTAM

GENERIC NAME	BRAND NAME	DOSAGE FORM
aztreonam	Azactam	IV

Tetracyclines

MOA: Inhibit protein synthesis in bacteria by binding ribosomes.

Indications: Acne, chronic bronchitis, Lyme disease, walking pneumonia, prophylaxis for traveler's diarrhea.

Adverse reactions: GI, such as nausea and vomiting; photosensitivity to sunlight, resulting in rashes and sunburns.

Special considerations: May bind to antacids and dairy products and therefore decrease the effectiveness of antibiotic. Tetracyclines should be taken several hours apart from antacids and dairy products because of the possibility of chelation. They should not be taken by pregnant women because of possibility of dental birth defects. Children younger than 9 years should not be given tetracyclines. Taking expired tetracycline may result in toxicity and possibly death. Tetracycline injection that has been reconstituted is stable at room temperature for 12 hours. Doxycycline should be protected from light, and reconstituted suspension can be stored at room temperature but will expire in 14 days.

EXAMPLES OF TETRACYCLINES

GENERIC NAME	BRAND NAME	DOSAGE FORMS
doxycycline hyclate	Vibramycin	Capsule, IV, oral suspension, tablet
doxycycline monohydrate	Monodox	Tablet
minocycline	Minocin	Capsule, IV, oral suspension, tablet
tetracycline	Achromycin, Sumycin	Capsule, oral suspension, topical

Macrolides

MOA: Inhibit protein synthesis by combining with ribosomes.

Indications: Pulmonary infections, chlamydia, *Haemophilus influenza*.

Adverse reaction: May cause GI distress.

Special considerations: Patient should take macrolides with food. Clarithromycin may leave a metallic taste in one's mouth. The first dose of azithromycin is a loading dose, which is twice the normal daily dose.

Reconstitution concerns: Reconstituted azithromycin injection is good for 24 hours when refrigerated; oral suspension will last 10 days if refrigerated. Clarithromycin does not need to be refrigerated after reconstitution but will expire in 14 days. Erythromycin for IV injection must be used within 8 hours of reconstitution.

EXAMPLES OF MACROLIDES

GENERIC NAME	BRAND NAME	DOSAGE FORMS
azithromycin	Zithromax	Capsule, oral suspension
clarithromycin	Biaxin	Granules for oral suspension, film-coated tablet
dirithromycin	Dynabac	Enteric coated tablet
erythromycin base	Eryc, E-Mycin, Ery-Tab	Capsule, tablet, enteric coated tablet, film-coated tablet
erythromycin estolate	Ilosone	Capsule, oral suspension, tablet
erythromycin ethylsuccinate	E.E.S.	Oral suspension, tablet, chewable tablet
erythromycin stearate	Erythrocin	Film-coated tablet, intramuscular, IV
erythromycin-sulfisoxazole	Pediazole	Oral suspension
erythromycin lactobionate	Erythrocin	IV

Ketolides

MOA: Block protein synthesis by binding to ribosomal subunits; may inhibit the formation of newly forming ribosomes.

Indications: Used to treat bacterial infections in the lungs and sinuses.

Adverse reactions: Blurred vision; side effects similar to those of macrolides.

EXAMPLE OF A KETOLIDE

GENERIC NAME	BRAND NAME	DOSAGE FORM
telithromycin	Ketek	Tablet

Quinolones

MOA: Antagonize the enzyme responsible for collecting and replicating DNA, therefore causing DNA breakage and finally death.

Indications: Bone and joint infections, dental work, infectious diarrhea, URIs, and UTIs.

Adverse reactions: Nausea and vomiting, joint swelling, dizziness.

Special considerations: Antacids interfere with absorption. Potentiate the effect of theophylline products and may cause toxicity. Cause phototoxicity. Should not be prescribed to individuals younger than 18 years because of possible tendon damage. Should not be given to pregnant women. Ciprofloxacin injection should be protected from light. Ofloxacin injection needs to be protected from light.

EXAMPLES OF QUINOLONES

GENERIC NAME	BRAND NAME	DOSAGE FORMS
cinoxacin	Cinobac	Capsule
ciprofloxacin	Cipro	Tablet, oral suspension, ophthalmic, intramuscular, IV
gatifloxacin	Tequin	Tablet, intramuscular, IV
levofloxacin	Levaquin	IV, tablet
lomefloxacin	Maxaquin	Tablet
moxifloxacin	Avelox, Vigamox	Tablet
norfloxacin	Noroxin	Tablet
ofloxacin	Floxin, Ocuflox	Tablet, IV, ophthalmic

Streptogramins

MOA: Inhibit protein synthesis within bacterial ribosomes.

Indications: Gram-positive infections, *Enterococcus faecium*, and vancomycin- and methicillin-resistant infections.

Adverse reactions: Nausea, vomiting, joint swelling, dizziness. There is a possibility of an adverse reaction occurring at site of infusion.

Special considerations: IV lines must be flushed with D5W. Synercid should not come into contact with saline or other medications. It must be stored in the refrigerator.

EXAMPLE OF A STREPTOGRAMIN

GENERIC NAME	BRAND NAME	DOSAGE FORM
quinupristin-dalfopristin	Synercid	IV

Aminoglycosides

MOA: Inhibit bacterial protein synthesis by binding to ribosomal subunits.

Indications: Life-threatening infections, sepsis, immunocompromised patients.

Adverse reactions: Nephrotoxicity, ototoxicity, tinnitus, permanent deafness.

Special considerations: Doses need to be adjusted for each patient after first dose. Once-per-day dosage has tendency to reduce toxicity.

EXAMPLES OF AMINOGLYCOSIDES

GENERIC NAME	BRAND NAME	DOSAGE FORMS
amikacin	Amikin	Injection
gentamicin	Garamycin	Cream, intramuscular, IV, ophthalmic
neomycin	Mycifradin	Tablet, solution, intramuscular, cream, ointment
streptomycin	Streptomycin	Intramuscular, IV
tobramycin	Nebcin	IV, ophthalmic

Cyclic Lipopeptides

MOA: Bind to bacterial membranes and cause the cell membrane to depolarize, resulting in an inhibition of DNA and RNA synthesis.

Indications: Used to treat complicated skin infections and aerobic gram-positive bacterial infections.

Adverse reactions: Hypotension, headache, insomnia, allergic site reactions.

Special consideration: Should not be taken with 3-hydroxy-3-methylglutaryl coenzyme A (HMG-CoA) reductase inhibitors.

EXAMPLE OF A CYCLIC LIPOPEPTIDE

GENERIC NAME	BRAND NAME	DOSAGE FORM
daptomycin	Cubucin	IV

Miscellaneous Antibiotics

Clindamycin (Cleocin)

MOA: Inhibits protein synthesis.

Indications: Acne, dental prophylaxis for penicillin-allergic patients, anaerobic pneumonia, bone infections, female genital infections.

Adverse reaction: Bloody diarrhea.

Metronidazole (Flagyl)

MOA: Destroys parts of the bacteria's DNA nucleus.

Indications: *Trichomonas* infections of vaginal canal, cervix, and male urethra; amebic dysentery, intestinal infections.

Adverse reactions: Metallic taste, diarrhea, rash, and "Antabuse-like reaction" when alcohol is consumed. An Antabuse-like reaction results in blurred vision, confusion, difficult breathing, hot and scarlet face, an intense throbbing in the head and neck, and chest pains.

Special considerations: Take with food, and avoid any form of alcohol 1 day before, during, and 2 days after therapy with metronidazole.

Pentamidine (NebuPent, Pentam)

MOA: The MOA is unknown.

Indication: Indicated for the treatment of *Pneumocystis carinii* infection.

Adverse reactions: Hypotension, wheezing, coughing.

Special considerations: If the medication is inhaled, the dose must be diluted with sterile water and delivered at a rate of 6 mL/min by a nebulizer.

Linezolid (Zyvox)

MOA: Inhibits bacterial protein synthesis.

Indications: Used to treat methicillin-resistant *Staphylococcus aureus* and vancomycin-resistant *E. faecium* and other gram-positive infections.

Special considerations: The IV form must be protected from light and cannot be administered with other medications.

Vancomycin (Vancocin)

MOA: Interferes with bacterial wall formation.

Indications: Dialysis patients, endocarditis, *Staphylococcus* infections.

Adverse reactions: Ototoxicity, nephrotoxicity, neutropenia.

Special considerations: Potential for overuse prompted the Centers for Disease Control and Prevention (CDC) to issue specific guidelines for use. Patient needs to be kept hydrated.

ANTIFUNGALS

Fungus: A single-cell organism without chlorophyll; a cell wall is present; reproduction occurs by spores. Fungal infections occur when immune system has been compromised.

MOA: Prevent synthesis of ergosterol and inhibit fungal cytochrome P450.

Adverse reactions: Liver toxicities may develop; therefore liver function tests are recommended. GI distress may occur. Photosensitivity, rashes, and nausea are other common side effects.

Special considerations: Antifungals may be used as either topical or systemic agents. Pulse dosing is recommended for nail fungal infections. Consuming a cola before taking itraconazole is recommended. Fatty meals should be taken with griseofulvin. Fluconazole suspension should be refrigerated and expires in 14 days.

EXAMPLES OF ANTIFUNGAL AGENTS

GENERIC NAME	BRAND NAME	DOSAGE FORMS
amphotericin B	Amphotec, Fungizone, Amphocin	IV, topical
butenafine	Mentax	Topical cream
ciclopirox	Loprox	Topical
clotrimazole	Lotrimin	Oral troche, topical, vaginal
clotrimazole-betamethasone	Lotrisone	Cream
fluconazole	Diflucan	IV, tablet, oral suspension
griseofulvin	Grisactin, Fulvicin, Gris-PEG	Capsule, tablet, oral suspension
itraconazole	Sporanox	Capsule, oral suspension
ketoconazole	Nizoral	Tablet, topical cream, shampoo
miconazole	Monistat	Topical, vaginal

Continued

EXAMPLES OF ANTIFUNGAL AGENTS—Cont'd

GENERIC NAME	BRAND NAME	DOSAGE FORMS
nystatin	Nilstat	Tablet, oral suspension, topical, vaginal
oxiconazole	Oxistat	Cream, lotion
sertaconazole	Ertaczo	Cream
sulconazole	Exelderm	Cream
terbinafine	Lamisil	Tablet, topical cream, solution
terconazole	Terazol	Vaginal cream, suppository
voriconazole	Vfend	IV, oral liquid, tablet

ANTIVIRALS

Indications: Cytomegalovirus retinitis, genital herpes, herpes simplex, herpes simplex keratitis, herpes zoster (shingles), influenza prophylaxis, organ transplants, varicella, chickenpox.

Adverse reactions: Headaches, nausea, vomiting, diarrhea, constipation, renal disorders.

Special considerations: Oral products should be taken with plenty of water. When acyclovir is reconstituted, the injection solution should be used within 12 hours.

EXAMPLES OF ANTIVIRALS

GENERIC NAME	BRAND NAME	DOSAGE FORMS
acyclovir	Zovirax	Capsule, tablet, oral suspension, IV, ointment
amantadine	Symmetrel	Capsule, syrup
cidofovir	Vistide	IV
famciclovir	Famvir	Tablet
foscarnet	Foscavir	IV
ganciclovir	Cytovene	Capsule, IV
oseltamivir	Tamiflu	Capsule, oral liquid
penciclovir	Denavir	Cream
rimantadine	Flumadine	Tablet, syrup
ribavirin	Virazole	Aerosol inhalant
valacyclovir	Valtrex	Caplet
valganciclovir	Valcyte	Tablet
zanamivir	Relenza	Inhalant

ANTIRETROVIRALS

Indication: Limits the progression of the retrovirus that causes HIV, which may progress to AIDS.

Nucleoside Reverse Transcriptase Inhibitors (NRTIs)

MOA: Inhibit the release of neuraminidase, a viral enzyme, to prevent the spread of the virus to healthy cells. NRTIs bind and inhibit the action of neuraminidase. This results in the formation of a defective proviral nucleus, which is unable to become part of the host cell's nuclei.

Adverse reactions: Nausea, vomiting, peripheral neuropathy.

EXAMPLES OF NRTIs

GENERIC NAME	BRAND NAME	DOSAGE FORMS
abacavir (ABC)*	Ziagen	Solution, tablet
didanosine (ddI)*	Videx, Videx EC	Capsule, tablet, powder
emtricitabine (FTC)*	Emtriva	Tablet
lamivudine (3TC)*	Epivir	Tablet, solution
stavudine (d4T)*	Zerit	Capsule, powder
tenofovir (TDF)*	Viread	Tablet
zalcitabine (ddC)*	Hivid	Tablet
zidovudine (AZT)*	Retrovir	Capsule, syrup, IV
abacavir-lamivudine	Epzicom	Tablet
emtricitabine-tenofovir	Truvada	Tablet
zidovudine-lamivudine (CBV)*	Combivir	Tablet
zidovudine-lamivudine-abacavir (TRZ)*	Trizivir	Tablet

*Both TJC and the Institute for Safe Medication Practices are against the using of abbreviations for medications; however, physicians may still use these abbreviations.

Nonnucleoside Reverse Transcriptase Inhibitors (NNRTIs)

MOA: Inhibit the action of neuraminidase by preventing the formation of the proviral DNA.

Adverse reactions: Dizziness, headache, rashes, nightmares, hallucinations, hepatotoxicity.

Special considerations: Drug interactions are common; can induce or inhibit the cytochrome P450 systems; resistance to one NNRTI results in resistance to the others.

EXAMPLES OF NNRTIs

GENERIC NAME	BRAND NAME	DOSAGE FORMS
delavirdine (DLV)*	Rescriptor	Capsule, tablet
efavirenz (EFZ)*	Sustiva	Capsule
nevirapine (NVP)*	Viramune	Capsule, tablet

*Both TJC and the Institute for Safe Medication Practices are against the using of abbreviations for medications; however, physicians may still use these abbreviations.

Protease Inhibitors

MOA: Prevent the cleavage of certain HIV protein precursors, which are necessary for the replication of new viruses.

Adverse reactions: Redistribution of body fat ("protease paunch," humped back), facial atrophy, breast enlargement, hyperglycemia, hyperlipidemia.

EXAMPLES OF PROTEASE INHIBITORS

GENERIC NAME	BRAND NAME	DOSAGE FORMS
amprenavir	Agenerase	Capsule, oral liquid
atazanavir	Reyataz	Capsule
fosamprenavir (FPV)*	Lexiva	Tablet
indinavir (IDV)*	Crixivan	Capsule
lopinavir-ritonavir (LPV/r)*	Kaletra	Solution, capsule
nelfinavir (NFV)*	Viracept	Powder, tablet
ritonavir (RTV)*	Norvir	Solution, capsule
saquinavir (SQV-SGC)*	Invirase	Capsule
lopinavir-ritonavir	Kaletra	Capsule, oral solution, tablet

*Both TJC and the Institute for Safe Medication Practices are against the using of abbreviations for medications; however, physicians may still use these abbreviations.

Fusion Inhibitor

Enfuvirtide (Fuzeon)

MOA: Prevents AIDS virus from entering immune cells.

Special consideration: The product has a pregnancy category B rating. It is diluted with sterile water.

ANTIHISTAMINES, ANTITUSSIVES, DECONGESTANTS, AND EXPECTORANTS

Antihistamines

MOA: Block the release of histamine (H_1) in the respiratory system.

Indications: Treatment of allergies, insomnia, rashes, hay fever, dizziness; prophylaxis for drug reactions and allergies.

Adverse reactions: Drowsiness, anticholinergic reactions such as drying up of body fluids, possible hyperactivity in children.

Special considerations: Antihistamines have synergistic effect with alcohol.

Antitussives

MOA: Depression of the cough center or suppression of nerve receptors in respiratory system.

Indications: Cough suppression.

Adverse reactions: Central nervous system (CNS) depression, nausea, lightheadedness.

Special considerations: Dextromethorphan interacts with monoamine oxidase inhibitors (MAOIs); benzonatate should be swallowed but not chewed.

EXAMPLES OF ANTIHISTAMINES

GENERIC NAME	BRAND NAME	DOSAGE FORMS
azelastine	Astelin	Spray
brompheniramine	Dimetapp	Tablet, caplet, syrup
cetirizine	Zyrtec	Tablet
chlorpheniramine	Chlor-Trimeton	Tablet, capsule
ciclesonide	Omnaris	Nasal spray
clemastine	Tavist	Tablet, syrup
cyproheptadine	Periactin	Tablet, syrup
diphenhydramine	Benadryl	Capsule, tablet, topical, elixir, IV
fexofenadine	Allegra	Tablet
hydroxyzine HCl	Atarax	Tablet, capsule, syrup, intramuscular, IV
hydroxyzine pamoate	Vistaril	Capsule, syrup
loratadine	Claritin	Tablet, syrup
meclizine	Antivert, Bonine	Tablet, capsule, chewable tablet
promethazine	Phenergan	Tablet, syrup, suppository, intramuscular, IV

EXAMPLES OF ANTITUSSIVES

GENERIC NAME	BRAND NAME	DOSAGE FORMS
benzonatate	Tessalon Perles	Capsule
codeine	Codeine	Tablet, elixir
dextromethorphan	Benylin, Delsym, Hold, Robitussin DM	Syrup, lozenges
diphenhydramine	Benadryl	Capsule, tablet, syrup
hydrocodone-homatropine	Hycodan	Syrup, tablet
promethazine-dextromethorphan		Oral liquid

Decongestants

MOA: Stimulation of the alpha-adrenergic receptors, resulting in constriction of the dilated arteries within the nasal mucosa.

Indications: Temporary relief of nasal congestion from the common cold, sinusitis, and upper respiratory allergies.

Adverse reactions: CNS stimulation, increased blood pressure, increased heart rate, insomnia, anxiety, tremor, rhinitis medicamentosa, and headache.

Special considerations: Decongestants should be avoided if patient has diabetes, heart disease, hypertension, hyperthyroidism, prostatic hypertrophy, or Tourette's syndrome.

EXAMPLES OF DECONGESTANTS

GENERIC NAME	BRAND NAME	DOSAGE FORMS
oxymetazoline	Afrin	Nasal drops, spray/mist
phenylephrine	Neo-Synephrine, Neo-Synephrine II	Nasal drops and spray, IV
pseudoephedrine	Sudafed	Capsule, tablet, oral solution

EXAMPLES OF COMBINATION DECONGESTANTS

GENERIC NAME	BRAND NAME	DOSAGE FORMS
cetirizine-pseudoephedrine	Zyrtec-D	Tablet
fexofenadine-pseudoephedrine	Allegra-D	Tablet
loratadine-pseudoephedrine	Claritin-D	Tablet

Expectorants

MOA: Decrease thickness of mucus by decreasing the viscosity of the liquid.
Indications: To remove mucus from both lungs and airway passages during coughing.
Adverse reactions: Nausea and vomiting, drowsiness, GI distress.
Special considerations: Patient should consume plenty of water while taking medication.

EXAMPLES OF EXPECTORANTS

GENERIC NAME	BRAND NAME	DOSAGE FORMS
guaifenesin	Robitussin, Humibid	Capsule, caplet, liquid, tablet

EXAMPLES OF COMBINATION EXPECTORANTS

GENERIC NAME	BRAND NAME	DOSAGE FORMS
guaifenesin-codeine	Robitussin A-C	Liquid
guaifenesin-pseudoephedrine	Mucinex D	Tablet

DRUGS FOR TREATMENT OF AFFECTIVE DISORDERS

Anxiety

Anxiety is a state of uneasiness characterized by apprehension and worry about possible events.
Indications: To control anxiety resulting from either exogenous or endogenous stress.
Adverse reactions: May cause either physical or psychological dependence, drug accumulation, birth defects if taken during early pregnancy, muscle relaxation, sedation, and depression.

Special considerations: Many agents used to treat anxiety are controlled substances; therefore federal and state controlled substance laws must be obeyed. Antianxiety agents should be tapered on discontinuation.

EXAMPLES OF ANTIANXIETY AGENTs

GENERIC NAME	BRAND NAME	DOSAGE FORM	CONTROLLED SUBSTANCE
alprazolam	Xanax	Tablet	Yes
amoxapine	Asendin	Tablet	No
buspirone	BuSpar	Tablet	No
chlordiazepoxide	Librium	Capsule, injection	Yes
clorazepate	Tranxene	Capsule, tablet	Yes
diazepam	Valium	Tablet, injection	Yes
lorazepam	Ativan	Tablet, intramuscular, IV	Yes
meprobamate	Equanil	Tablet	Yes
oxazepam	Serax	Capsule, tablet	Yes

Depression

Depression is characterized by feelings of pessimism, worry, intense sadness, loss of concentration, slowing of mental process, and problems with eating and sleeping.

Selective Serotonin Reuptake Inhibitors (SSRIs)

MOA: Block the reuptake of serotonin.
Adverse reactions: Nervousness, insomnia, nausea, diarrhea, loss of weight, decreased libido, ejaculatory disturbances.
Indications: Major depression, obsessive-compulsive behavior, anxiety.
Special considerations: Delay of onset for SSRIs is 10 to 21 days; alcohol should be avoided. This drug interacts with phenytoin.

EXAMPLES OF SSRIs

GENERIC NAME	BRAND NAME	DOSAGE FORMS
citalopram	Celexa	Tablet, liquid
duloxetine	Cymbalta	Capsule
escitalopram	Lexapro	Tablet
fluoxetine	Prozac	Capsule, liquid
fluvoxamine	Luvox	Tablet
paroxetine	Paxil	Tablet
sertraline	Zoloft	Tablet
venlafaxine	Effexor	Tablet, timed-release capsule

Tricyclic Antidepressants (TCAs)

MOA: Block reuptake of norepinephrine or serotonin.
Indications: Depression, nocturia (bedwetting) in children.

Adverse reactions: Cardiotoxic in high doses, postural hypotension in the elderly, drowsiness, anticholinergic effects.

Special considerations: Noticeable results may not occur for several weeks.

EXAMPLES OF TCAs

GENERIC NAME	BRAND NAME	DOSAGE FORMS
amitriptyline	Elavil	Tablet, injection
clomipramine	Anafranil	Capsule
desipramine	Norpramin	Tablet
doxepin	Sinequan, Zonalon	Capsule, oral liquid, cream
imipramine	Tofranil	Capsule, tablet, injection
nortriptyline	Pamelor, Aventyl	Capsule, oral solution
protriptyline	Vivactil	Tablet

Tetracyclic Antidepressants

Indication: Depression accompanied by anxiety.

Adverse reaction: Have a high potential for seizures.

Special considerations: Effects of medication may be delayed, and discontinuing medication should be slow.

EXAMPLE OF A TETRACYCLIC ANTIDEPRESSANT

GENERIC NAME	BRAND NAME	DOSAGE FORM
Maprotiline	Ludiomil	Tablet

Monoamine Oxidase Inhibitors

MOA: Inhibit enzymes that break down catecholamines.

Indication: Atypical depression.

Adverse reaction: Possible hypertension.

Special considerations: If physician changes therapy, MAOIs should be discontinued for 2 weeks before new therapy begins. Patient should avoid certain foods containing tyramine (aged cheeses, certain wines, and certain yeast products); MAOIs should not be taken if patient is taking ephedrine, amphetamine, methylphenidate, levodopa, or meperidine.

EXAMPLES OF MAOIs

GENERIC NAME	BRAND NAME	DOSAGE FORMS
phenelzine	Nardil	Tablet
selegiline	Eldepryl	Tablet
tranylcypromine	Parnate	Tablet

Bipolar Disorder

Bipolar disorder is a depressive psychosis, alternating between excessive phases of mania and depression.

MOA: Not known.

Adverse reactions: Bloating and abdominal distress, bloody stools, acne, leucocytosis, hand tremor, increased body weight, polyuria, polydipsia, nocturia, and abnormal development of fetus during pregnancy.

Special considerations: Blood levels must be established for patients taking lithium and should be in the range of 0.6 to 0.8 mg/mL. Salt content must be monitored and alcohol avoided. Carbamazepine interacts with benzodiazepines, cimetidine, corticosteroids, cyclosporine, diltiazem, doxycycline, erythromycin, ethosuximide, isoniazid, MAOIs, oral contraceptives, phenytoin, propoxyphene, theophylline, thyroid medications, tricyclic antidepressants, valproic acid, verapamil, and warfarin.

EXAMPLES OF BIPOLAR AGENTS

GENERIC NAME	BRAND NAME	DOSAGE FORMS
carbamazepine	Tegretol	Tablet, chewable tablet, suspension
divalproex	Depakote	Tablet
lamotrigine	Lamictal	Tablet
lithium	Eskalith, Lithonate	Capsule, tablet
olanzapine-fluoxetine	Symbyax	Capsule
valproic acid	Depakene	Capsule, syrup, IV

Psychosis

Psychosis is a chronic psychotic disorder manifested by a retreat from reality, delusions, hallucinations, ambivalence, withdrawal, and bizarre or regressive behavior.

Indications: Used to reduce the symptoms associated with psychosis, such as hallucinations, delusions, and thought disorders.

Adverse reactions: Sedation, anticholinergic responses, postural hypotension, excessive tanning, hyperglycemia, lack of menses, nonreversible bone marrow depression, dystonia, akathisia, and pseudoparkinsonism. The following drugs may minimize the side effects: dimenhydrinate, benztropine, diphenhydramine, trihexyphenidyl.

Special considerations: Gains in reducing symptoms may take anywhere from 6 to 12 weeks. Discontinuing medication may lead to relapse of symptoms. Thioridazine has a ceiling dose of 800 mg/day, and promazine dosage should not exceed 1000 mg/day.

EXAMPLES OF ANTIPSYCHOTIC AGENTS

GENERIC NAME	BRAND NAME	DOSAGE FORMS
aripiprazole	Abilify	Tablet
clozapine	Clozaril	Tablet
fluphenazine	Prolixin	Tablet, liquid, intramuscular, IV
haloperidol	Haldol	Tablet, liquid, intramuscular
loxapine	Loxitane	Capsule, liquid, intramuscular
olanzapine	Zyprexa	Tablet
prochlorperazine	Compazine	Tablet, capsule, liquid, suppository, intramuscular, IV
promazine	Sparine	Tablet, intramuscular
quetiapine	Seroquel	Tablet
paliperidone	Invega	Extended-release tablet
risperidone	Risperdal	Tablet, liquid
thioridazine	Mellaril	Tablet, liquid
thiothixene	Navane	Capsule, intramuscular
trifluoperazine	Stelazine	Tablet, liquid, intramuscular
ziprasidone	Geodon	Capsule, injection

DRUGS FOR TREATMENT OF INSOMNIA

Insomnia is difficulty in falling and remaining asleep.

Adverse reactions: CNS depression, dizziness, confusion, impaired reflexes.

Special consideration: Potential for abuse.

EXAMPLES OF AGENTS TO TREAT INSOMNIA

GENERIC NAME	BRAND NAME	DOSAGE FORMS
alprazolam	Xanax	Oral liquid, tablet
chlordiazepoxide	Librium	Capsule
clorazepate	Tranxene	Tablet
diazepam	Valium	Injection, IV, oral liquid, tablet
eszopiclone	Lunesta	Tablet
flurazepam	Dalmane	Capsule
lorazepam	Ativan	Injection, IV, oral liquid, tablet
ramelteon	Rozerem	Tablet
temazepam	Restoril	Capsule
zaleplon	Sonata	Capsule
zolpidem	Ambien, Ambien CR	Tablet

DRUGS FOR TREATMENT OF CENTRAL NERVOUS SYSTEM DISORDERS

Convulsions and Epilepsy

Epilepsy is a neurologic disorder defined as paroxysmal, recurring seizures. It involves disturbances of neuronal electrical activity. Seizures can be partial, generalized (grand mal, petit mal, myoclonic, and atonic), or status epilepticus.

MOA: Blocks the firing of neurotransmitters, resulting in a raised level of depolarization.

Adverse reactions: Sedation and loss of cognitive processes.

Special considerations: Monotherapy is preferred over polytherapy unless patient is not responding to monotherapy. A large number of drug interactions may occur with anticonvulsants because of induction or inhibition. Divalproex should be taken with water, not with carbonated drinks.

EXAMPLES OF ANTICONVULSANT AGENTS

GENERIC NAME	BRAND NAME	DOSAGE FORMS
carbamazepine	Tegretol	Tablet, chewable tablet, suspension
clonazepam	Klonopin	Tablet
diazepam	Valium	Injection, IV, oral liquid, tablet
divalproex	Depakote	Tablet
fosphenytoin	Cerebyx	IV
gabapentin	Neurontin	Capsule, suspension
lamotrigine	Lamictal	Tablet
levetiracetam	Keppra	Tablet
oxcarbazepine	Trileptal	Oral liquid, tablet
phenobarbital	Luminal	Tablet, solution, intramuscular, IV
phenytoin	Dilantin	Tablet, capsule, suspension, IV
pregabalin	Lyrica	Capsule
primidone	Mysoline	Tablet, suspension
tiagabine	Gabitril	Capsule
topiramate	Topamax	Tablet
valproic acid	Depakene	Capsule, syrup, IV
zonisamide	Zonegran	Capsule

Parkinson's Disease

Parkinson's disease is a group of disorders resulting from pathologic alterations of the basal ganglia.

Adverse reactions: Nausea, vomiting, cardiac arrhythmias, drowsiness, postural hypotension, insomnia, constipation, diarrhea.

Special considerations: Therapy is aimed at symptomatic relief. Numerous side effects may occur, resulting in a continual change of therapy. Alcohol should be avoided.

EXAMPLES OF ANTIPARKINSONIAN AGENTS

GENERIC NAME	BRAND NAME	DOSAGE FORMS
amantadine	Symmetrel	Capsule, syrup
apomorphine	Apokyn	Injection (subcutaneous)
benztropine	Cogentin	Tablet, intramuscular, IV
bromocriptine	Parlodel	Tablet, capsule
entacapone	Comtan	Tablet
levodopa	Larodopa	Tablet
levodopa-carbidopa	Sinemet	Tablet
levodopa-carbidopa-entacapone	Stalevo	Tablet
pergolide	Permax	Tablet
rasagiline	Azilect	Tablet
ropinirole	Requip	Tablet
rotigotine transdermal system	Neupro	Transdermal
selegiline	Eldepryl	Tablet
tolcapone	Tasmar	Tablet
trihexyphenidyl	Artane	Capsule, elixir, tablet

Attention Deficit–Hyperactivity Disorder

ADHD is characterized by hyperactivity, impulsivity, and distractibility.

Special considerations: Schedule II drugs with high potential for abuse. Patients taking methylphenidate should have complete blood counts performed periodically. Caffeine should be avoided because of its ability to decrease the effectiveness of the medication.

EXAMPLES OF ADHD AGENTS

GENERIC NAME	BRAND NAME	DOSAGE FORMS
amphetamine-dextroamphetamine	Adderall	Tablet
atomoxetine	Strattera	Capsule
clonidine	Catapres	Tablet, transdermal patch
desipramine	Norpramin	Tablet
dexmethylphenidate	Focalin	Tablet
imipramine	Tofranil	Capsule
lisdexamfetamine dimesylate	Vyvanse	Capsule
methylphenidate	Ritalin, Concerta	Tablet, timed-release tablet
pemoline	Cylert	Tablet

Multiple Sclerosis

Multiple sclerosis is an autoimmune disease in which the myelin sheaths around nerves degenerate. Results in loss of muscles and eyesight.

Adverse reaction: Photosensitivity.
Special considerations: Products require special storage. Copaxone is given daily, Betaseron is administered every other day, and Avonex is administered once weekly.

EXAMPLES OF MULTIPLE SCLEROSIS AGENTS

GENERIC NAME	BRAND NAME	DOSAGE FORMS
baclofen	Lioresal	Tablet
glatiramer acetate	Copaxone	Injection, subcutaneous
interferon beta-1a	Avonex	Single-dose vial, subcutaneous
interferon beta-1b	Betaseron	Injection, subcutaneous
mitoxantrone	Novantrone	IV
tizanidine	Zanaflex	Tablet

Alzheimer's Disease

Alzheimer's disease is a degenerative disease of the brain that leads to dementia; depression and agitation may occur during the course of the disease.
Adverse reactions: Nausea, vomiting, diarrhea.
Special consideration: No drugs can reverse the cognitive abnormalities of Alzheimer's disease.

EXAMPLES OF AGENTS USED TO TREAT ALZHEIMER'S DISEASE

GENERIC NAME	BRAND NAME	DOSAGE FORMS
donepezil	Aricept	Tablet
galantamine	Reminyl	Oral liquid, tablet
gingko	Gingko	Tablet
memantine	Namenda	Tablet
rivastigmine	Exelon	Capsule, oral liquid
tacrine	Cognex	Tablet

RESPIRATORY AGENTS

Asthma

Asthma is an inflammation in the lungs that causes the airways to constrict and is characterized by wheezing, dyspnea, and cough.

Bronchodilators

MOA: Cause the β_2 receptors to relax the smooth muscles, resulting in a decrease of bronchospasms.
Indications: Airway obstruction, chronic obstructive pulmonary disease, reversible bronchospasms associated with bronchitis and emphysema.
Adverse reactions: CNS stimulation, which may result in nervousness, tremors, anxiety, nausea, palpitations, tachycardia, arrhythmias.
Special considerations: Patients may overmedicate themselves to control their asthma. Ipratropium solution needs to be protected from light. Salmeterol needs to be stored at room temperature and

protected from freezing temperatures and direct sunlight. A salmeterol canister should be stored with the nozzle end down.

EXAMPLES OF BRONCHODILATORS

GENERIC NAME	BRAND NAME	DOSAGE FORMS
albuterol	Proventil HFA, Ventolin	Aerosol, capsule, solution, syrup, tablet, inhaler
bitolterol	Tornalate	Inhaler, inhalation solution
epinephrine	Primatene and Bronkaid Mist, Adrenalin	Aerosol, subcutaneous, intramuscular, IV
formoterol fumarate	Foradil	Capsule
ipratropium	Atrovent	Inhaler, nasal spray
ipratropium-albuterol	Combivent	Aerosol
pirbuterol	Maxair	Inhaler
salmeterol	Serevent	Inhaler, inhalant disks
terbutaline	Brethine	Injection, tablet
tiotropium	Spiriva	Powdered capsule placed in a handihaler

Xanthine derivatives

MOA: Reverse bronchospasm associated with antigens and irritants. Improve contractility of diaphragm.

Indications: Used to treat lung disease that is unresponsive to other medications. Used as a bronchodilator in reversible airway obstruction caused by asthma, chronic bronchitis, or emphysema.

Special considerations: Blood levels need to be maintained at 8 to 20 mcg/mL. Theophylline may interact with macrolide and fluoroquinolone antibiotics.

EXAMPLES OF XANTHINE DERIVATIVES

GENERIC NAME	BRAND NAME	DOSAGE FORMS
aminophylline	Truphylline	Tablet, liquid, intramuscular, IV
theophylline	Theo-Dur, Slo-Phyllin	Capsule, tablet, solution

Leukotriene inhibitors

MOA: Block the effects of leukotrienes, resulting in blocking of tissue inflammatory responses such as edema.

Indications: Prophylaxis and long-term treatment of asthma.

Adverse reaction: Headache.

Special consideration: Patients using Singulair must be older than 6 years.

EXAMPLES OF LEUKOTRIENE INHIBITORS

GENERIC NAME	BRAND NAME	DOSAGE FORM
montelukast	Singulair	Tablet
zafirlukast	Accolate	Tablet
zileuton	Zyflo	Tablet

Corticosteroids

MOA: Stimulate adenylate cyclase and inhibit inflammatory cells.

Adverse reactions

Inhaled corticosteroids: Oral candidiasis, irritation and burning of the nasal mucosa, hoarseness, and a dry mouth

Oral corticosteroids: Facial hair on females, breast development in males, "buffalo hump" or "moon face," edema, weight gain, and easy bruising

Special considerations: Long-term oral dosing needs to be tapered off to avoid nightmares.

EXAMPLES OF CORTICOSTEROIDS

GENERIC NAME	BRAND NAME	DOSAGE FORMS
beclomethasone	Beclovent, Vanceril, Vancenase	Inhaler
budesonide	Rhinocort	Inhaler
dexamethasone	Decadron	Solution, tablet
flunisolide	AeroBid	Inhaler
fluticasone	Flovent, Flonase	Inhaler
fluticasone-salmeterol	Advair	Inhaler
methylprednisolone	Medrol	Tablet
mometasone furoate	Nasonex	Nasal spray
prednisolone	Orapred, Pediapred	Oral liquid, tablets
prednisone	Deltasone	Oral liquid, tablet
triamcinolone	Azmacort	Inhaler

Mast cell stabilizers

MOA: Inhibit inflammatory cells.

Indications: Prophylaxis; has no use in an acute attack.

Adverse reactions: Patients using cromolyn may experience an unpleasant taste after inhalation, hoarseness, dry mouth, and stuffy nose.

Special considerations: Airway passages must be open before use; therefore a bronchodilator is used first in conjunction with mast cell stabilizers. Patient compliance is an obstacle because of dosing four times per day.

EXAMPLES OF MAST CELL STABILIZERS

GENERIC NAME	BRAND NAME	DOSAGE FORMS
cromolyn	Intal, NasalCrom	Inhaler
nedocromil	Tilade	Inhaler

EXAMPLE OF A MAST CELL STABILIZER—COMBINATION PRODUCT

GENERIC NAME	BRAND NAME	DOSAGE FORM
fluticasone-salmeterol	Advair Diskus	Inhalation

Emphysema

Emphysema is characterized by the destruction of the tiny alveoli, walls, or air sacs of the lungs. Major risk factors include cigarette smoking, air pollution, occupational exposure, and genetic factors.

Bronchitis

Bronchitis is an obstruction of the airflow during expiration. May be caused by cigarette smoke, exposure to occupational dusts, fumes, environmental pollution, and bacterial infection. Characterized by a cough that produces a purulent, green, or blood-soaked sputum. The lungs' defense mechanism has been destroyed, and there is excessive mucus expectoration with at least 30 mL of sputum every 24 hours for 3 months. Mucolytics are used for the treatment of bronchitis.

Cystic Fibrosis

Cystic fibrosis is a fatal disease involving the GI and respiratory systems. An increased secretion of viscous mucus results in hypoxia.

Mucolytic agents

MOA: Break apart glycoprotein, resulting in a reduction of viscosity and easier movement and removal of secretions.
Adverse reactions: Mucomyst has an unpleasant odor and taste that may cause noncompliance.

EXAMPLES OF MUCOLYTIC AGENTS

GENERIC NAME	BRAND NAME	DOSAGE FORM
acetylcysteine	Mucomyst	Solution
dornase alfa	Pulmozyme	Solution

Tuberculosis

Tuberculosis is a slow, progressive respiratory disease with symptoms of weight loss, fever, night sweats, malaise, and loss of appetite. A major issue with tuberculosis is patient compliance because of the length of therapy and number of medications a patient may be taking. Asymptomatic patients will receive isoniazid daily for 12 months; patients with clinical symptoms are treated with at least two medications.
Special considerations: Patients should avoid alcohol.

EXAMPLES OF TUBERCULOSIS AGENTS

GENERIC NAME	BRAND NAME	DOSAGE FORMS
capreomycin	Capastat	Injection
ciprofloxacin	Cipro	Intramuscular, IV, suspension, tablet
cycloserine	Seromycin	Capsule
ethambutol	Myambutol	Tablet
isoniazid (INH)	Laniazid, Nydrazid	Tablet
isoniazid-pyrazinamide-rifampin	Rifater	Tablet
isoniazid-rifampin	Rifamate	Tablet
ofloxacin	Floxin	IV, tablet
rifampin	Rifadin	Capsule, IV
rifapentine	Priftin	Tablet
streptomycin	—	Injection, IV

Smoking

Smoking increases the risk of heart disease, chronic obstructive pulmonary disease, and stroke. Acute risks include shortness of breath, aggravation of asthma, impotence, infertility, and increased serum carbon monoxide concentration. Smoking cessation results in a reduced risk of lung, laryngoesophageal, oral, pancreatic, bladder, and cervical cancer and coronary artery disease.

EXAMPLES OF SMOKING CESSATION AGENTS

GENERIC NAME	BRAND NAME	DOSAGE FORMS
bupropion	Zyban	Tablet
nicotine	Habitrol, Nicoderm, Nicotrol, Nicorette, Nicotrol NS	Transdermal patch, gum, spray, tablet
varenicline	Chantix	Tablet

GASTROINTESTINAL AGENTS

Antacids

MOA: Neutralize stomach acid to prevent reflux.
Adverse effects: Constipation, diarrhea.
Special considerations: Increased frequency of administration may result in poor patient compliance; reduce the effectiveness of tetracycline; are available OTC.

EXAMPLES OF ANTACIDS

GENERIC NAME	BRAND NAME	DOSAGE FORMS
aluminum hydroxide	Amphojel	Tablet, liquid
aluminum hydroxide–magnesium hydroxide	Maalox, Mylanta	Tablet, liquid
magnesium hydroxide	Milk of Magnesia	Tablet, liquid
magnesium trisulcate	Gelusil	Tablet

H₂ Antagonists

MOA: Block gastric acid and pepsin secretion from histamine, gastrin, certain foods, caffeine; cholinergic stimulation through competitive inhibition at H_2 receptors of the gastric parietal cells.
Adverse reactions: Constipation, drowsiness.
Special considerations: Bedtime dose is extremely important in therapy. Drug interactions include aspirin, alcohol, caffeine, and cough and cold preparations. Available OTC in lower doses. Famotidine IV should be stored at room temperature; reconstituted oral suspension can be stored at room temperature and expires in 30 days.

EXAMPLES OF H₂ ANTAGONISTS

GENERIC NAME	BRAND NAME	DOSAGE FORMS
cimetidine	Tagamet (OTC form available)	Tablet, liquid, intramuscular, IV
nizatidine	Axid (OTC form available)	Tablet, capsule
ranitidine	Zantac (OTC form available)	Tablet, liquid, intramuscular, IV, oral solution
famotidine	Pepcid (OTC form available)	Tablet, suspension, intramuscular, IV

Proton Pump Inhibitors

MOA: Inhibit the parietal cell adenosine triphosphate pump.
Indications: Gastroesophageal reflux disease, erosive esophagitis; taken with other agents in treatment of *Helicobacter pylori.*
Adverse reactions: Diarrhea, dehydration.
Special considerations: Capsules may be opened and the contents placed in applesauce if patient has difficulty swallowing.

Coating Agents

MOA: Form a protective coat over ulcer against gastric acid, pepsin, and bile salts.

EXAMPLES OF PROTON PUMP INHIBITORS

GENERIC NAME	BRAND NAME	DOSAGE FORMS
esomeprazole	Nexium	Capsule
lansoprazole	Prevacid	Capsule, oral powder packets
omeprazole	Prilosec	Capsule
pantoprazole	Protonix	Tablet, IV
rabeprazole	AcipHex	Tablet

EXAMPLES OF COATING AGENTS

GENERIC NAME	BRAND NAME	DOSAGE FORMS
alginic acid	Gaviscon	Tablet, chewable tablet, liquid
sucralfate	Carafate	Tablet, liquid suspension

Antiinflammatory Agents

Indications: Crohn's disease and ulcerative colitis.
Adverse reactions: Nausea, vomiting, headache.
Special considerations: Sulfasalazine is contraindicated in patients allergic to sulfa drugs and aspirin. Will bind to iron tablets. Patient needs to be kept hydrated, and the drug should be taken after meals. Will stain urine orange-yellow and permanently stain soft contact lenses yellow.

EXAMPLES OF ANTIINFLAMMATORY AGENTS

GENERIC NAME	BRAND NAME	DOSAGE FORMS
mesalamine	Rowasa, Asacol, Pentasa	Suppository, enema, tablet, capsule
sulfasalazine	Azulfidine	Tablet, liquid

Antidiarrheals

Adverse reactions: Constipation, respiratory depression, drowsiness.
Special considerations: Diarrhea may lead to dehydration of the individual and may mask more serious conditions, including malabsorption of drugs and nutrients.

EXAMPLES OF ANTIDIARRHEALS

GENERIC NAME	BRAND NAME	DOSAGE FORMS
attapulgite	Kaopectate	Liquid, tablet
bismuth subsalicylate	Pepto Bismol	Tablet, caplet, liquid
diphenoxylate with atropine	Lomotil	Tablet, liquid
loperamide	Imodium, Imodium AD (OTC)	Caplet, capsule, liquid

Drugs for Treatment of Constipation

Emollients, Lubricants, Saline Laxatives

MOA: Emollient laxatives draw water into colon, resulting in bowel evacuation.
Adverse reactions: Nausea, vomiting, diarrhea.

EXAMPLES OF EMOLLIENTS, LUBRICANTS, AND SALINE LAXATIVES

GENERIC NAME	BRAND NAME	DOSAGE FORMS
dioctyl calcium sulfosuccinate	Surfak	Tablet, capsule, liquid
docusate sodium	Colace	Tablet, capsule, microenema
lactulose	Cephulac	Solution
mineral oil		Solution
magnesium hydroxide	Milk of Magnesia	Liquid
sodium phosphate	Fleet Phospho-Soda	Liquid

Stimulant Laxatives

MOA: Increase gut activity from mucosal stimulation.
Adverse reactions: Diarrhea, allergic reactions such as hives, and peripheral swelling.

EXAMPLES OF STIMULANT LAXATIVES

GENERIC NAME	BRAND NAME	DOSAGE FORMS
bisacodyl	Dulcolax	Tablet, suppository
senna	Senokot	Tablet, syrup, granules

Bulk-Forming Laxatives

MOA: Increase fiber in the diet, resulting in intestinal peristalsis.
Special considerations: Considered the safest to use; patient should drink plenty of water.

EXAMPLES OF BULK-FORMING LAXATIVES

GENERIC NAME	BRAND NAME	DOSAGE FORMS
methylcellulose	Citrucel, Fiber Trim	Tablet, powder
psyllium hydrophilic mucilloid	Metamucil	Powder

Bowel Evacuant Laxatives

MOA: Increase osmolarity of bowel fluids.
Indication: Bowel cleansing before GI examination.
Special considerations: Patient should fast for at least 3 hours before administration. Eight ounces should be taken every 10 minutes until 4 L is consumed.
Example: Polyethylene glycol–electrolyte solution (e.g., GoLYTELY or NuLYTELY).

RECENTLY APPROVED BOWEL EVACUANT LAXATIVE

GENERIC NAME	BRAND NAME	DOSAGE FORM
lubiprostone	Amitiza	Capsule

Antiemetics

MOA: Inhibit the impulse going from the chemotrigger zone to the stomach.
Indication: Used to treat side effect of nausea, which may be associated with various medications.
Adverse reaction: Drowsiness.
Special considerations: Phenothiazines may cause hypotension and must be used cautiously in children because of the potential for overdosage, resulting in seizures. Promethazine suppositories need to be refrigerated and protected from light.

EXAMPLES OF ANTIEMETICS

GENERIC NAME	BRAND NAME	DOSAGE FORMS
chlorpromazine	Thorazine	Tablet, capsule
dimenhydrinate	Dramamine	Tablet, chewable tablet, oral solution
granisetron	Kytril	Tablet, IV
hydroxyzine HCl	Atarax	Tablet, syrup, intramuscular, IV
meclizine	Antivert, Bonine (OTC)	Tablet
metoclopramide	Reglan	Tablet, syrup, intramuscular, IV
ondansetron	Zofran	Tablet, IV
prochlorperazine	Compazine	Tablet, capsule, syrup, IV, suppository
promethazine	Phenergan	Tablet, syrup, intramuscular, IV, suppository
thiethylperazine	Torecan	Tablet, suppository, intramuscular, IV
trimethobenzamide	Tigan	Capsule, intramuscular, suppository

Antiflatulents

MOA: Reduce surface tension, resulting in gas bubbles being released more easily.
Indications: Flatulence, gastric bloating, postoperative gas pains.
Example: Simethicone (Gas-X, Mylicon, Phazyme).

Obesity Drugs

Obesity: Males: 25% of total body weight over ideal body weight. Females: 35% of total body weight over ideal body weight.
Adverse reactions: CNS stimulation, dizziness, fatigue, insomnia, dry mouth, nausea, abdominal discomfort,

constipation, hypertension, palpitations, arrhythmias.

Special considerations: All are controlled substances, except Xenical. Both federal and state controlled substance regulations must be followed regarding processing, filling, and record keeping.

EXAMPLES OF DRUGS USED TO TREAT OBESITY

GENERIC NAME	BRAND NAME	DOSAGE FORMS
diethylpropion	Tenuate	Tablet
mazindol	Mazanor	Tablet
phentermine	Fastin, Ionamin	Capsule
orlistat	Xenical	Capsule
sibutramine	Meridia	Capsule

TREATMENT FOR OTHER GI DISEASES

GENERIC NAME	BRAND NAME	DOSAGE FORMS
azathioprine	Imuran	Tablet
balsalazide	Colazal	Capsule
mesalamine	Asacol, Pentasa, Rowasa	Capsule, enema, tablet
infliximab	Remicade	IV
olsalazine	Dipentum	Capsule
pancrelipase	Pancrease, Viokase	Capsule, tablet

URINARY SYSTEM DRUGS

Diuretics: Maintain balance of water, electrolytes, acids, and bases in the body.

Thiazide Diuretics

MOA: Promote sodium and water excretion in the urine, resulting in lower sodium levels in blood vessels and a reduction in vasoconstriction.

Indications: Adjunctive therapy in cardiovascular diseases, such as hypertension.

Adverse reactions: Hypokalemia, hypomagnesemia, hyperuricemia, hyperglycemia, hypercalcemia, photosensitivity.

Special considerations: Patients may be advised to take potassium supplements or to add bananas or oranges to their diet.

EXAMPLE OF A THIAZIDE DIURETIC

GENERIC NAME	BRAND NAME	DOSAGE FORM
hydrochlorothiazide	Hydrodiuril, Esidrix	Tablet

Loop Diuretics

MOA: Inhibit reabsorption of sodium and chloride in the ascending loop of Henle and distal renal tubules, resulting in urinary excretion of water.

Indications: Adjunctive therapy in cardiovascular diseases, hypertension.

Adverse reactions: Low levels of sodium, chloride, magnesium, calcium, potassium.

Comments: Diuretics should be taken early in the day to avoid nocturia (frequent urination during the night). Discolored furosemide tablets or solution should be discarded.

EXAMPLES OF LOOP DIURETICS

GENERIC NAME	BRAND NAME	DOSAGE FORMS
bumetanide	Bumex	Tablet, injection
ethacrynic acid	Edecrin	Injection
furosemide	Lasix	Tablet, oral solution, intramuscular, IV
torsemide	Demadex	Tablet, IV

Potassium-Sparing Diuretics

MOA: Exchange of sodium excreted in urine to returning potassium to the body.

Indications: Adjunctive therapy in cardiovascular issues, hypertension.

Adverse reactions: Hyperkalemia, arrhythmias, gynecomastia in males.

Special considerations: Should be avoided in patients taking angiotensin-converting enzyme (ACE) inhibitors owing to potassium-sparing effect.

EXAMPLES OF POTASSIUM-SPARING DIURETICS

GENERIC NAME	BRAND NAME	DOSAGE FORMS
amiloride	Midamor	Tablet
spironolactone	Aldactone	Tablet
triamterene	Dyrenium	Capsule

Combination Diuretic Products

Adverse reactions: Hyperkalemia; patients taking Maxzide may experience a change in their urine color to blue-green.

Special considerations: Should not be given to patients taking ACE inhibitors.

EXAMPLES OF COMBINATION DIURETIC PRODUCTS

GENERIC NAME	BRAND NAME	DOSAGE FORMS
bisoprolol-hydrochlorothiazide	Ziac	Tablet
triamterene-hydrochlorothiazide	Dyazide, Maxzide	Capsule, tablet

Alpha-Blockers Used in the Treatment of Prostatic Disease

MOA: Relax smooth muscles, especially in the prostatic tissue, resulting in a reduction of urinary symptoms.

Adverse reactions: Headache, orthostatic hypotension, dizziness.

EXAMPLES OF ALPHA-BLOCKERS

GENERIC NAME	BRAND NAME	DOSAGE FORMS
alfuzosin	Uroxatral	Tablet
doxazosin	Cardura	Tablet
dutasteride	Avodart	Capsule
finasteride	Proscar	Tablet
prazosin	Minipress	Capsule
tamsulosin	Flomax	Tablet
terazosin	Hytrin	Capsule, tablet

RENAL DISEASE AGENTS

GENERIC NAME	BRAND NAME	DOSAGE FORMS
cinacalcet	Sensipar	Tablet
darbepoetin	Aranesp	Injection
epoetin alfa	Epogen, Procrit	Injection, IV
iron dextran	InFeD	Injection, IV
sevelamer	Renagel	Tablet

DRUGS USED TO TREAT PROSTATIC CARCINOMAS

GENERIC NAME	BRAND NAME	DOSAGE FORMS
flutamide	Eulexin	Capsule
goserelin	Zoladex	Implant
leuprolide	Eligard, Lupron, Viadur	Implant
megestrol	Megace	Oral liquid, tablet
nilutamide	Nilandron	Tablet

URINARY TRACT AGENTS

Urex or Hiprex (Methenamine)

Bactericidal agent used to treat UTIs. Citrus products and antacids should be avoided when this medication is taken. Sulfonamides are contraindicated.

Pyridium or Azo-Standard (Phenazopyridine)

Local anesthetic that should be taken with an antibiotic for 2 days.

Elmiron (Pentosan Polysulfate Sodium)

Oral preparation for interstitial cystitis.

Ditropan (Oxybutynin)

Antispasmodic used to decrease frequent urination.

Detrol (Tolterodine)

Used to treat frequent urination with strong anticholinergic effects.

CARDIOVASCULAR AGENTS

Arrhythmias

Contractions of ventricle and atria are not synchronized. Premature contractions include tachycardia, atrial flutter, and atrial fibrillation.

Membrane-stabilizing agents

MOA: Slow the movement of ions into the cardiac cells, resulting in a reduction of the action potential.
Adverse reactions: Nausea, vomiting, dizziness.
Special considerations: Procainamide and quinidine are extremely similar and have been interchanged in therapy. Lidocaine is drug of choice for emergency IV therapy.

EXAMPLES OF MEMBRANE-STABILIZING AGENTS

GENERIC NAME	BRAND NAME	DOSAGE FORMS
disopyramide	Norpace	Capsule
flecainide	Tambocor	Tablet
lidocaine	Xylocaine	IV
procainamide	Pronestyl	Tablet, capsule, intramuscular, IV
mexiletine	Mexitil	Tablet
procainamide	Procanbid, Pronestyl	Capsule, injection, IV, tablet
propafenone	Rythmol	Tablet
quinidine	Quinaglute	Tablet, intramuscular, IV
tocainide	Tonocard	Tablet

Inhibitors of neurotransmitter release and reuptake

MOA: Prevent the release of various transmitters and prolong the action potential.
Adverse reactions: Hypotension, bradycardia, mental depression, decreased sexual ability.
Special considerations: IV amiodarone must be mixed in a glass container with D5W.

EXAMPLES OF INHIBITORS OF NEUROTRANSMITTER RELEASE AND REUPTAKE

GENERIC NAME	BRAND NAME	DOSAGE FORMS
amiodarone	Cordarone	Tablet, IV
bretylium	—	Injection, IV
sotalol	Betapace	Tablet

Calcium channel blockers

MOA: Prevent movement of calcium ions through slow channels, resulting in a reduction through the atrioventricular node, reduction in sinoatrial node action, and relaxation of coronary artery smooth muscle.

Adverse reactions: Bradycardia, hypotension, heart block, cardiac failure, constipation, headache, dizziness.

Comments: Diltiazem must be stored in a light-resistant container.

EXAMPLES OF CALCIUM CHANNEL BLOCKERS

GENERIC NAME	BRAND NAME	DOSAGE FORMS
diltiazem	Cardizem	Capsule, tablet, intramuscular, IV
verapamil	Isoptin, Calan, Verelan	Tablet, capsule, IV

Congestive Heart Failure

The pumping ability of the heart is unable to meet the metabolic needs of the body's tissues, resulting in the heart pumping less blood than it receives; blood accumulates in the chambers of the heart.

Antiarrhythmics

Lanoxin is the drug of choice because it increases the force of contraction; increases the effective refractory period of the atrioventricular node; and affects the sinoatrial node through direct stimulation.

Adverse reactions: Nausea, vomiting, arrhythmias.

Special considerations: Concern for digoxin toxicity. A symptom of digoxin toxicity is seeing a green-blue halo.

Angiotensin-converting enzyme inhibitors

MOA: Inhibit the conversion of angiotensin I to angiotensin II. Lower quantities of angiotensin II increase plasma renin activity and reduce aldosterone secretion.

Adverse reactions: A dry, unproductive cough; dizziness occurs during the first few days of therapy; angioedema and possible postural hypotension.

Special considerations: ACE inhibitors have a potassium-sparing effect; therefore one must be aware of possibility of hyperkalemia. Should be avoided in patients receiving lithium.

EXAMPLES OF ACE INHIBITORS

GENERIC NAME	BRAND NAME	DOSAGE FORMS
benazepril	Lotensin	Tablet
captopril	Capoten	Tablet
enalapril	Vasotec	Tablet, IV
fosinopril	Monopril	Tablet
lisinopril	Prinivil, Zestril	Tablet
perindopril	Aceon	Tablet
quinapril	Accupril	Tablet
ramipril	Altace	Capsule
trandolapril	Mavik	Tablet

Angiotensin II antagonists

MOA: Block the action of angiotensin II at its receptors.

Adverse reactions: Angioedema, cough.

EXAMPLES OF ANGIOTENSIN II ANTAGONISTS

GENERIC NAME	BRAND NAME	DOSAGE FORMS
candesartan	Atacand	Tablet
eprosartan	Teveten	Tablet
irbesartan	Avapro	Tablet
losartan	Cozaar	Tablet
olmesartan	Benicar	Tablet
telmisartan	Micardis	Tablet
valsartan	Diovan	Capsule

Myocardial Infarction

The heart muscle does not receive enough oxygen because of a reduced blood supply, and muscle cells die. MI can be prevented through behavior modifications, which include eliminating smoking, controlling diabetes, reducing hypertension through diet and lifestyle modification, exercising three times per week, reducing calories to meet ideal weight, decreasing alcohol consumption, reducing cholesterol and triglycerides, and using aspirin therapy if appropriate. Beta-blockers are used and should be tapered appropriately after the occurrence of MI.

Beta-blockers

MOA: Block response to beta stimulation, resulting in a reduction in the heart rate, myocardial contractility, blood pressure, and myocardial demand.

Adverse reactions: Heart depression, bronchoconstriction, impotence, fatigue, depression, bradycardia.

Special considerations: Discontinuation should be tapered to reduce likelihood of angina.

EXAMPLES OF BETA-BLOCKERS

GENERIC NAME	BRAND NAME	DOSAGE FORMS
acebutolol	Sectral	Capsule
atenolol	Tenormin	Tablet, IV
betaxolol	Kerlone	Tablet
carvedilol	Coreg	Tablet
esmolol	Brevibloc	IV
labetalol	Normodyne, Trandate	Tablet
metoprolol	Lopressor	Tablet, IV
nadolol	Corgard	Tablet
propranolol	Inderal	Tablet, capsule, IV, intramuscular
sotalol	Betapace	Tablet

Angina Pectoris

Angina pectoris is an imbalance between the oxygen supply and oxygen demand in the body.

Nitrates

MOA: Relax vascular smooth muscle, resulting in lower venous return and cardiac filling and therefore decreased tension in cardiac walls. Coronary vessels are dilated.

Adverse reactions: Orthostatic hypotension, flushing.

Comments: Nitroglycerin inhalant is flammable. Nitroglycerin injection needs to be protected from light. Medication should not be stopped abruptly, but tapered.

EXAMPLES OF NITRATES

GENERIC NAME	BRAND NAME	DOSAGE FORMS
isosorbide dinitrate	Isordil, Dilatrate-SR, Sorbitrate	Tablet, capsule, sublingual tablet
isosorbide mononitrate	Imdur	Tablet
nitroglycerin	Nitrobid, Nitro-Dur, Nitrostat, Transderm-Nitro	Spray, tablet, capsule, ointment, injection, IV, transdermal patch

Calcium channel blockers

MOA: Inhibit calcium ions from entering "slow channels" of the vascular smooth muscle and the myocardium, resulting in relaxation of the coronary smooth muscle and coronary vasodilation and a decrease in oxygen demand.

Adverse reactions: Constipation, drowsiness.

Special considerations: Should be taken with food; caffeine should be limited in quantity. Nifedipine liquid-filled capsules need to be protected from light.

EXAMPLES OF CALCIUM CHANNEL BLOCKERS

GENERIC NAME	BRAND NAME	DOSAGE FORMS
amlodipine	Norvasc	Tablet
diltiazem	Cardizem, Dilacor XR	Capsule, tablet, IV
felodipine	Plendil	Tablet
isradipine	DynaCirc	Capsule
nicardipine	Cardene	Capsule, injection
nifedipine	Procardia, Adalat	Capsule, IV
nisoldipine	Sular	Tablet
verapamil	Calan, Isoptin, Verelan, Covera-HS	Tablet, capsule, IV

Beta-blockers

MOA: Slow the heart rate, causing decreased myocardial contractility and lowered blood pressure, resulting in a decrease in oxygen demand.

Adverse reaction: Bradycardia.

Special considerations: May mask symptoms of hypoglycemia and hyperthyroidism. Medication should be tapered off when therapy is discontinued.

EXAMPLES OF BETA-BLOCKERS

GENERIC NAME	BRAND NAME	DOSAGE FORMS
acebutolol	Sectral	Capsule
atenolol	Tenormin	Tablet, IV
metoprolol	Lopressor, Toprol XL	Tablet, IV
nadolol	Corgard	Tablet
propranolol	Inderal	Capsule, tablet, solution, IV

RECENTLY APPROVED AGENT FOR ANGINA

GENERIC NAME	BRAND NAME	DOSAGE FORM
ranolazine	Ranexa	Extended-release tablet

Hypertension

Diuretics

MOA: Reduce total peripheral resistance.

Adverse reaction: Possible hypokalemia depending on agent used.

Special consideration: Should be taken early in the day to eliminate the possibility of nocturia.

EXAMPLES OF DIURETICS

GENERIC NAME	BRAND NAME	DOSAGE FORMS
chlorothiazide	Diuril	Tablet, intramuscular, IV
furosemide	Lasix	Tablet, oral solution, intramuscular, IV
hydrochlorothiazide	Esidrix, Hydrodiuril	Tablet
spironolactone	Aldactone	Tablet
triamterene-hydrochlorothiazide	Dyazide, Maxzide	Capsule, tablet

Calcium channel blockers

MOA: Dilate arterioles, resulting in a reduction in total peripheral resistance, energy consumption, and oxygen requirement.

Adverse reactions: Drowsiness.

EXAMPLES OF CALCIUM CHANNEL BLOCKERS

GENERIC NAME	BRAND NAME	DOSAGE FORMS
amlodipine	Norvasc	Tablet
bepridil	Vascor	Tablet
diltiazem	Cardizem	Capsule, tablet, IV
felodipine	Plendil	Tablet
isradipine	DynaCirc	Capsule
nicardipine	Cardene	Capsule, injection
nifedipine	Procardia, Adalat	Capsule, IV
verapamil	Calan, Isoptin, Verelan, Covera-HS	Tablet, capsule, IV

Angiotensin-converting enzyme inhibitors

MOA: Block ACE to prevent the conversion of angiotensin I to angiotensin II, resulting in a reduction in total peripheral resistance and improved elasticity of arteries.

EXAMPLES OF ACE INHIBITORS

GENERIC NAME	BRAND NAME	DOSAGE FORMS
benazepril	Lotensin	Tablet
captopril	Capoten	Tablet
enalapril	Vasotec	Tablet, IV
fosinopril	Monopril	Tablet
lisinopril	Prinivil, Zestril	Tablet
quinapril	Accupril	Tablet
perindopril	Aceon	Tablet
ramipril	Altace	Capsule
trandolapril	Mavik	Tablet

Angiotensin II–receptor antagonists

MOA: Bind to angiotensin II receptors and block vasoconstrictive effects of the arteries.

EXAMPLES OF ANGIOTENSIN II RECEPTOR ANTAGONISTS

GENERIC NAME	BRAND NAME	DOSAGE FORMS
losartan	Cozaar	Tablet
valsartan	Diovan	Capsule

Beta-blockers

MOA: Block beta-receptor response to adrenergic response, resulting in decreased heart rate, myocardial contractibility, blood pressure, and myocardial response.

EXAMPLES OF BETA-BLOCKERS (CARDIOSELECTIVE)

GENERIC NAME	BRAND NAME	DOSAGE FORMS
acebutolol	Sectral	Capsule
atenolol	Tenormin	Tablet, IV
metoprolol	Lopressor, Toprol XL	Tablet, IV

EXAMPLES OF BETA-BLOCKERS

GENERIC NAME	BRAND NAME	DOSAGE FORMS
carvedilol	Coreg	Tablet
labetalol	Normodyne, Trandate	Tablet, IV
nadolol	Corgard	Tablet
propranolol	Inderal	Capsule, tablet, solution, IV
timolol	Blocadren	Tablet

Central nervous system agents

MOA: Stimulate alpha-2 adrenergic responses in the brain and reduce sympathetic outflow from the vasomotor center in the brain, resulting in decreased heart rate, cardiac output, and total peripheral resistance.
Adverse reactions: Drowsiness, fatigue, depression, fluid retention.

EXAMPLES OF CNS AGENTS

GENERIC NAME	BRAND NAME	DOSAGE FORMS
clonidine	Catapres	Tablet, patch, IV
guanfacine	Tenex	Tablet, liquid
methyldopa	Aldomet	Tablet, oral suspension, IV

Peripherally acting agents

MOA: Block alpha stimulation to peripheral nerves, resulting in vasodilation and hypotension.
Adverse reactions: Hypotension.

EXAMPLES OF PERIPHERALLY ACTING AGENTS

GENERIC NAME	BRAND NAME	DOSAGE FORMS
doxazosin	Cardura	Tablet
prazosin	Minipress	Capsule
terazosin	Hytrin	Capsule

Vasodilators

MOA: Reduce arteriole smooth muscle, resulting in lower peripheral resistance.
Adverse reactions: Tachycardia, palpitations, flushing, headache.

EXAMPLES OF VASODILATORS

GENERIC NAME	BRAND NAME	DOSAGE FORMS
fenoldopam	Corlopam	IV
hydralazine	Apresoline	Tablet
minoxidil	Loniten	Tablet

Combination products

MOA: An additive effect to lower blood pressure and reduce the number of side effects.

Special considerations: Fewer side effects because medications are in lower dosages.

EXAMPLES OF COMBINATION PRODUCTS

GENERIC NAME	BRAND NAME	DOSAGE FORMS
amlodipine-benazepril	Lotrel	Capsule
benazepril-hydrochlorothiazide	Lotensin HCT	Tablet
enalapril-diltiazem	Teczem	Tablet
enalapril-hydrochlorothiazide	Vaseretic	Tablet
irbesartan-hydrochlorothiazide	Avalide	Tablet
losartan-hydrochlorothiazide	Hyzaar	Tablet
trandolapril-verapamil	Tarka	Tablet
valsartan-hydrochlorothiazide	Diovan HCT	Tablet

ANTICOAGULANT THERAPY

MOA: Prevent proper clot formation while maintaining adequate coagulation.

Adverse reactions: Bleeding; urine may turn red-orange; feces may turn red or black.

Special considerations: Warfarin injection must be protected from light. Patient should avoid foods rich in vitamin K if warfarin is taken. Many drug interactions occur with warfarin. Mephyton is given to treat an overdose of warfarin. Blood clotting must be monitored through prothrombin time or international normalized ratio testing. Heparin is to be given either IV or subcutaneously, never intramuscularly. Protamine sulfate is used to treat overdoses of heparin.

EXAMPLES OF ANTICOAGULANTS

GENERIC NAME	BRAND NAME	DOSAGE FORMS
argatroban	Argatroban	Injection
bivalirudin	Angiomax	IV
dalteparin	Fragmin	Subcutaneous
enoxaparin	Lovenox	Subcutaneous
fondaparinux	Arixtra	Injection
heparin	Heparin	IV
lepirudin	Refludan	IV
tinzaparin	Innohep	Subcutaneous
warfarin	Coumadin	Tablet

ANTIPLATELET AGENTS

MOA: Interfere with chemical reactions that cause platelets to clot.

EXAMPLES OF ANTIPLATELET AGENTS

GENERIC NAME	BRAND NAME	DOSAGE FORMS
abciximab	ReoPro	IV
alteplase	Activase	IV
aspirin	—	Tablet
clopidogrel	Plavix	Tablet
eptifibatide	Integrilin	IV
reteplase	Retavase	IV
streptokinase	Streptase	IV
tenecteplase	TNKase	IV
ticlopidine	Ticlid	Tablet
tirofiban	Aggrastat	IV
urokinase	Abbokinase	IV

HYPERLIPIDEMIA

Hyperlipidemia is an elevation of one or more of the lipoprotein levels.

- Blood cholesterol levels per 100 mL of blood:
  - 240 mg: at risk
  - Less than 200 mg: desirable
  - 135 mg: more desirable
- Blood low-density lipoprotein levels per 100 mL of blood:
  - 160 mg: high risk
  - 139 to 159 mg: borderline risk
  - Less than 139 mg: desirable

HMG-CoA Reductase Inhibitors

MOA: Inhibit the enzyme that catalyzes the rate-limiting step in cholesterol synthesis.

Adverse reactions: GI upset, headache, muscle pain, and fever.

Special considerations: Liver function tests should be conducted every 6 months.

EXAMPLES OF HMG-COA REDUCTASE INHIBITORS

GENERIC NAME	BRAND NAME	DOSAGE FORMS
atorvastatin	Lipitor	Tablet
fluvastatin	Lescol	Capsule
lovastatin	Mevacor	Tablet
pravastatin	Pravachol	Tablet
rosuvastatin	Crestor	Tablet
simvastatin	Zocor	Tablet

Fibric Acid Derivatives

MOA: Unknown.

Adverse reactions: Headache, nausea, vomiting, diarrhea, skin rash, alteration in liver and kidney function.

EXAMPLES OF FIBRIC ACID DERIVATIVES

GENERIC NAME	BRAND NAME	DOSAGE FORMS
clofibrate	Atromid-S	Capsule
fenofibrate	TriCor	Capsule
gemfibrozil	Lopid	Tablet, capsule

Bile Acid Sequestrants

MOA: Form a nonabsorbable complex with bile acids in the intestine.

Adverse reactions: Nausea and vomiting.

EXAMPLES OF BILE ACID SEQUESTRANTS

GENERIC NAME	BRAND NAME	DOSAGE FORMS
cholestyramine	Questran	Powder
colesevelam	Welchol	Tablet
colestipol	Colestid	Tablet, granule

OTHER CHOLESTEROL-LOWERING AGENTS

GENERIC NAME	BRAND NAME	DOSAGE FORMS
amlodipine-atorvastatin	Caduet	Tablet
ezetimibe	Zetia	Tablet
ezetimibe-simvastatin	Vytorin	Tablet
omega-3 acid ethyl esters capsules	Omacor	Capsule
niacin-lovastatin	Advicor	Tablet

NARCOTIC AND OPIOID ANALGESICS

Narcotics and opioids: May provide analgesia, sedation, euphoria, or dysphoria during pain management.

MOA: Narcotic and opioid analgesics interact with specific receptor sites and have an effect on the CNS. The body produces endorphins, enkephalins, and dynorphins. These substances are released by the brain after the release of stimuli caused by pain. An increase in the level of pain results in an increase in the release of these substances. There is a decrease in the nerve transmission to the CNS, resulting in a decrease in the sensation of pain. Narcotic and opioid analgesics respond to the same receptors as endorphins, enkephalins, and dynorphins.

Adverse reactions: Respiratory depression, constipation, mental confusion, nausea, and vomiting.

Special considerations: Have a potential for tolerance and addiction. All opiates are controlled substances, and one must adhere to both federal and state laws regarding processing, dispensing, and maintaining proper records of controlled substances. Increased fluid intake is recommended along with stool softeners to combat constipation.

EXAMPLES OF NARCOTICS AND OPIOIDS

GENERIC NAME	BRAND NAME	DOSAGE FORMS	CONTROLLED SUBSTANCE SCHEDULE
acetaminophen with codeine	Tylenol with Codeine	Capsule, tablet, intramuscular, IV, subcutaneous, elixir	III
butorphanol	Stadol, Stadol NS	Nasal spray, intramuscular	IV
codeine	Codeine	Tablet, intramuscular, oral solution	II
fentanyl	Duragesic	Transdermal patch, IV	II
hydrocodone	Hycodan	Tablet, syrup	III
hydrocodone-acetaminophen	Lortab, Vicodin	Tablet, expectorant, elixir	III
hydromorphone	Dilaudid	Tablet, syrup, liquid, intramuscular, IV, subcutaneous, suppository	II
meperidine	Demerol	Tablet, syrup, intramuscular, IV, subcutaneous	II
methadone	Dolophine	Oral concentrate, oral solution, tablet	II
morphine	MS Contin	Tablet	II
oxycodone	OxyContin	Capsule, liquid, tablet	II
oxycodone-acetaminophen	Percocet, Tylox	Tablet, capsule	II
oxycodone-aspirin	Percodan	Tablet	II
pentazocine	Talwin	Tablet, intramuscular, IV, subcutaneous	IV
pentazocine-naloxone	Talwin Nx	Tablet	IV
propoxyphene-acetaminophen	Darvocet-N	Tablet	IV
propoxyphene HCl	Darvon	Capsule	IV

NONNARCOTIC ANALGESICS

Nonsteroidal Antiinflammatory Drugs (NSAIDs)

MOA: Inhibit prostaglandin synthesis, preventing the sensitization of the pain receptors.

Indications: Conditions for which antipyretic, analgesic, and antiinflammatory agents are used.

Adverse reactions: Stomach irritation, drowsiness, nausea, abdominal cramps, jaundice, rash.

EXAMPLES OF NSAIDS

GENERIC NAME	BRAND NAME	DOSAGE FORMS
diclofenac	Voltaren, Cataflam	Tablet, ophthalmic drops
diclofenac-misoprostol	Arthrotec	Tablet
diflunisal	Dolobid	Tablet
etodolac	Lodine	Tablet, capsule
fenoprofen	Nalfon	Tablet, pulvule
flurbiprofen	Ansaid, Ocufen	Tablet, ophthalmic drops
ibuprofen	Motrin, Advil, Nuprin	Tablet, liquid, drops, chewable tablets
indomethacin	Indocin	Capsule, IV, suppository
ketorolac	Toradol	Tablet, intramuscular, IV
nabumetone	Relafen	Tablet
naproxen	Anaprox, Naprosyn	Tablet, caplet
oxaprozin	Daypro	Caplet
piroxicam	Feldene	Capsule

Cyclooxygenase-2 Inhibitors

MOA: Block cyclooxygenase-2 (COX-2) enzymes produced during inflammation.
Indications: Rheumatoid arthritis, osteoarthritis, menstrual cramps, acute pain.
Adverse effects: GI distress and fluid retention.

EXAMPLE OF A COX-2 AGENT

GENERIC NAME	BRAND NAME	DOSAGE FORM
celecoxib	Celebrex	Capsule

Aspirin

MOA: Reduce fever by increasing blood flow to the skin and inhibiting prostaglandin synthesis.
Indications: Conditions treated with analgesics, antipyretics, antiinflammatories, antirheumatics.
Adverse reactions: Stomach ulceration, anemia, prolonged pregnancy and labor, tinnitus, dizziness, headache, mental confusion.
Special considerations: Should not be given to children who have been exposed to chickenpox; may result in Reye syndrome. Should not be given to patients who are taking warfarin.

Acetaminophen

MOA: Mechanism has not been established.
Indications: Conditions treated with analgesics and antipyretics.
Adverse reactions: May increase bleeding in patients taking warfarin; may damage liver and therefore should not be given to patients with liver disease or alcoholics.

Selective 5-HT receptor agonists

MOA: Stimulate serotonin receptors in the cerebral and temporal arteries, which causes vasoconstriction, which in turn inhibits neural transmission, resulting in excessive vasodilation of the cranial arteries.
Adverse reactions: Tingling warm sensation, chest discomfort, dizziness, vertigo.
Comment: Sumatriptan injection needs to be protected from light.

EXAMPLES OF SELECTIVE 5-HT RECEPTOR AGONISTS

GENERIC NAME	BRAND NAME	DOSAGE FORMS
almotriptan	Axert	Tablet
eletriptan	Relpax	Tablet
frovatriptan	Frova	Tablet
naratriptan	Amerge	Tablet
rizatriptan	Maxalt	Sublingual tablet, tablet
sumatriptan	Imitrex	Subcutaneous, tablet, nasal spray, intramuscular
zolmitriptan	Zomig	Tablet

Disease-Modifying Antirheumatic Agents

MOA: Inhibit lymphocytes and cytokine activity.
Indication: Rheumatoid arthritis.

EXAMPLES OF DMARDs

GENERIC NAME	BRAND NAME	DOSAGE FORMS
abatacept	Orencia	IV
adalimumab	Humira	Injection
anakinra	Kineret	Injection
auranofin	Ridaura	Capsule
aurothioglucose	Solganal	Injection
azathioprine	Imuran	Tablet
cyclophosphamide	Cytoxan	Injection, IV, tablet
etanercept	Enbrel	Injection
hydroxychloroquine	Plaquenil	Tablet
infliximab	Remicade	IV
leflunomide	Arava	Tablet
methotrexate	Rheumatrex	Injection, IV, tablet
penicillamine	Cuprimine	Capsule

THYROID HORMONES

Hypothyroidism

Iodine deficiency disease in children results in cretinism. The symptoms in adults include apathy, decreased heart rate, and depression; symptoms in children include short stature, thick tongue, possible enlarged thyroid, lowered voice pitch, myxedema, puffy face, reduced mental acuity, and weight gain.

Indications: Thyroid replacement therapy.

Adverse reactions: Cardiotoxicity and hyperthyroidism.

Special notation: Patient should undergo thyroid-stimulating hormone tests. Levothyroxine injection needs to be used promptly after reconstitution.

EXAMPLES OF HYPOTHYROID AGENTS

GENERIC NAME	BRAND NAME	DOSAGE FORMS
levothyroxine	Synthroid, Levothroid, Levoxyl	Tablet, injection
liothyronine	Cytomel	Tablet
liotrix	Thyrolar	Tablet
thyroid	Armour Thyroid	Tablet

Hyperthyroidism (Graves' Disease)

Hyperthyroidism is an excessive secretion of thyroid hormones that may be caused by thyroid nodules, an excessive iodine intake, or a tumor causing overproduction of thyroid-stimulating hormone. Symptoms include decreased menses, diarrhea, exophthalmos, heat intolerance, nervousness, perspiration, tachycardia, and possible weight loss.

MOA: Therapy includes hormone replacement or surgery.

Adverse reactions: Fever, sore throat, unusual bleeding or bruising, headache, malaise.

EXAMPLES OF HYPERTHYROID AGENTS

GENERIC NAME	BRAND NAME	DOSAGE FORMS
methimazole	Tapazole	Tablet
propylthiouracil	PTU	Tablet
radioactive iodine	—	Capsule, oral solution

HORMONE REPLACEMENT THERAPY

Estrogen Replacement Therapy

Relieves symptoms of estrogen deficiency. The deficiency results in symptoms of vasomotor instability, drying and atrophy of vaginal mucosa, insomnia, irritability, and mood changes.

MOA: Suppress follicle-stimulating hormone secretion, which blocks follicular development and ovulation.

Adverse reactions: Nausea, bloating, weight gain, breast tenderness, possible breakthrough bleeding.

Comments: All estrogen products should be dispensed with a patient package insert. Conjugated estrogen therapy is cyclic. Estraderm and Vivelle are applied twice weekly, whereas Climara is applied weekly.

EXAMPLES OF ESTROGENS

GENERIC NAME	BRAND NAME	DOSAGE FORMS
conjugated estrogen	Premarin	Tablet, cream
conjugated estrogen-medroxyprogesterone	Prempro, Premphase	Tablet
estradiol-levonorgestrel	Climara Pro	Patch
estradiol-norethindrone	Activella, CombiPatch	Tablet, transdermal patch
estradiol-norgestimate	Ortho-Prefest	Tablet
estropipate	Ogen	Tablet, cream
ethinyl estradiol	Estinyl	Tablet
ethinyl estradiol–norethindrone acetate	Estinyl	Tablet

Progestins

Indications: Treatment of menstrual dysfunction, such as uterine bleeding, amenorrhea, dysmenorrhea, and endometriosis.

MOA: Inhibit luteinizing hormone secretion by means of a negative feedback on the hypothalamic anterior pituitary axis.

Adverse reactions: Weight gain, depression, fatigue, acne, hirsutism.

EXAMPLES OF PROGESTINS

GENERIC NAME	BRAND NAME	DOSAGE FORMS
levonorgestrel	Norplant	Implant
medroxyprogesterone	Amen, Cycrin, Provera	Tablet
norethindrone	Micronor	Tablet

Oral Contraceptives

Normally are a combination of progestin and estrogen.

MOA: Suppress ovulation by interfering with production of hormones that regulate the menstrual cycle and alter the cervical mucus.

Adverse reactions: Potential for heart attack, stroke, and thromboembolic disease. Other side effects include nausea, weight gain, breast tenderness, and depression.

Comments: Oral contraceptives must be dispensed with a patient package insert.

EXAMPLES OF ORAL CONTRACEPTIVES

GENERIC NAME	BRAND NAME	DOSAGE FORMS
Biphasic		
estradiol cypionate–medroxyprogesterone	Lunelle	Injection
ethinyl estradiol–desogestrel	Cyclessa, Desogen, Kariva, Mircette, Ortho-Cept	Tablet

Continued

EXAMPLES OF ORAL CONTRACEPTIVES—Cont'd

GENERIC NAME	BRAND NAME	DOSAGE FORMS
ethinyl estradiol–drospirenone	Yasmin	Tablet
ethinyl estradiol–ethynodiol diacetate	Demulen	Tablet
ethinyl estradiol–etonogestrel	NuvaRing	Ring
ethinyl estradiol–levonorgestrel	Levlen, Tri-Levlen, Triphasil	Tablet
ethinyl estradiol–norelgestromin	Ortho Evra	Patch
ethinyl estradiol–norethindrone	Estrostep Fe, Femhrt, Loestrin Fe, Ovcon	Tablet
ethinyl estradiol–norgestimate	Ortho Tri-Cyclen, Ortho Tri-Cyclen Lo	Tablet
ethinyl estradiol–norgestrel	Lo/Ovral, Low-Ogestrel, Ovral	Tablet
Emergency Contraceptives		
levonorgestrel	Plan B	Tablet
norgestrel	Ovrette	Tablet
Progestin		
norgestrel	Ovrette	Tablet
Parenteral		
estradiol cypionate–medroxyprogesterone	Lunelle	Injection
medroxyprogesterone	Depo-Provera	Injection
Implant		
levonorgestrel	Norplant	Capsule

EXAMPLES OF ORAL CONTRACEPTIVE INTERACTIONS

CLASS	DRUGS	TYPE OF INTERACTION
Antibiotics	Erythromycin, griseofulvin, penicillin, rifampin, tetracycline	May decrease effectiveness of oral contraceptive from interference with enterohepatic cycling of estrogen, resulting in a fluctuation of hormone levels
Anticonvulsants	Tegretol, Dilantin, Mysoline, phenobarbital	Decrease contraceptive action from increased metabolism of hormones
Antifungals	Diflucan, Nizoral, Sporanox	May decrease effectiveness of oral contraceptives
Benzodiazepines	Dalmane, Halcion, Librium, Valium, Xanax	Metabolism of benzodiazepine may be decreased, resulting in an increase in side effects
Bronchodilator	Theophylline	Increased side effects of theophylline resulting from decreased theophylline metabolism
Corticosteroids	Hydrocortisone, methylprednisolone, prednisolone, prednisone	Increased effects from inhibition of metabolism by oral contraceptives
Lipid-lowering agents	Atromid-S	Decreased oral contraceptive effect
Tricyclic antidepressants	Elavil, Tofranil	Increased side effects of tricyclic antidepressants

BONE DISEASE AGENTS

Fosamax (Alendronate) and Fosamax with Vitamin D

Bisphosphate approved for osteoporosis. Inhibits bone reabsorption by osteoclasts. It should be taken 30 minutes before the first meal, beverage, or medication of the day. The medication should be taken with 6 to 8 ounces of water to avoid esophageal burning. The patient should not lie down for at least 30 minutes after taking the medication.

Miacalcin (Calcitonin-Salmon)

A nasal spray for estrogen replacement therapy. One should alternate nostrils each day. Patient may experience local nasal side effects.

Evista (Raloxifene)

Inhibits estrogen receptors.

OTHER BONE DISEASE AGENTS

GENERIC NAME	BRAND NAME	DOSAGE FORMS
etidronate	Didronel	Tablet
risedronate	Actonel	Tablet
teriparatide	Forteo	IV
tiludronate	Skelid	Tablet
zoledronic acid	Zometa	IV

CORTICOSTEROIDS

Addison's Disease

Addison's disease is a deficiency of glucocorticoids and mineralocorticoids that is treated with corticosteroids. Symptoms of Addison's disease include debilitating weakness, weight loss, hyperpigmentation of the skin, reduced blood pressure, low sodium and glucose levels, and hyperkalemia.

Cushing's Disease

Cushing's disease results from an overproduction of steroids or excessive administration of corticosteroids over an extended period. Symptoms include a protruding abdomen and fat over the shoulder blades.

Indications: Used to inhibit inflammation.

Adverse reactions: Stomach irritation, hypertension from sodium retention, slow wound healing, thinning of skin, peptic ulcer disease, increased infections, reduced white blood cell function, truncal obesity, moon face, buffalo hump, hyperglycemia, hypokalemia, osteoporosis, alterations in mood, manic-depressive behavior, and cataracts.

EQUIVALENCY OF CORTICOSTEROIDS COMPARED WITH THE DAILY SECRETION OF HYDROCORTISONE (20 MG)

CORTICOSTEROID	BRAND NAME	EQUIVALENCY (MG)	ANTIIN-FLAMMA-TORY POTENCY
betamethasone	Diprolene	0.6	25.0
cortisone	Cortone	25.0	0.8
dexamethasone	Decadron	0.75	30.0
hydrocortisone	Hydrocortisone	20.0	1.5
methylprednisolone	Medrol	4.0	5.0
prednisolone	Pediapred	5.0	4.0
prednisone	Deltasone	5.0	3.0
triamcinolone	Aristocort	4.0	5.0

SIDE EFFECTS OF CORTICOSTEROIDS

TYPE OF EFFECT	SIDE EFFECT
Cardiovascular	Hypertension
Dermatologic	Impaired wound healing, thinning of the skin, petechiae, purpura
Gastrointestinal	Peptic ulcer disease, pancreatitis
Immune system	Infections and reduction of white blood cell function
Metabolic	Redistribution of fat deposits, acne, hirsutism, growth suppression, hyperglycemia, hypokalemia, sodium and water retention
Musculoskeletal	Osteoporosis, vertebral compression
Neuropsychiatric	Alterations in mood; manic-depressive, psychotic, suicidal, or schizophrenic tendencies
Ophthalmic	Cataracts and glaucoma

HYPOGLYCEMIC AGENTS

Diabetes

Type 1 diabetes: Body is unable to produce insulin, and individual is insulin-dependent.

Type 2 diabetes: Impaired insulin secretion.

Gestational diabetes: Diabetes resulting from pregnancy.

Secondary diabetes: Diabetes caused by other medications.

Oral hypoglycemic agents

First-generation sulfonylureas: Increase insulin release.

Second-generation sulfonylureas: Promote release of insulin from the beta cells of the pancreas; increase insulin sensitivity and lower blood glucose levels.

Comment: Adjunct to exercise and diet.

Enzyme inhibitors

Inhibit intestinal wall enzymes that convert saccharides into glucose, resulting in lowering of postprandial hyperglycemia.

Adverse reactions: Abdominal pain, diarrhea, and flatulence.

Contraindications: Patients with cirrhosis, inflammatory bowel disease, colon ulceration, intestinal obstruction.

Biguanides

Decrease intestinal absorption of glucose and improve insulin sensitivity.

MOA: Decrease intestinal absorption of glucose and improve insulin sensitivity.

Adverse reactions: Nausea, metallic aftertaste, weight loss.

Comment: Need to be titrated upward over a period of weeks.

Glitazones

Improve cellular response to glucose.

MOA: Improve cellular response to insulin.

Adverse reactions: Increased plasma volume, elevated high-density lipoprotein levels.

EXAMPLES OF HYPOGLYCEMIC AGENTS

GENERIC NAME	BRAND NAME	AGENT TYPE	DOSAGE FORMS
acarbose	Precose	Enzyme inhibitor	Tablet
glimepiride	Amaryl	Second-generation sulfonylureas	Tablet
glipizide	Glucotrol, Glucotrol XL	Second-generation sulfonylureas	Tablet
glyburide	DiaBeta, Glynase, Micronase	Second-generation sulfonylureas	Tablet

Continued

EXAMPLES OF HYPOGLYCEMIC AGENTS—Cont'd

GENERIC NAME	BRAND NAME	AGENT TYPE	DOSAGE FORMS
metformin	Glucophage	Biguanide	Tablet
miglitol	Glyset	Enzyme inhibitor	Tablet
nateglinide	Starlix	Meglitinide	Tablet
repaglinide	Prandin	Meglitinide	Tablet
pioglitazone	Actos	Glitazone	Tablet
rosiglitazone	Avandia	Glitazone	Tablet
Combination Products			
sitagliptin phosphate	Januvia		Tablet
glipizide-metformin	Metaglip		Tablet
glyburide-metformin	Glucovance		Tablet
rosiglitazone-metformin	Avandamet		Tablet
pramlintide	Symlin		Injection

Injectable hypoglycemic agents

Comments: Humulin insulin can be stored at room temperature for 1 month. Regular insulin can be used IV only.

EXAMPLES OF INJECTABLE HYPOGLYCEMIC AGENTS

GENERIC NAME	BRAND NAME	DURATION OF ACTION
exenatide injection	Byetta	Long acting
insulin detemir injection	Levemir	Long acting
insulin injection	Regular Iletin I	Rapid
	Regular Iletin II	Rapid
	Novolin R	Rapid
isophane insulin	NPH Iletin I	Intermediate
	Humulin N	Intermediate
isophane insulin suspension and insulin injection	Humulin 70/30	Intermediate
isophane insulin suspension and insulin injection	Humulin 50/50	Intermediate
insulin glulisine	Apidra	Rapid
insulin zinc suspension	Lente I Humulin L	Intermediate
insulin zinc suspension; extended lente	Humulin Ultralente	Long acting
insulin analog injection	Humalog	Rapid
insulin glargine	Lantus	Long acting

TOPICAL, OPHTHALMIC, AND OTIC AGENTS

Drugs Used for Treatment of Psoriasis

Psoriasis consists of patches of red, scaly skin, usually on the elbows and knees. May be caused by illness, injury, or emotional stress.

MOA: Regulate skin cell production and proliferation.

EXAMPLES OF AGENTS TO TREAT PSORIASIS

GENERIC NAME	BRAND NAME	DOSAGE FORMS	SPECIAL CONSIDERATIONS
acitretin	Soriatane	Capsule	
alefacept	Amevive	Injection	
calcipotriene	Dovonex	Cream, ointment	Patient should wash hands after each application
coal tar	Tegrin	Shampoo	
cyclosporine	Neoral	Capsule, oral liquid	
methotrexate	Rheumatrex	Tablet, intramuscular, IV	May inhibit normal cell growth
pimecrolimus	Elidel	Cream	
tacrolimus	Protopic	Ointment	

Drugs Used for Treatment of Acne Vulgaris

MOA: Remove keratinocytes in the sebaceous follicle. They loosen the horny cells at the mouth of the ducts, resulting in easy sloughing.

Special considerations: Hands should be washed after each application.

EXAMPLES OF AGENTS TO TREAT ACNE VULGARIS

GENERIC NAME	BRAND NAME	DOSAGE FORMS	SPECIAL CONSIDERATIONS
adapalene	Differin	Gel	Water based—causes less irritation than Retin-A
azelaic acid	Azelex	Cream	Thin film should be applied to affected area twice per day
clindamycin-benzoyl peroxide	BenzaClin	Gel	
furfuryladenine	Kinerase	Cream	Alternative to Retin-A or Renova; causes less irritation
tretinoin	Retin-A	Cream, gel, lotion	Avoid exposure to sun; hands should be washed after each use; may cause severe irritation
tretinoin	Renova	Cream	Has a more moisturizing effect than Retina-A
benzoyl peroxide	Brevoxyl	Lotion	

Drugs Used for Treatment of Actinic Keratoses

Indications: Antiproliferative agents for skin cancer.

Special considerations: May cause transient burning of the skin.

Topical Corticosteroids

MOA: Able to penetrate the skin and suppress the hypothalamic-pituitary axis.

Special considerations: Creams and ointments should not be considered interchangeable. A thin layer should be applied sparingly to the affected area.

Ointments are more potent than creams. Superpotent corticosteroids should not be used for more than 2 weeks, and patients should not receive more than 50 g in 1 week.

Topical Antifungals

MOA: Prevent the synthesis of ergosterol, which is needed for fungal cell membranes. Inhibit fungal cytochrome P450.

Special considerations: Pulse dosing is effective in treating fungal infections in toenails and fingernails.

EXAMPLES OF AGENTS TO TREAT ACTINIC KERATOSES

GENERIC NAME	BRAND NAME	DOSAGE FORMS	SPECIAL CONSIDERATIONS
aminolevulinic acid	Levulan	Topical solution	
diclofenac	Solaraze	Gel	
fluorouracil	Efudex	Cream, solution	Proper hand washing should be followed; avoid direct sunlight; needs to be disposed of properly because it is an antineoplastic agent
masoprocol	Actinex	Cream	Area needs to be washed, and cream must be massaged in properly; should be used for 4 weeks

EXAMPLES OF TOPICAL ANTIFUNGAL AGENTS

GENERIC NAME	BRAND NAME	DOSAGE FORMS	SPECIAL CONSIDERATIONS
amphotericin B	Fungizone	Cream, lotion, ointment, injection	Used to treat patients with a progressive fungal infection
butenafine	Mentax	Cream	Used to treat athlete's foot, jock itch, and ringworm; used daily for 4 weeks
ciclopirox	Loprox	Cream, lotion	Available OTC
clotrimazole	Lotrimin, FemCare, Mycelex	Cream, lotion, vaginal, troche	Available OTC
clotrimazole-betamethasone	Lotrisone	Cream, lotion	
econazole	Spectazole	Cream	
griseofulvin	Fulvicin	Tablet, capsule, oral suspension	Fungal infections of the hair, skin, and nails; avoid exposure to sun; take with a fatty meal
miconazole	Monistat	Cream, vaginal, IV, spray	OTC; used to treat vulvovaginal candidiasis
nystatin	Mycolog, Mycostatin	Cream, ointment, oral suspension, capsule	Commonly used to treat children with candidiasis; patients are told to swish and swallow
oxiconazole	Oxistat	Cream, lotion	
sertaconazole	Ertaczo	Cream	
sulconazole	Exelderm	Cream	
terbinafine	Lamisil	Cream, tablet	Taken orally once per day for 6 weeks for fingernail infections and for 12 weeks for toenail infections; may be pulse dosed
tolnaftate	Tinactin	Liquid, powder, cream, solution	OTC

EXAMPLES OF TOPICAL CORTICOSTEROIDS

GENERIC NAME	BRAND NAME	DOSAGE FORMS
amcinonide	Cyclocort	Cream, lotion, ointment
betamethasone 0.05%	Diprolene	Cream, gel, ointment
ciclopirox	Loprox	Cream, gel, shampoo
clobetasol 0.05%	Temovate	Cream, ointment
desoximetasone 0.25%	Topicort	Cream, ointment
diflorasone 0.05%	Florone	Ointment
fluocinolone	—	Cream, ointment
fluocinonide 0.05%	Lidex	Cream, ointment, solution
halobetasol 0.05%	Ultravate	Cream, ointment
hydrocortisone butyrate	Locoid	Cream, ointment, solution
hydrocortisone valerate	Westcort	Cream, ointment
mometasone 0.1%	Elocon	Ointment
triamcinolone	Kenalog	Cream, lotion, ointment

EXAMPLES OF TOPICAL ANTIBIOTICS

GENERIC NAME	BRAND NAME	DOSAGE FORMS
bacitracin-neomycin-polymyxin B	Triple Antibiotic	Ointment
clindamycin	Cleocin T	Cream, gel, lotion, solution
doxycycline	Vibramycin	Capsule, IV, oral liquid, tablet
erythromycin	T-Stat, A/T/S, Eryderm	Gel, roll-on, solution
mafenide	Sulfamylon	Cream, topical solution
metronidazole	MetroGel, MetroCream	Gel, cream
mupirocin	Bactroban	Ointment
neomycin-polymyxin B	Neosporin	Ointment
silver sulfadiazine	Silvadene	Cream
tetracycline	Topicycline	Solution

Glaucoma

Glaucoma is a chronic disorder characterized by abnormally high internal eye pressure that destroys the optic nerve and may cause loss of vision. Three types of glaucoma exist: open-angle, narrow-angle, and secondary glaucoma.

Glaucoma agents

MOA: Reduce intraocular pressure.
Special consideration: Drug treatment cannot cure the disease but can control it.

EXAMPLES OF OPHTHALMIC AGENTS USED IN THE TREATMENT OF GLAUCOMA

GENERIC NAME	BRAND NAME	DOSAGE FORMS	COMMENTS
apraclonidine	Iopidine	Solution	
betaxolol	Betoptic	Solution, suspension	
bimatoprost	Lumigan	Solution	
brimonidine	Alphagan	Solution	Reduces fluid production in the eye
brinzolamide	Azopt	Solution	Should not be taken with carbonic anhydrase inhibitors
dipivefrin	Propine	Solution	
dorzolamide	Trusopt	Solution	Bitter taste may be present after administration
latanoprost	Xalatan	Solution	May cause light-colored eyes to turn brown; should be stored in the refrigerator
timolol	Timoptic	Solution	
travoprost	Travatan	Solution	
unoprostone	Rescula	Solution	

EXAMPLES OF OTHER OPHTHALMIC AGENTS

GENERIC NAME	BRAND NAME	DOSAGE FORMS	CLASSIFICATION
bacitracin	—	Ointment	Antibiotic
ciprofloxacin	Ciloxan	Solution	Antibiotic
cromolyn sodium	Crolom	Solution	Mast cell stabilizer
cyclosporine	Restasis	Solution	NSAID
dexamethasone	Ak-Dex	Ointment	Corticosteroid
diclofenac	Voltaren	Solution	NSAID
flurbiprofen	Ocufen	Solution	NSAID
gatifloxacin	Zymar	Solution	Antibiotic
gentamicin	Garamycin	Solution	Antibiotic
ketorolac	Acular	Solution	NSAID
levofloxacin	IQUIX	Solution	Antibiotic
naphazoline	Naphcon	Solution	Decongestant
ofloxacin	Ocuflox	Solution	Antibiotic
olopatadine	Patanol	Solution	Antihistamine
sulfacetamide-prednisolone	Blephamide	Ointment, solution, suspension	Corticosteroid
sulfacetamide sodium	Bleph-10	Ointment, solution	Antibiotic
tobramycin-dexamethasone	Tobradex	Ointment, solution	Corticosteroid
trifluridine	Viroptic	Solution	Antiviral
vidarabine	Vira-A	Ointment	Antiviral

EXAMPLES OF OTIC AGENTS

GENERIC NAME	BRAND NAME	DOSAGE FORMS	COMMENTS
antipyrine-benzocaine	Auralgan	Solution	Analgesic
carbamide peroxide	Auro, Debrox	Solution	Wax dissolver
neomycin–polymyxin B–hydrocortisone	Cortisporin	Suspension, solution	Antibiotic
triethanolamine-polypeptide–oleate condensate	Cerumenex	Solution	Wax dissolver

CHEMOTHERAPY AGENTS

Alkylating Agents

MOA: Bind irreversible cross-links in DNA, resulting in cells unable to reproduce.
Adverse reaction: Myelosuppression.

Antibiotics

MOA: Inhibit DNA-dependent RNA synthesis; delay or inhibit mitosis.
Adverse reaction: Cardiotoxicity.

Antimetabolites

MOA: Blend into normal cell constituents, causing them to become nonfunctional, or prevent the normal function of a key enzyme.
Adverse reactions: Nausea, vomiting, diarrhea.

Nitrogen Mustards

MOA: Bind irreversible cross-links in DNA and RNA, preventing normal nucleic acid function.

Plant Alkaloids

MOA: Prevent formation of spindle fibers.

EXAMPLES OF CHEMOTHERAPY AGENTS

GENERIC NAME	BRAND NAME	DOSAGE FORMS	CLASSIFICATION
bleomycin	Blenoxane	IV, intramuscular, subcutaneous	Antibiotic
busulfan	Myleran	Tablet	Alkylating
chlorambucil	Leukeran	Tablet	Nitrogen mustard
cisplatin	Platinol	IV, tablet	Alkylating
cyclophosphamide	Cytoxan	Tablet, injection	Alkylating
cytarabine	Cytosar-U	Subcutaneous, intramuscular, IV	Antimetabolite
daunorubicin	Cerubidine	IV	Antibiotic
doxorubicin	Adriamycin	IV	Antibiotic
epirubicin	Ellence	IV	Antimetabolite
etoposide	VePesid	Capsule, IV	Plant alkaloid
fluorouracil (5-FU)*	Efudex	Cream, IV, topical solution	Antimetabolite
hydroxyurea	Hydrea	Capsule	Antimetabolite
lomustine (CCNU)*	CeeNU	Capsule	Alkylating
melphalan	Alkeran	IV	Nitrogen mustard
mercaptopurine	Purinethol	Tablet	Antimetabolite
methotrexate	Rheumatrex	Intramuscular, IV, tablet	Antimetabolite
mitomycin C	Mutamycin	IV	Antibiotic
temozolomide	Temodar	Capsule	Antibiotic
thioguanine (6TG)*	Tabid	Tablet	Antimetabolite
thiotepa	Thioplex	IV	Nitrogen mustard
valrubicin	Valstar	Injection into the bladder	Antimetabolite
vinblastine	Velban	IV	Plant alkaloid
vincristine	Oncovin	IV	Plant alkaloid

*Both TJC and the Institute for Safe Medication Practices are against using abbreviations for medications; however, physicians may still use these abbreviations.

Hormones

MOA: Inhibit synthesis of adrenal steroids.

EXAMPLES OF HORMONE AGENTS

GENERIC NAME	BRAND NAME	DOSAGE FORMS	TARGET
aminoglu-tethimide	Cytadren	Tablet	Breast, prostate
flutamide	Eulexin	Capsule	Prostate
goserelin	Zoladex	Implant, subcutaneous	Prostate, endometriosis, metastatic breast cancer
leuprolide	Lupron Depot	Subcutaneous	Prostate carcinoma, endometriosis
megestrol	Megace	Suspension, tablet	Breast, endometriosis
tamoxifen	Nolvadex	Tablet	Breast

EXAMPLES OF BIOLOGIC RESPONSE MODIFIERS

GENERIC NAME	BRAND NAME	DOSAGE FORMS	ADVERSE EFFECTS
aldesleukin	Proleukin	IV	
interferon alfa-2a	Roferon	Intramuscular, IV, subcutaneous	Weight loss, metallic taste, nausea, vomiting, abdominal cramps
interferon alfa-2b	Intron	Intramuscular, IV, subcutaneous	Changes in mental status, sore throat, fever, fatigue, unusual bleeding
interferon beta-1a	Avonex	Intramuscular	Myalgia, fever, chills, malaise, fatigue
interferon beta-1b	Betaseron	Subcutaneous	Myalgia, fever, chills, malaise, fatigue

RECENTLY APPROVED AGENTS FOR THE TREATMENT OF CARCINOMAS

GENERIC NAME	BRAND NAME	TREATMENT
bevacizumab injection	Avastin	Treatment of metastatic colorectal disease
cetuximab injection	Erbitux	Treatment of metastatic colorectal disease
clofarabine injection	Clolar	Treatment of relapsed or refractory pediatric acute lymphoblastic leukemia
dasatinib	Sprycel	Treatment for adults with chronic myeloid leukemia
erlotinib	Tarceva	Treatment of advanced and non–small cell lung cancer
panitumumab	Vectibix	Treatment for metastatic colorectal carcinoma
pemetrexed disodium injection	Alimta	Treatment of mesothelioma and non–small cell lung cancer

Continued

RECENTLY APPROVED AGENTS FOR THE TREATMENT OF CARCINOMAS—Cont'd

GENERIC NAME	BRAND NAME	TREATMENT
sorafenib tosylate	Nexavar	Treatment of advanced renal cell carcinoma
vorinostat	Zolinza	Treatment of patients with cutaneous T-cell lymphomas
nelarabine	Arranon	Treatment of T-cell lymphoblastic leukemia

VITAMINS, ELECTROLYTES, AND NUTRITIONAL SUPPLEMENTS

Vitamins

Vitamins are essential organic constituents found in many food products and necessary for normal metabolic functions. May be either water soluble or fat soluble. Fat-soluble vitamins accumulate in large stores, primarily in the liver. Deficiencies may lead to disease after periods of restricted intake. Excessive intake may result in toxicity. Water-soluble vitamins are easily eliminated by the kidneys on a daily basis.

EXAMPLES OF WATER-SOLUBLE VITAMINS

VITAMIN	GENERIC NAME	FUNCTIONS AND INDICATIONS	SOURCES
B_1	Thiamine	Coenzyme in carbohydrate metabolism; deficiency results in beriberi	Pork, liver, kidney, whole cereal, grains, beans, and yeast
B_2	Riboflavin	Maintains integrity of mucous membranes and metabolic energy pathways	Milk, liver, kidney, cereals, and green vegetables
B_3	Nicotinic acid	Involved in fat synthesis, electron transport, and protein metabolism; deficiencies result in diarrhea, dementia, and dermatitis; prevents pellagra	Liver, yeast, lean meats, peanuts, beans
B_5	Pantothenic acid	Deficiencies may result in fatigue, headache, sleepiness, nausea, GI pain, and disturbances of coordination	Vegetables, cereals, yeast, and liver

Continued

EXAMPLES OF WATER-SOLUBLE VITAMINS—Cont'd

VITAMIN	GENERIC NAME	FUNCTIONS AND INDICATIONS	SOURCES
B$_6$	Pyridoxine	Coenzyme in amino acid and fatty acid metabolism	All plants and animals
B$_9$	Folic acid	Needed for the production of healthy red blood cells	Liver and fresh green vegetables
B$_{12}$	Cyanocobalamin	Intrinsic factor for the production of red blood cells; deficiency is seen in pernicious anemia	Animal tissue
Biotin		Deficiency is characterized by dermatitis and anorexia	Yeast, egg yolk, vegetables, nuts, and cereals
C	Ascorbic acid	Maintaining normal cell membrane permeability promotes wound healing and antiinflammatory ability; prevents scurvy	Green plants, tomatoes, citrus fruits

EXAMPLES OF FAT-SOLUBLE VITAMINS

VITAMIN	GENERIC NAME	INDICATIONS	SOURCES
A	Retinol	Prevents keratomalacia	Milk, butter, cheese, liver, and fish oils
D$_2$	Ergocalciferol	Prevents rickets in small children and prevents osteomalacia in adults	Butter, milk, cheese, egg yolk, and fish oils
D$_3$	Cholecalciferol		
E	Tocopherols	Antioxidant for unsaturated fatty acids; deficiency is characterized by irritability, edema, and hemolytic anemia	Soybean oil, wheat germ, rice germ, nuts, corn, butter, eggs, and leafy green vegetables
K	Phytonadione	Formation of prothrombin	Leafy green vegetables, wheat bran, soybeans

Minerals

- Calcium—needed for proper muscle and nerve function; necessary for proper bone and tooth formation; prevention of osteoporosis
- Chromium—aids in metabolism of sugars
- Copper—needed for proper blood formation
- Iodine—needed for proper thyroid function
- Iron—needed for red blood cell formation
- Magnesium—needed for muscle function
- Potassium—needed for heart and nerve function: cellular homeostasis
- Sodium—needed for nerve and muscle formation; cellular homeostasis
- Sulfur—needed for energy production and cellular function
- Zinc—needed for proper immune function

RELATIVE ROLE OF DRUG AND NONDRUG THERAPY

EXAMPLES OF HERBAL MEDICATIONS

NAME	INDICATIONS
Aloe vera	Wound and burn healing
American ginseng	Energy, stress, immune system builder
Basil	Reducing gas
Bilberry	Eye and vascular disorders
Black cohosh	Menopause, premenstrual syndrome, mild depression, arthritis
Cascara sagrada	Laxative
Cat's claw	Antiinflammatory, antimicrobial, antioxidant, immunosupportive
Catnip tea	Diarrhea
Cayenne	Eliminates chills and discomfort from colds; promotes the healing of ulcers
Chamomile	Calming agent, sedative
Chasteberry	Premenstrual syndrome
Chondroitin	Osteoarthritis
Cinnamon	Gas, diarrhea, upset stomach
Cramp bark	Menstrual cramping
Cranberry	UTI
Dandelion	Water retention associated with premenstrual syndrome
Dill	Gas and indigestion
Dong quai	Anemia, energy (females), menopause, dysmenorrhea, premenstrual syndrome
Echinacea	Boosts immune system
Evening primrose oil	Premenstrual syndrome
Fennel	Stomach cramps and gas
Feverfew	Headaches; prophylaxis for migraine
Ginger	Antiemetic, antiinflammatory, GI distress
Glucosamine	Osteoarthritis and rheumatoid arthritis
Goldenseal	Boosts immune system
Grapeseed	Antioxidant, allergies, circulation

Continued

EXAMPLES OF HERBAL MEDICATIONS—Cont'd

NAME	INDICATIONS
Green tea	Anticancer, antioxidant, lowers cholesterol
Hop tea	Sleeping aid
Isoflavones	Cancer prevention, decreased bone loss, lower cholesterol, menopausal symptoms
Kava	ADD, ADHD, anxiety, sedation
Lomatium	Antiviral agent for the flu, immunostimulant
Lungwort	URI
Marshmallow root	Scratchy throat, ulcers, colitis
Melatonin	Insomnia
Milk thistle	Antioxidant, liver disease
Panax	Energy, stress, immune system builder
Passionflower	Tranquilizer
Peppermint	Upset stomach
Saw palmetto	Benign prostatic hyperplasia
Siberian ginseng	Athletic performance, stress, immune builder
Skullcap	Tension headaches, irritability and anxiety associated with premenstrual syndrome, stress
Slippery elm bark	Sore throat
St. John's wort	Depression, improves immune system
Valerian	Sedative, analgesic, nervous tension
White willow bark	Aspirin substitute (analgesic, antipyretic, and antiinflammatory)
Wild yam	Female vitality

LIFESTYLE AND BEHAVIORAL MODIFICATIONS AND THEIR IMPACT ON SPECIFIC DISEASE STATES

ASTHMA

Remove factors from life that may trigger attacks, such as pets, dust, and smoke-filled areas. Yearly flu shots are recommended.

DIABETES

Type 2 diabetes (formerly known as adult-onset diabetes) can be modified through weight reduction; oral contraceptives may cause gestational diabetes; secondary diabetes may be caused by oral contraceptives, beta-blockers, diuretics, calcium channel blockers, glucocorticoids, and phenytoin.

HYPERLIPIDEMIA

Modify types of fat consumed, especially saturated fat.

HYPERTENSION

Modify detrimental lifestyle factors by lowering sodium intake; reducing consumption of calories to reduce weight; increasing regular aerobic activity; lowering alcohol consumption; eliminating nicotine usage; and lowering stress levels.

OBESITY

Weight loss occurs when calories consumed are fewer than calories expended. Strategies include changing the amount of protein, carbohydrates, and fat consumed in daily diet; keeping records of what is eaten; restricting cues that stimulate eating; eating smaller portions; avoiding skipping meals; and avoiding eating late at night.

SMOKING CESSATION

Set a date to stop; inform family and close associates of decision to stop smoking; remove cigarettes and other tobacco products from environment; avoid areas where smoking occurs; if attempts have failed in the past, look for causes and make plans for dealing with these situations; may be difficult at first to stop, but remain persistent.

STROKE

Modify smoking behavior, coronary artery disease, diabetes, alcohol intake, hyperlipidemia, hypertension, obesity, and physical inactivity.

PRACTICE SITE POLICIES AND PROCEDURES REGARDING PRESCRIPTIONS OR MEDICATION ORDERS

- **ASAP order:** An order that is not as urgent as a STAT order but should be given special preference in filling
- **PRN order:** Medication on an as-needed basis in a hospital
- **Standing order:** Order to administer a specific drug at a specific time each day in a hospital
- **STAT order:** Order requiring a medication to be filled within 15 minutes in a hospital

INFORMATION TO BE OBTAINED FROM PATIENT OR PATIENT'S REPRESENTATIVE

Information collected from either the patient or his or her representative by the pharmacy technician is maintained on a patient profile. Every patient has a profile. This information is necessary for the pharmacist to ensure that the patient receives the proper medication and to reduce potential adverse effects. This information includes the following:

- **Patient Information:** Name, sex, address, and age of patient. Obtaining the telephone number of the patient is highly recommended.

- **Billing Information:** Who is responsible for payment of prescription, whether it is the patient or a third-party provider. The third-party provider information includes a group number and subscriber number (e.g., Social Security number) and the individual's relationship to the cardholder.
- **Disease States or Health Conditions:** Specific medications can have an adverse effect on a disease state or condition; drug-disease interactions.
- **Medications Patient Is Taking:** Either prescription or OTC medications. Information is used to prevent drug-drug interactions.
- **Drug Allergies:** Any medication allergies the patient is known to possess. This information is necessary to ensure that the patient does not receive a medication that can have an adverse effect on the patient.

REQUIRED PRESCRIPTION ORDER REFILL INFORMATION

Information required for refilling a prescription includes patient's name, patient's home telephone number, and prescription number. Some systems require the name, strength, and quantity of medication. Pharmacies may be able to locate a prescription by reviewing the patient's profile.

FORMULA TO VERIFY THE VALIDITY OF A PRESCRIBER'S DRUG ENFORCEMENT AGENCY NUMBER

Drug Enforcement Agency Number

A DEA number consists of two letters and seven numbers assigned to a physician. A physician is required to have a DEA number if he or she wishes to write prescriptions for controlled substances. Institutions, such as hospitals and pharmacies, are required to have a DEA number if controlled substances are dispensed from these locations.

Verifying a Drug Enforcement Agency Number

- The first letter is an A, B, F, or M.
- The second letter is the first letter of the physician's last name when he or she applied for a DEA number.
- Add the numbers in the first, third, and fifth positions together.
- Add the numbers in the second, fourth, and sixth positions together. Multiply the sum by two.
- Add both sums of numbers together. The number in the last column farthest from the right should be the same as the seventh digit of the DEA number. For example, what should be the seventh digit in

Dr. Andrew Shedlock's DEA number if it begins with BS452589____?

$$\text{Add } 4 + 2 + 8 = 14$$
$$\text{Add } 5 + 5 + 9 = 19; \text{ multiply 19 by 2 and get 38}$$
$$\text{Add 14 to 38 and get 52; the last number}$$
$$\text{should be a 2}$$

Therefore the correct DEA number for Dr. Andrew Shedlock is BS4525892.

TECHNIQUES FOR DETECTING FORGED OR ALTERED PRESCRIPTIONS

Types of Fraudulent Prescriptions

- Legitimate prescription pads are stolen from physicians' offices, and prescriptions are written for fictitious patients.
- Drug abusers may alter the physician's prescription to obtain larger quantities of medications.
- Drug abusers may have prescription pads from legitimate physicians printed with a different callback number that is answered by an accomplice to verify the prescription.
- Drug abuser will call in prescriptions and give his or her own telephone number as a callback number.
- Computers may be used to create prescriptions for nonexistent physicians or to copy legitimate physicians' prescriptions.

Signs Indicating a Prescription Was Not Issued for a Legitimate Medical Purpose

- Prescriber writes significantly more prescriptions or in larger quantities compared with other practitioners in the area.
- The patient appears to be returning too frequently. For example, a prescription that should last for a month is being refilled biweekly or more frequently.
- The prescriber writes prescriptions for antagonistic drugs, such as stimulants and depressants simultaneously.
- The patient is presenting prescriptions written in the names of other people.
- A number of people appear simultaneously or within a short time bearing similar prescriptions from the same physician.
- "Strangers," individuals who are not regular residents of the community, show up with prescriptions from the same physician.
- The medication prescribed is not within the scope of practice of the doctor.

- Patients may appear to be very talkative and therefore may prevent you from verifying the prescription.

Characteristics of Forged Prescriptions

- Prescription looks "too good"; the prescriber's handwriting is too legible.
- Quantities, directions, or dosages differ from usual medical usage.
- Prescription does not comply with the acceptable standard abbreviations or appears to be textbook presentation.
- Prescription appears to be photocopied.
- Directions written in full with no abbreviations.
- Prescriptions written in different colored inks, different pens, or different handwriting.

PREVENTION TECHNIQUES FOR FRAUDULENT PRESCRIPTIONS

- Know the prescriber and his or her signature.
- Know the prescriber's DEA registration number.
- Know the patient. Check the date of when the prescription was written.
- If there is a discrepancy, the patient must have a plausible reason before the medication is dispensed.
- Anytime there is doubt, request proper identification.
- If you believe that you have a forged, altered, or counterfeited prescription, do not dispense the medication. Contact the local police.
- If you discover a pattern of prescription abuses, contact the state board of pharmacy or the local DEA office.

Knowledge of Techniques for Detecting Prescription Errors

- Verify that the patient information is correct, including birth date, home address, and telephone number. Some patients with very common names may appear several times in the pharmacy system. Choosing the incorrect patient may result in an incorrect drug utilization review. Incorrect patient information may lead to incorrect billing to an insurance carrier.
- Make sure that the dose is appropriate for the age of the patient.
- Check the label on the stock bottle and the NDC number in the computer against the original for confirmation of the order. If it does not seem right, bring it to the attention of the pharmacist.
- Pull the appropriate medication from the shelf. Take the label with you when you are retrieving the medication. Do not make assumptions about dosage forms; creams and ointments are different;

capsule and spansules are not the same; dosage forms with CR, XL, and SA are not the same as normal tablets or capsules.
- Place stock bottles back on shelf when the prescription has been verified by the pharmacist. Extra bottles and clutter on the counter can contribute to errors.
- Place correct auxiliary label on top of container so the pharmacist can check it before placing it on the bottle for dispensing.
- If counting out medication manually, count in multiples of fives.

EFFECTS OF PATIENTS' DISABILITIES ON DRUG AND NONDRUG THERAPY

- As patients age, their eyesight may begin to deteriorate. This may increase the possibility of misreading the label and not taking medication properly.
- As patients age, their hearing may decline; they may not properly hear questions being asked and thus provide incorrect information to the pharmacy, or they may not thoroughly understand how they are to take their medication.
- An individual's dexterity may worsen as he or she ages, which may cause difficulty in removing the lid of the container, resulting in the possibility of missed doses.
- As individuals age, they may experience several conditions resulting in additional medications to be taken. The possibility of side effects will increase. Treatment of these side effects may result in additional side effects.
- An individual's mental sharpness may decrease, resulting in missed doses from forgetfulness.

TECHNIQUES, EQUIPMENT, AND SUPPLIES FOR DRUG ADMINISTRATION

- Home infusion supplies, including IV starter kits, central venous catheter starter kits, catheters, IV tubing, extension tubing, IV connectors, IV filters, injection caps, syringes and needles, IV poles, sterile dressings, antibacterial cleansing solutions, sharps containers, infectious waste containers, tape, masks, gloves, batteries (for battery-operated infusion kits), and chemotherapy spill kits
- Infusion pumps
- Insulin syringes: 30, 50, 100 units/mL
- Oral syringes: may be used for pediatric medications
- Radiopharmaceuticals (nucleotide and carrier drugs, such as macroaggregated albumin, medronic acid (e.g., Choletec, Cardiolite, TechniScan)

- Vaginal inserters, vaginal creams and suppositories

MONITORING AND SCREENING EQUIPMENT

Pharmacy technicians should be familiar with various types of monitoring and screening equipment. These may include the following:

- **AIDS testing kits:** Detect HIV antibodies in the blood
- **Air purifiers:** Remove dust, pollen, spores, secondhand smoke, and other irritants from room air
- **Blood glucose monitors (Glucometer):** Used to determine glucose in the blood
- **Blood pressure monitors:** Used to determine blood pressure of an individual
- **Echocardiogram:** Used to measure the functionality of the heart valves
- **Electrocardiogram:** Used to measure cardiac rates and rhythms
- **Nebulizers:** Generate very fine particles of liquid in a gas and are used in providing inhalation therapy
- **Oxygen therapy:** Supplemental oxygen is used to treat both respiratory and nonrespiratory clinical disorders
- **Peak flow meter:** Used to measure and manage asthma in an individual
- **Phototherapy:** Used in the treatment of neonatal jaundice; consists of an illuminator, fiberoptic cable, and fiberoptic panel
- **Pneumograms:** Two-channel recording of heart rate and respiration in the monitoring of apnea
- **Pregnancy testing kits:** Used to diagnose pregnancy based on the ability to detect human chorionic gonadotropin in the urine
- **Sphygmomanometer:** Used to measure vital capacity
- **Steam vaporizers:** Provide relief for upper respiratory illness, such as colds and sinusitis
- **Thermometers:** Used to measure body temperature; one of three types—oral, rectal, or stubby; basal thermometers are used to determine whether a women is ovulating

MEDICAL AND SURGICAL APPLIANCES AND DEVICES

- **Bedpans:** Used for the collection of feces
- **Breast pumps:** Allow women to continue breastfeeding their babies on return to work; may be either manual or electrical
- **Bulb syringes:** A nonsterile irrigation method for the nose, ear, wounds, or vagina
- **CADD-Plus pump:** Infusion pump for antibiotics
- **CADD Prizm PCS:** Pump for patient-controlled analgesia (PCA)
- **CADD-TPN:** Infusion pump for total parenteral nutrition (TPN)
- **Cane:** A walking device that provides a means to transfer weight off the weak limb and provides balance over the supporting limb
- **Catheters:** Used to collect urine from a patient unable to urinate naturally
- **Commode:** A portable toilet used when a patient is unable to ambulate from the bed to the bathroom
- **Crutches:** Provide support for the patient's wrist and elbow; provide more support than a cane
- Cushions and supplies for pressure sores
- **Elastometric balloon system:** Pressurized balloon; infusion results when device is deflated
- **Electric heating pads:** Used to apply dry heat to an individual; does not result in the leaking or spilling of hot water on an individual; temperature is kept constant
- **Enema syringes:** Used for irrigating with water, salt solution, soapsuds, or special medications
- **Enteral feeding tubes** include nasogastric tube, nasoduodenal tube, nasojejunal tube, percutaneous endoscopic tube (PEG), and percutaneous endoscopic jejunostomy tube
- **Gravity infusion system:** Medication in a minibag is infused by gravity; patient controls the number of drops
- **Hospital beds:** May be either manual or electrical; fixed or variable height; may come with a mattress, safety rails, bed handles, alternating pressure pads, and trapeze bars
- **Hot water bottles:** A method of applying dry heat to an area; should have a cover to prevent the skin from becoming burned
- **IV push system:** manually depressing syringe
- **Moist heat packs:** Known as *hydrocollators*; can be heated by boiling water or by being placed in a microwave; reusable and can be stored in the freezer when not in use
- **Ostomy appliance for solid waste:** Known as a *colostomy bag*
- **Ostomy appliance for urine and semisolids:** Used for urinary diversions and ileostomies
- **Patient lifter:** May be either hydraulic or a screw-type lifter; enables a patient to be lifted up and down into a chair
- **Syringe infusion system:** Medication is infused by a special syringe pump
- **Traction:** May be either flexion or hyperextension; can be used for cervical or pelvic traction

- **Transcutaneous electrical nerve stimulation:** Delivers electrical signals throughout the skin to control pain
- **Urinals:** Used to collect urine; male and female urinals differ in shape
- **Vacuum constriction device:** A nonsurgical solution to impotence in men; the penis is placed in a patented vacuum cylinder, which generates blood flow in the penis, resulting in an erection
- **Walker:** Provides steadier support than a cane but requires good arms, wrists, and hands
- **Wheelchairs:** Should be individualized for the patient based on the patient's physical limitations and lifestyle; should provide good body alignment

PROPER STORAGE CONDITIONS

All medications have specific storage conditions determined by the manufacturer, which include the type of container (such as a light-resistant container) and temperature. The following definitions indicate the proper temperature at which a drug is to be stored.

- **Cold:** Not to exceed 8°C (46°F)
- **Cool:** Any temperature between 8° and 15°C (46° and 59°F)
- **Room temperature:** Any temperature between 15° and 30°C (59° and 86°F)
- **Warm:** Any temperature between 30° and 40°C (86° and 104°F)
- **Excessive heat:** Any temperature above 40°C (104°F)

Specific packaging requirements include the following:

- **Light-resistant container:** Protects contents from the effects of light through the use of special materials or by an opaque covering
- **Tamper-resistant packaging:** Sealed in a manner that would alert an individual that the package had been opened
- **Tight container:** Protects contents from contamination by liquids, solids, or vapors during normal shipping, handling, storage, and distribution
- **Hermetic container:** The container is impermeable to air under normal handling, shipment, storage, and distribution
- **Single-unit container:** The container holds a specific quantity of drug for a single dose
- **Single-dose container:** Single-unit container intended for parenteral administration only
- **Unit-dose container:** A single-unit container for articles intended for administration other than the parenteral route as a single dose, directly from the container

AUTOMATED DISPENSING TECHNOLOGY

Automated Dispensing Systems

An automated dispensing system is a drug storage device or cabinet that electronically dispenses medications in a controlled fashion and tracks medication use. Automatic dispensing allows a nurse to obtain medication for inpatients at the point of use. The systems require user identifiers and passwords, and internal electronic devices track nurses accessing the system, track the patients for whom medications are administered, and provide usage to the hospital's financial office for the patients' bills. The system may be centralized or decentralized.

Robotics

Robotics refers to machinery that increases productivity in the pharmacy and results in fewer prescription errors.

Outpatient Dispensing System

Baker Cells (McKesson Corp., San Francisco, Calif.): Can accurately count and dispense up to 600 tablets per minute. A flexible, lockable system that can adapt to various space requirements and can be expanded if necessary. Can interface with pharmacy host system.

Inpatient Dispensing Systems

AcuDose-Rx (McKesson Corp.): A decentralized medication distribution center. Operational after a physician's order has been entered into the patient's profile. Authorized users choose the patient's profile and select the appropriate drug.

Baxter ATC 212 (Baxter B.V., Utrecht, The Netherlands): The system uses a microcomputer to pack unit-dose tablets and capsules for oral administration. It is installed at the pharmacy. Medications are stored in calibrated canisters that are designed specifically for each medication. The canisters are assigned a numbered location to reduce mix-up errors on dispensing. An order is sent to the microcomputer, and a tablet is dispensed from a particular canister. The drug is ejected into a strip-packing device, in which it is labeled and hermetically sealed.

McLaughlin Dispensing System: Includes a bedside dispenser, a programmable magnetic card, and a pharmacy computer. It is a locked system that is loaded with the medications for a specific patient. At the correct dosing time the bedside dispenser drawer unlocks automatically to allow a dose to be removed and administered to the patient. A light above the patient's door illuminates at the appropriate dosing time.

MedCarousel (McKesson Corp.): A medication and storage system and retrieval system for hospital pharmacies with vertically rotating shelves; bar code scannable.

Physician's Order Entry System

- **MedDirect (Grand Rapids, Mich.):** An automated system for communicating medication ordering for managing documents.
- **OmniLinkRx (Omnicell, Mountain View, Calif.):** An advanced patient safety solution for the management of handwritten physician orders; it simplifies the communication of orders from remote nursing stations to the pharmacy. Improves communication between nursing and pharmacy, resulting in improved efficiency and productivity.
- **Medstation and Medstation Rx (Pyxis):** Automated dispensing devices kept on the nursing unit. The Medstation interfaces with the pharmacy computer. Physician orders are entered into the pharmacy computer and then transferred to the Medstation, where patient profiles are displayed to the nurse who accesses the medications for verified orders. Each nurse is provided with a password that must be used to access the Medstation. Charges are made automatically for drugs dispensed by the unit.
- **Robot-Rx (McKesson Corp.):** A centralized, robotic drug distribution system that automates storage, dispensing, returning, restocking, and crediting bar-coded inpatient medications.
- **Saf-T-Pak (Edmonton, Canada):** An automated bar code medication packaging system. Can be used for unit-dose and multidose oral solid medications. Automates the replenishment of decentralized cabinets and the filling of individual patient medication bins.

PACKAGING REQUIREMENTS

Packaging is determined by the manufacturer's specification to ensure the effectiveness and shelf life of the drug. The packaging will be affected by how a medication is to be stored in the pharmacy. A pharmacy technician must be familiar with the packaging of each medication. The packaging conditions take into consideration temperature, humidity, light, and incompatibilities with other medications and various types of packaging materials.

All medications, whether prescription or OTC, are subject to the Poison Prevention Act of 1970. Exceptions to this law include the following:

- Single-time dispensing of product in noncompliant container as ordered by the physician
- Single-time or blanket dispensing of product in noncompliant container as requested by patient or customer in a signed statement
- One noncompliant size of OTC product for elderly or handicapped patients, provided the label contains the warning "This Package for Households Without Young Children," or "Package Not Child Resistant"
- Drugs dispensed to institutionalized patients, provided that they are to be administered by an employee of the institution

SPECIFIC DRUGS

- Betamethasone with no more than 12.6 mg per package
- Erythromycin ethylsuccinate tablets in packages containing no more than 16 g
- Inhalation aerosols
- Mebendazole tablets with no more than 600 mg per package
- Methylprednisolone tablets with no more than 85 mg per package
- Oral contraceptives taken cyclically in manufacturer's dispensing package
- Pancrelipase preparations
- Powdered anhydrous cholestyramine
- Powdered colestipol up to 5 g per packet
- Prednisone tablets with no more than 105 mg per package
- Sodium fluoride tablets with no more than 264 mg of sodium fluoride per package
- Sublingual and chewable isosorbide dinitrate, in doses of 10 mg or less
- Sublingual nitroglycerin tablets

NATIONAL DRUG CODE NUMBER COMPONENTS

Each drug is assigned a specific 11-digit number to identify it. The first five numbers identify the manufacturer, the next four numbers identify the drug product, and the final two numbers represent the package size and packaging. If a medication is reformulated, it will be given a new NDC number. If a drug manufacturer purchases another drug company, the NDC number will also change.

PURPOSE OF LOT NUMBERS AND EXPIRATION DATES

Lot numbers are assigned by the drug manufacturer to identify a given batch of medication. Expiration dates are assigned by the manufacturer and ensure the amount of time a product will be pure, safe, and effective for use by a patient. The expiration date is the last day of a particular month of a given year. Both of these pieces of information are used in the recall of a drug, whether by the manufacturer or the FDA.

INFORMATION FOR PRESCRIPTION OR MEDICATION ORDER LABEL(S)

A prescription is filled in an outpatient pharmacy for a patient. A medication order is filled for an individual who has been assigned a bed in a hospital or long-term care facility.

Required Prescription Label Information

- Date when the prescription was filled
- Serial (prescription) number of the prescription
- Name and address of the pharmacy
- Name of the patient
- Name of the prescribing physician
- All directions for use of the prescription
- Generic or brand name of the prescription
- Strength of the medication
- Name of the drug manufacturer
- Quantity of the drug
- Expiration date of the drug
- Initials of the licensed pharmacist
- Number of refills allowed

Auxiliary (Ancillary) Labels

Auxiliary labels provide additional information, such as special instructions, warnings, or storage conditions, to the patient. They may provide information on the administration of the drug.

Required Medication Order Label Information

- Name and location of patient
- Trade or generic name of drug
- Strength of drug
- Quantity of drug
- Expiration date of medication
- Lot number of medication

REQUIREMENTS REGARDING PATIENT PACKAGE INSERTS

A patient package insert is an informational leaflet written for the lay public describing the benefits and risks of medications. Information found on a package insert includes the following:

- Description
- Clinical pharmacology
- Indications and usage
- Contraindications
- Warnings
- Precautions
- Adverse reactions
- Drug abuse and dependence
- Overdosage
- Dosage and administration
- How supplied
- Date of the most recent revision of the labeling

A pharmacy is required to provide patient package inserts to all patients receiving metered-dose inhalers, oral contraceptives, estrogen, progesterone, and Accutane.

SPECIAL DIRECTIONS AND PRECAUTIONS FOR PATIENT OR PATIENT'S REPRESENTATIVE REGARDING PREPARATION AND USE OF MEDICATIONS

The following information can be given to either the patient or the patient's representative. This information may be considered as counseling, and therefore it is the pharmacist's responsibility rather than a pharmacy technician's:

- Name of medication
- Dosage form
- Dosage
- Route of administration
- Duration of therapy
- Action to be taken if a dose is missed
- Common or severe side effects
- Interactions and contraindications of the medication (to include food)
- Self-monitoring of medication
- Proper storage of medication
- Special directions

TECHNIQUES FOR ASSESSING A PATIENT'S COMPLIANCE WITH PRESCRIPTION OR MEDICATION ORDER

- Calculate how many days the prescriptions should last (i.e., day's supply = quantity dispensed/quantity taken each day).
- If the patient is seeking a refill early or the prescription is lasting longer than it should last, the pharmacist should seek information from the patient. If the directions have changed, a new prescription should be issued from the physician.
- The pharmacist should ascertain the reason for possible noncompliance of the patient in an empathetic manner. The patient may have received professional samples from the physician, or the patient may admit he or she has been experiencing financial difficulties, resulting in noncompliance.

- Pharmacists should attempt to persuade physicians not to use "as directed" for directions to the patient.
- If the patient has forgotten to take medication, the pharmacist should work with the patient to find a way to resolve the issue.
- Finally, the pharmacist should emphasize the importance of compliance to the patient in a caring and understanding manner.

ACTION TO BE TAKEN IN THE EVENT OF A MISSED DOSE

Patients need to check with the pharmacist regarding what to do if they forget a dose. Situations vary depending on the medication and frequency of dosing. Providing this information is part of counseling and can be done only by a pharmacist.

MEDICATION DISTRIBUTION

REQUIREMENTS FOR MAILING MEDICATIONS

The U.S. Post Office will not allow the mailing of controlled substances with the exception of the Veterans Administration. Other postal services (such as FedEx or UPS) are not governed by these regulations, but the outside label of the package is to be unmarked so the contents cannot be identified. Medications mailed from a drug manufacturer must be sent by registered mail with a return request form.

DELIVERY SYSTEMS FOR DISTRIBUTING MEDICATIONS

Drug Distribution System

A drug distribution system is a safe and economic method of distributing a medication. A drug distribution system includes the packaging that holds the medication during the transfer of the drug from the pharmacy to the patient.

Centralized dispensing: A system of distribution in which all functions—processing, preparation, and distribution—occur in the main area. Medications are transported to the floors on a daily basis at predetermined times. Multiple deliveries may be needed for certain IV preparations for stability issues. The pharmacist is responsible for visually checking the work of the technicians. Centralized dispensing has greater management control.

Decentralized dispensing (satellite pharmacy): A system of distribution in which all functions (processing, preparation, and distribution) occur on or near the nursing unit. A decentralized pharmacy may service multiple nursing units. An advantage of a decentralized pharmacy is the pharmacist-physician-nurse-patient relationship.

Floor stock system: Storage of medication on the patient care units of a hospital. The nursing staff is responsible for all aspects of preparation and administration of medications. Disadvantages of this system include the following:

- Increased potential for medication errors—pharmacist does not review medication orders
- Increased drug inventory needed because of multiple inventories; poor inventory control
- Storage and control problems because of limited storage on nursing floors
- Greater possibility of drug diversion and misappropriation of medications

Individual prescription system: Medications are dispensed in multiple-dose vials. A 3- to 5-day supply is provided by the pharmacy. Time management issues occur.

Unit dose: Provides the medication in its final "unit of use." Improves productivity and reduces errors during ordering, distribution, storage, and administration of the medication. Advantages of unit dose include a reduction in medication errors, improved drug control, a decrease in the overall cost of medication distribution, improved medication billing and decreased medication credits, and a reduction in drug inventories. Variations in the unit-dose system include a modified unit-dose system and a blended unit-dose system.

> **Modified unit dose:** Combines unit-dose medications in blister packaging (punch cards, bingo cards, or blister cards) instead of a box. Packaged in quantities of 30, 60, or 90.
>
> **Blended unit dose:** Combines unit of use with non–unit-dose drug distribution system.
> - *Multiple medication package:* All medications for a specific administration time are packaged together.
> - *Modular cassette:* Combination of drawer exchange with unit dose (7-day system).

Dumbwaiter: An in-house elevator used to transport medications and supplies. Major disadvantage of dumbwaiters is that they move vertically only.

Robotics: A mobile, computerized mechanical device programmed to move throughout the hospital and deliver medications. In certain situations, robotics can be programmed to scan and pick medications for specific patients.

Pneumatic tube: A method of sending medication orders through the hospital by placing them in a tube and sending them to a dispatcher who then forwards them to a specific location.

REQUIREMENTS FOR DISPENSING INVESTIGATIONAL DRUGS

Investigational drugs are dispensed for a controlled study only, which is sponsored by a drug manufacturer or agency. The FDA may allow dispensing of a particular drug for a particular situation when all other methods of treatment have been exhausted. The Pharmacy and Therapeutic Committee asks the pharmacy to maintain administrative control over the clinical investigation. Duties of the hospital pharmacy include the following:

- Distribution and control of investigational drugs, which includes drug procurement, storage, inventory management, packaging, labeling, distribution, and disposition
- Clinical services, such as patient education, staff in-service training, and the monitoring and reporting of adverse drug reactions
- Research activities, such as participation in the preparation or review of research proposals and protocols and assisting in data collection and research
- Clinical study management; writing reports to drug sponsor

Physicians initiate the process of prescribing investigational drugs. They must do the following:

- Obtain approval for any study of investigational agents from the Institutional Review Board
- Complete the Investigational Drug Data Form and return it to the pharmacy
- Provide the pharmacy with a copy of the signed consent form
- Instruct the manufacturer to supply the pharmacy with all pharmacologic and stability data
- Make arrangements for the transfer of the drug to the pharmacy
- Arrange for the pharmacy to maintain a minimum level of the medication

In controlled studies the investigational drugs are received from the sponsoring company. Accurate dispensing records must be kept for the sponsor.

These medications need to be kept separately in the pharmacy from other medications. After the study has been completed, the leftover drugs are returned to the sponsor.

RECORD-KEEPING REQUIREMENTS FOR MEDICATION DISPENSING

CONTROLLED SUBSTANCES

All controlled substance prescriptions in System 2, File II should be stamped with a red C, 1 inch in height, in the lower right corner (Table 1-4). All controlled substance records must be maintained for a minimum of 2 years and must be readily retrievable. Readily retrievable means that one must provide the records within 48 hours of a request to view them.

- **Biennial inventory of narcotics:** Must be maintained in the pharmacy.
- **Change of pharmacist-in-charge inventory:** Must be maintained in the pharmacy.
- **Controlled substance invoices:** Must be maintained in the pharmacy. Schedule II invoices should be attached to pharmacy's copy of the DEA Form 222 with the appropriate dating and signature. Schedule III to V invoices need to be stamped with a red C, dated, and signed by the individual checking the invoice. Schedule III to V invoices need to be kept separate from Schedule II invoices.
- **Exempt narcotic log:** Requires name and address of purchaser (must be at least 18 years of age), name of product and date sold, seller's signature, and price of product. The pharmacist must be present for any transaction involving "exempt narcotics."
- **Master formula record:** Work sheets are considered permanent records. Provides directions for compounding and uniform record keeping. Quantities and lot numbers of ingredients used; initials of the preparer and pharmacist who checked the work; and calculations performed to determine how long the compound must be kept.
- **MSDS:** Documentation required by OSHA; a facility must receive this sheet time every time a haz-

TABLE **1-4** Filing of Prescriptions

SYSTEM	FILE I	FILE II	FILE III
1	CII Separate	CIII-CV	All other prescriptions
2	CII Separate	CIII-CV and all other legend drugs	
3	CII-CV	All other prescriptions	

ardous chemical is provided to it. Hazardous chemicals may be either physical or health hazards.

- **Medication administration record:** Provides documentation that a drug has actually been dispensed in a hospital or long-term facility. Medication administration records are found in hospitals and long-term care facilities.
- **Nonsterile compounded products:** All recipe information is copied and shows the step-by-step process. The following information is documented: date prepared, name of ingredients, manufacturers of ingredients, lot number and expiration date of each ingredient, amount or weight of each ingredient, dosage form of each ingredient, pharmacy lot number assigned, technician's initials, pharmacist's initials, date dispensed, patient's name, and medical record number. This information must be maintained for a minimum of 2 years.
- **Poison log:** Requires name and address of purchaser (must be at least 18 years of age), name of product and date sold, intended use, seller's signature, and price of product.
- **Prescription hard copy:** On the back of the hard copy of the prescription is a copy label with the initials of the pharmacist or technician who filled the prescription. Prescriptions are filed numerically. Backup copies are made at the end of the day. They must be maintained for a minimum of 2 years.
- **Repackaged medications:** All repackaged medications must be maintained on a log with the following information: date, drug, dosage form, manufacturer, manufacturer's lot number, manufacturer's expiration date, pharmacy lot number, pharmacy expiration date, technician, and pharmacist. The information must be readily retrievable.

AUTOMATIC STOP ORDERS

Automatic stop orders are used for specific classifications of medications; prescriptions are active for only a limited period, after which a new medication order is required if the medication is to be continued. These medications will automatically be stopped after a given period unless otherwise specified by a physician. Examples include the following:

- Analgesics: 30 days
- Antianemia drugs: 30 days
- Antibiotics: 7 days
- Antiemetics: 4 days
- Anticoagulants: 30 days
- Antihistamines: 7 days
- Antineoplastics: 30 days

- Barbiturates: 30 days
- Cardiovascular agents: 30 days
- Cathartics: 30 days
- Cold preparations: 5 days
- Dermatologic agents: 30 days
- Diuretics: 30 days

RESTRICTED MEDICATION ORDERS

Restricted drug: A therapeutic agent, admitted to a formulary, that is authorized for a specific doctor or group of doctors by a committee. Guidelines for use include that a drug in this category will be dispensed only if prescribed by a full-time faculty member of the designated group of physicians. Other members of the medical staff may prescribe the drug for an individual patient if the drug order is authorized by one of the designated doctors.

QUALITY IMPROVEMENT METHODS

- Adequate lighting can prevent errors from occurring.
- Bar code scanning for ordering medications maintains appropriate stock levels.
- Be aware of look-alike drug names.
- Confirm illegible prescriptions with the physician.
- Digital images of what the medication should look like and the manufacturer's container with NDC number are useful.
- Double counts of narcotics.
- If medications are being counted manually, count in multiples of fives.
- Make sure the prescribed agent is appropriate for the clinical situation.
- Order should be transcribed and read back to the party giving the order.
- Perpetual inventories can reduce possible theft.
- Scanning prescriptions can reduce prescription errors.
- "Tech check tech" is a method to catch prescription errors.
- Verbal orders should be taken only by authorized personnel.
- Workflow allows for processing prescriptions in a systematic manner, resulting in speedier processing and fewer prescription errors.

PHARMACY CALCULATIONS

ROMAN NUMERALS

Many doctors continue to use Roman numerals when writing quantities in a prescription or directions to the pharmacist. It is imperative that the pharmacy technician be able to correctly interpret these numerals in a prescription. Listed below are the more commonly used Roman numerals.

$$Ss = \tfrac{1}{2}$$
$$I \text{ or } i = 1$$
$$V \text{ or } v = 5$$
$$X \text{ or } x = 10$$
$$L \text{ or } l = 50$$
$$C \text{ or } c = 100$$
$$D \text{ or } d = 500$$
$$M \text{ or } m = 1000$$

Rules for Interpreting Roman Numerals

1. When a smaller numeral is repeated or follows a larger numeral, the numbers are added. For example:

$$iii = 1 + 1 + 1 = 3$$
$$vii = 5 + 1 + 1 = 7$$
$$xvi = 10 + 5 + 1 = 16$$

2. If a smaller numeral precedes a larger numeral, the smaller numeral is subtracted from the larger numeral. The smaller numeral in front of the larger number must not be smaller than one tenth of the larger numeral. For example:

$$iv = 5 - 1 = 4$$
$$ix = 10 - 1 = 9$$

3. Numerals are never repeated more than three times (e.g., iii = 3, XXX = 30); 4 should be written iv, not iiii; 40 should be written XL instead of XXXX.

4. If a smaller numeral is between two larger numerals, the smaller numeral is subtracted from the numeral following it. For example:

$$XIV = 10 + (5 - 1) = 14$$
$$XXIX = 10 + 10 + (10 - 1) = 29$$

RATIOS AND PROPORTIONS

A ratio is a relationship between two parts of a whole or between one part and the whole. A ratio can be written either as 1/2 or 1:2. A proportion is a relationship between two ratios. A proportion may be written as 1/2 = 2/4 or 1:2::2:4. The majority of all pharmaceutical calculations performed in either retail or institutional settings can be accomplished by using proportions.

There are two ways to solve proportion problems. The first involves cross-multiplying and dividing. The second method is described as the mean and extremes. Both methods will yield the same answer if set up correctly. Solve the following problem using both methods, where X is the value we are seeking.

$$\frac{4}{7} = \frac{X}{28}$$

Method 1: Cross-Multiply and Divide

$$\frac{4}{7} = \frac{X}{28}$$

Multiply the numerator on the left side of the equation by the denominator on the right side ($4 \times 28 = 112$).

Multiply the denominator on the left side of the equation by the numerator on the right side of the equation ($7 \times X = 7X$).

Divide both sides of the equation by the side where a number is represented by a number multiplied by X. For example:

$$\frac{112}{7} = \frac{7X}{7}$$
$$16 = X$$

Always make sure that units in the numerator correspond and the units in the denominator are the same. If they are not, the likelihood of an incorrect answer increases.

Method 2: Means and Extremes
4:7::X:28, where the first and last numbers in the series are considered the extremes and the two numbers in the middle are considered the means. In this situation, the 4 and the 28 represent the extremes and the 7 and X represent the means. One multiplies the extremes (4×28) and then multiplies the means ($7 \times X$).

$$4 \times 28 = 7 \times X$$
$$12 = 7X$$

Divide both sides of the equation by the side where a number is represented by a number multiplied by X.

$$\frac{112}{7} = \frac{7X}{7}$$
$$16 = X$$

Always make sure the units in the first and third positions are the same and the units in the second and fourth position are the same. If they are not, the likelihood of an incorrect answer increases.

REDUCING OR ENLARGING A FORMULA

When a formula specifies a specific total quantity, one may determine how much of each ingredient is needed to prepare a different total quantity by using this equation:

Total quantity of formula (specified) = Quantity of an ingredient (specified) in formula

Total quantity of formula (desired) = X

METRIC-HOUSEHOLD-APOTHECARY CONVERSION

The practice of pharmacy uses the metric system, the household system, and the apothecary system. A pharmacy technician must be able to calculate doses of medication in any of these systems and to convert them from one system to another system. It is essential that a technician memorize the basic conversions. Using proportions can solve any conversion.

Prefixes

Nano: one billionth of the basic unit
Micro: one millionth of the basic unit
Milli: one thousandth of the basic unit
Centi: one hundredth of the basic unit
Deci: one tenth of the basic unit
Deka: 10 times the basic unit
Hecto: 100 times the basic unit
Kilo: 1000 times the basic unit

Metric

Length (meter): Commonly used measurements in the practice of pharmacy are millimeter (mm), centimeter (cm), and meter (m).

1000 millimeters (mm) = 100 centimeters (cm)
100 centimeters (cm) = 1 meter (m)

Weight (gram): Commonly used measurements in the practice of pharmacy are microgram (mcg), milligram (mg), gram (g), and kilogram (kg).

1000 micrograms (mcg) = 1 milligram (mg)
1000 milligrams (mg) = 1 gram (g)
1000 grams (g) = 1 kilogram (kg)

Volume (liter): Commonly used measurements in the practice of pharmacy are milliliter (mL) and liter (L).

1000 milliliters (mL) = 1 liter (L)

Household

Weight

2.2 lb = 1 kg

Volume

5 mL = 1 teaspoon (tsp)
3 tsp = 1 tablespoon (tbsp)
2 tbsp = 1 fluid ounce (fl oz)
8 fl oz = 1 cup
2 cups = 1 pint (pt)
2 pt = 1 quart (qt)
4 qt = 1 gallon (gal)

Apothecary

Weight

20 grains (gr) = 1 scruple
3 scruples = 1 dram
8 drams = 1 ounce
16 ounces = 1 pound

Volume

60 minims = 1 fluid dram
8 fluid drams = 1 fl oz
16 fl oz = 1 pint
2 pints = 1 quart
4 quarts = 1 gallon

Apothecary Metric

16.23 minims = 1 mL
1 fl dram = 5 mL
1 fl oz = 29.57 mL (30 mL)
1 pt = 480 mL
1 gal = 3840 mL
1 g = 15.432 gr
1 gr = 60 or 65 mg
1 lb (avoirdupois) = 454 g
1 oz (apothecary) = 31.1 g
1 oz (avoirdupois) = 28.35 g

Units and Milliequivalents (mEq)

Several pharmaceutical products made from biologic products are expressed as "units" or International Units. Examples of these products include insulin, heparin, and vitamin E. Units represent an amount of activity within a particular system. Each pharmaceutical product is unique in determining the amount of activity of that product. Units represent a concentration and may be expressed as units/tablet or units/mL.

CALCULATION OF DOSES

There are two methods to determine a dose. The first looks at what one has in stock and what is needed, which can be expressed as

$$(Have) = (Need)$$

in the form of a proportion.

The second method uses the desired dose (D), the drug in stock (H), and the quantity in stock (Q) to calculate the amount of medication to give to the patient.

$$D/H \times Q = \text{Amount of medication to give}$$

PERCENTAGES AND STRENGTH OF MEDICATION

Percentages are another method of showing a relationship between parts and the whole. Percent means "parts per 100." A number less than 1 is considered less than 100%, whereas a number greater than 1 is greater than 100%. A percent can be calculated using ratios, fractions, or decimals.

Rules

- To convert a decimal to a percent, multiply the number by 100 and add a percent (%) sign (e.g., 0.45 × 100 = 45%; 1.00 × 100 = 100%; 1.25 × 100 = 125%).
- To convert a percent to a decimal, remove the % sign and divide by 100 (e.g., 95%/100 = 0.95; 50%/100 = 0.50; 100%/100 = 1.0).
- To convert a fraction to a percent, divide the numerator by the denominator, multiply by 100, and add a % sign (e.g., 95/100 = 0.95, then multiply by 100 = 95%).
- To convert a percent to a fraction, drop the % sign and write the value of the number as the numerator. Place it over a denominator of 100 and reduce it to its lowest terms (e.g., 75% = 75/100, reduce to lowest terms where both 75 and 100 are divisible by 25, resulting in an answer of ¾).
- To convert a ratio to a percent, divide the first number by the second number, multiply by 100, and add a % sign (e.g., 1:10 is the same as 1/10 = 0.1; next, multiply 0.1 by 100 = 10%).

Percents can be calculated by setting up a proportion. The numerator represents parts and the denominators wholes. The left side of the equation can be expressed as follows:

$$\frac{\text{Parts of the whole}}{\text{Whole}}$$

The right side of the equation is expressed in a percentage form, where the numerator is a percent of the whole; meanwhile, the denominator is considered 100%.

$$\frac{\text{Percent}}{100\%}$$

The equation would look like this:

$$\frac{\text{Parts of the whole}}{\text{Whole}} = \frac{\text{Percent}}{100\%}$$

To solve this type of problem, one needs two of the three variables, parts of the whole, the whole, or the percent. Identify the term as a part of the whole, the whole, or a percent. After identifying the values and placing them in the equation, cross-multiply and divide to find the missing term.

CONCENTRATION AND DILUTION

A concentration is a strength. It can be expressed as a fraction (e.g., mg/mL, mEq/mL, or units/mL), as a ratio (e.g., 1:100, 1:1000, or 1:10,000), or as a percentage (e.g., 10%, 25%, or 50%). Percents are found in solids (%w/w) and in solutions (%w/v or %v/v); %w/w is the number of grams per 100 g, %w/v is the number of grams per 100 mL, and %v/v is the number of milliliters per 100 mL.

The majority of all problems involving concentrations result in a dilution of a substance. In a daily application, a pharmacist receives an order to prepare a product of a given strength and volume (weight). These are known as the *final strength* (FS) and *final volume* (FV). The pharmacist must go to the shelf, choose the product at a given strength (initial strength [IS]), and determine the amount (initial volume [IV]) needed to prepare the compound. The same process would be done in preparing solids, except an initial weight (IW) and final weight (FW) would substituted for initial and final volumes.

One can use the following equation for this type of situation:

$$\begin{aligned}\text{Initial volume (IV)} \times \text{Initial strength (IS)} = \\ \text{Final volume (FV)} \times \text{Final strength (FS)}\end{aligned}$$

Hints to prevent errors in solving dilution problems include the following:

- Initial strength must be larger than final strength.
- Initial volume must be less than final volume.
- Final volume minus initial volume equals amount of diluent (inert substance) to be added to make the final volume.

POWDER VOLUME

$$\text{Powder volume} = \text{Final volume} - \text{Diluent volume}$$

This equation is used in calculations for reconstituting a solution.

ALLIGATION

Alligations are used in pharmacy when a pharmacist or pharmacy technician is compounding either a solution or a solid. The strength being prepared is different from the strength of the substance on the shelf. In this situation, there are substances of at least two different concentrations on the shelf—one that is greater than the desired concentration and one that is less than the desired concentration.

For example, a pharmacist receives an order to prepare 4 ounces of a 10% solution using a 25% and 5% solution. How much of each these should the pharmacist use?

Step 1: Draw a tic-tac-toe table.

Step 2: Place the highest concentration in the upper left corner, the lowest concentration in the lower left corner, and the desired concentration in the middle.

25%		
	10% (4 oz)	
5%		

Step 3: Subtract the desired concentration from the highest concentration, and place that number in the lower right corner and express the answer as parts. Next, subtract the lowest concentration from the desired concentration and place that number in the upper right corner and label it as parts.

25%		5 parts
	10% (4 oz)	
5%		15 parts

Step 4: Total the number of parts: 5 + 15 parts = 20 parts.

Step 5: Set up a proportion using the parts of the highest and lowest concentration and the total quantity to be prepared.

$$25\%: \frac{5 \text{ parts}}{20 \text{ parts}} \times 4 \text{ ounces} = 1 \text{ oz of } 25\% \text{ needed}$$

$$5\%: \frac{15 \text{ parts}}{20 \text{ parts}} \times 4 \text{ ounces} = 3 \text{ oz of } 5\% \text{ needed}$$

Step 6: Check your work by adding the amounts of each concentration to see if they equal the amount to be compounded.

SPECIFIC GRAVITY

Specific gravity is a ratio expressed as the weight of a substance to the weight of an equal volume of a substance as a standard. Water is the standard that is used and has a specific gravity of 1. Specific gravity can be expressed as follows:

$$\text{Weight of substance/Weight of an equal volume of water}$$

FLOW RATES

Pharmacy technicians must be aware of calculations associated with IV fluids. A pharmacy technician must be able to determine the flow rates of IV infusions; calculate the volume of fluids administered over a period; and control the total volume of fluids administered to a patient over a period of time.

A variety of IV sets are available to the pharmacist and are identified by the number of drops of a fluid per milliliter. Common IV sets include 10 drops/mL, 15 drops/mL, and 60 drops/mL (minidrip set).

Time of infusion = Volume of fluid (or amount of drug)/Rate of infusion

Rate of infusion = Volume of fluid (or amount of drug)/Time of infusion

Infusion rate: Drops/min = (Number of mL/hr) × (Number of drops/mL)/60 min/hr

CALCULATION OF CHILDREN'S DOSES

Children require different amounts of medication than adults. These doses are affected by the individual's age, weight, body surface area (BSA), organ development, sex, and disease state. An individual's age is placed into one of several categories.

Neonates: Birth to 1 month of age
Infant: 1 month to 1 year of age
Early childhood: 1 to 5 years of age
Late childhood: 6 to 12 years of age
Adolescence: 13 to 17 years of age

To calculate the appropriate dose for children, one of several methods may be used. Young's rule uses age as a guide; Clark's rule uses weight as the determining factor; mg/kg uses weight in kilograms for a patient, and BSA uses both height and weight as the basis for choosing a dose.

$$\textbf{Young's rule} = \frac{\text{Age of child (expressed in years)}}{\text{Age of child (in years) 12}} \times \text{Adult dose}$$

$$\textbf{Clark's rule} = \frac{\text{Weight of child (expressed in pounds)}}{150} \times \text{Adult dose}$$

All four of the these methods require the adult dose and the given parameter to be provided to the practitioner for calculation of the appropriate dose. The adult dose may be measured in milligrams, milliliters, units, milliequivalents, or even tablets.

A more accurate method of determining the appropriate dose is based on BSA. This method takes into account both the height and weight of the individual (Figure 1-4). If one knows both of these variables, a nomogram (a specialized graph) is referenced. BSA is measured in square meters (m^2). The dosage is calculated as follows:

BSA of child (in square meters)/1.73 m^2 (average adult BSA) × Adult dose = Approximate dose for child

TEMPERATURE CONVERSION

To solve math problems converting degrees Fahrenheit to Celsius or degrees Celsius to Fahrenheit, the following formula can be used:

$$9C = 5F - 160$$

where *C* represents the temperature in Celsius and *F* represents the Fahrenheit temperature. Only one of

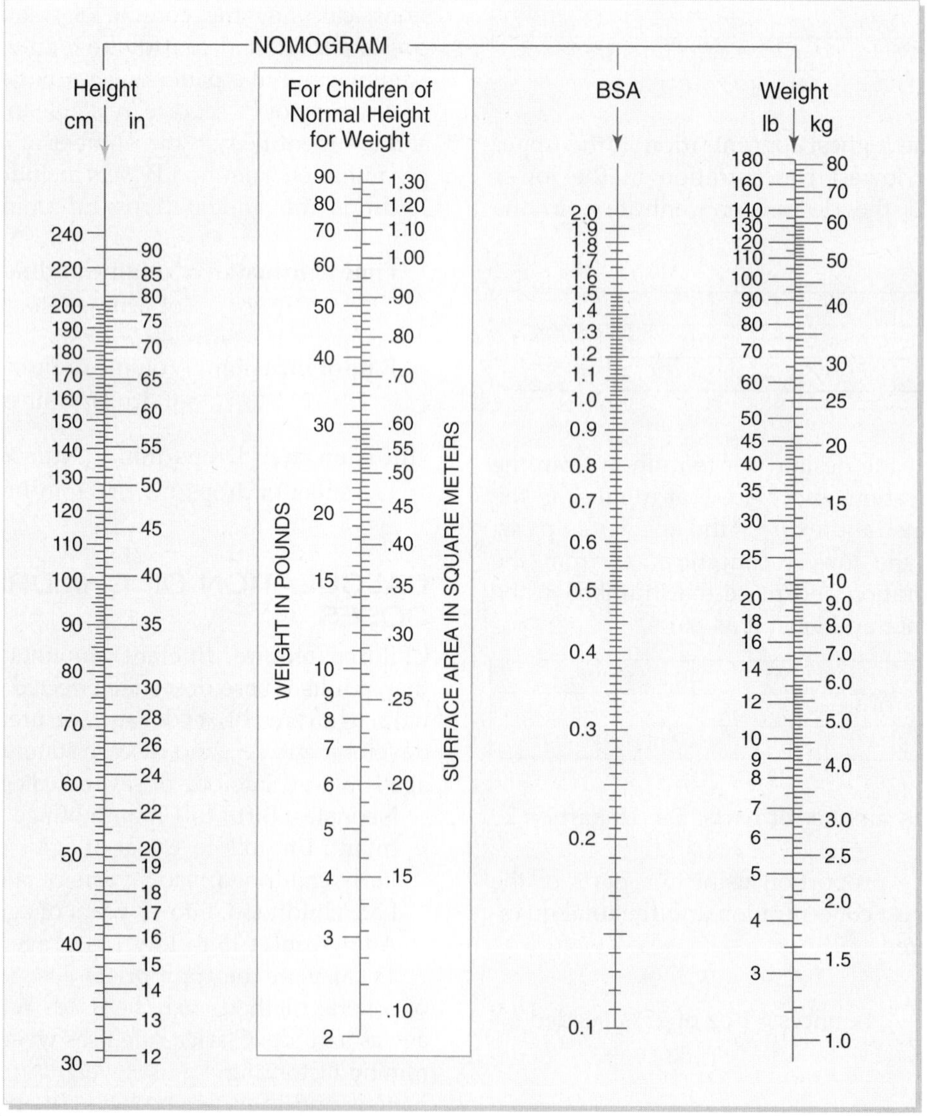

Fig. 1-4 Body surface area chart.

the two variables is required for this problem to be solved. For example, given a temperature of 75° F, 75 would be multiplied by 5, 160 subtracted from the result, and the result divided by 9. The answer would be 23.8° C. On the other hand, if one were told that the temperature is 20° C, 20 would be multiplied by 9, 160 added to the result, and the result divide by 5, resulting in an answer of 68° F.

Another way to solve this problem is to use the following equations:

$$F = (C \times 1.8) + 32$$

$$C = \frac{F - 32}{1.8}$$

Either method will yield the same answer.

COMMERCIAL MATH

Cost: Purchase price + cost to dispense
Discount: Purchase price × discount rate
Discounted price: Purchase price − discount
Gross profit: Selling price − purchase price
Inventory turnover rate: Annual dollar purchase/ average inventory value
Markup: Selling price − purchase price
Net profit: Overall cost × desired percent profit
Overhead: Sum of all expenses
Profit: Selling price − overall cost

DRUG STABILITY

FACTORS AFFECTING DRUG STABILITY

- Dosage form
- Humidity
- Ingredients used in a compound
- Light
- Material of the container
- Order and method of preparation
- Temperature

PHYSICAL AND CHEMICAL INCOMPATIBILITIES

Physical incompatibilities: Occur from changes in solubility, which may result in changes in color or the formation of a precipitate. A change in the pH of a solution, the use of buffers, and the type of solvent used may create problems.

Chemical incompatibilities: Chemical reaction occurs between one or more of the ingredients. Incompatibilities may not be noticeable. Changes in pH or chemical decomposition may occur. The presence of light may cause deterioration of the ingredients. IV

medications are normally prepared using D5W, except ampicillin, ampicillin-sulbactam, erythromycin lactobionate, imipenem-cilastatin, and oxacillin, which must be mixed with normal saline.

Therapeutic incompatibilities: The mixing together of two or more ingredients, resulting in a change in the therapeutic response of the drugs.

PROCEDURES TO PREPARE INTRAVENOUS ADMIXTURES

- Flow hood should be on for at least 30 min.
- Wear protective clothing.
- Clean laminar flow hood with 70% isopropyl alcohol or other suitable disinfectant, the pole to hang IV bags, then sides of hood by moving from the back to the front, and finally the bottom of the hood by moving side to side from the back to the front.
- Collect supplies. Check expiration dates and bags for leaks. Remove dust coverings before placing supplies in the hood. Use presterilized needles, syringes, and filters.
- Position supplies in the hood.
- Sterilize puncture surfaces with an alcohol wipe.
- Prevent coring by placing the vial on a flat surface, and insert needle into rubber closure at a 45- to 60-degree angle. Use downward pressure on the needle and move needle to a 90-degree angle.
- **Using vials with solutions:** Draw into syringe a volume of air equal to amount of volume being replaced (Figure 1-5). Penetrate vial without coring. Invert vial upside down and pull back on plunger to fill the syringe. Tap to bring air bubbles to the top of the syringe. Transfer solution to final container.
- **Vials with lyophilized powder:** Determine the correct volume of diluent and withdraw it. Transfer diluent into vial containing powder. Remove more air from vial than amount of diluent injected. Whirl vial until powder is dissolved. Use new syringe and needle, and proceed as if using a vial with solution.
- **Using ampules:** If the ampule is not prescored, then score the neck of the ampule with a fine file. Hold ampule upright and tap it. Wipe neck of ampule with alcohol swab. Wrap gauze around the neck and gently snap neck. Inspect and use a filter needle to withdraw. Hold ampule downward at a 20-degree angle, and withdraw solution with a filter syringe. Exchange old filter needle with a new filter needle, and transfer solution into the final container.

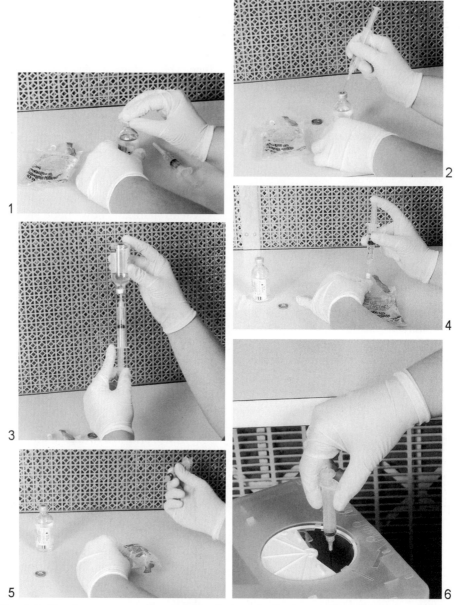

Fig. 1-5 Six-step process of aseptic technique in the hood. (Reprinted from Hopper T: *Mosby's pharmacy technician: principles and practice*, ed 2, St Louis, 2007, Saunders.)

PROCEDURES TO PREPARE CHEMOTHERAPY DRUGS

The same aseptic techniques used in preparing IV solutions are used in preparing chemotherapy medications, with a few exceptions. Chemotherapy requires a vertical laminar airflow hood, which is smaller than a horizontal laminar flow hood. Special chemotherapy clothing is worn. The hands in a vertical flow hood should not be over the top of any needle, vial, or IV bag.

PREPARING PARENTERAL ANTINEOPLASTICS

- The safety cabinet work surface should be covered with a plastic-backed absorbent paper, which is disposed of in a biohazard container after use.
- Personnel should wear surgical gloves and a closed-front surgical gown with knit cuffs. Contaminated gloves or outer gloves should be removed and replaced. If the skin comes in contact with antineoplastics, one should wash the area with soap and water.

- Reconstituted vials should be vented to reduce the possibility of spraying and spillage.
- A sterile alcohol pledget should be wrapped around the needle and vial top during withdrawal of solution.
- External surfaces of syringes and IV bags (bottles) should be wiped clean of contamination.
- When using ampules, wrap neck of ampule with sterile alcohol pledget to protect fingers from being cut by the glass.
- Syringes and IV bottles should be properly identified and dated. Cautionary labels should be affixed to containers.
- Safety cabinet should be wiped down with 70% alcohol on completion of compounding.
- Contaminated needles and syringes should be placed in the sharps container. Disposable gowns, gloves, masks, and head and shoe covers should be placed in red biohazard bags.
- Wash hands.
- Dispose of remaining antineoplastic agents according to federal and state regulations.

PROCEDURES TO PREPARE TOTAL PARENTERAL NUTRITION SOLUTIONS

TPN normally contains 50% dextrose, 10% amino acids, and 20% fat. Aseptic technique is required because TPN is infused into the right atrium of the heart. TPN compounders have been developed that include a multichannel pump for the amino acids, dextrose, fats, and other additives that is connected to a personal computer. The computer assists in the calculations and drives the pump. Micro compounding pumps are used for the electrolytes and other additives (Figure 1-6).

Peripheral parenteral nutrition (PPN) normally contains 25% dextrose, 10% amino acids, and 10% fat. PPN is a short-term therapy.

TPN and PPN are premixed from the manufacturer, but electrolytes, vitamins, and medications may be added to the nutrients at the pharmacy.

COMPOUNDING TECHNIQUES

Compounding techniques require aseptic technique.
Method 1: Amino acids and dextrose are mixed first. Fat emulsion is added next, followed by the additives.
Method 2: Amino acids are added to the fat emulsion. Dextrose is added next, followed by the additives.
Method 3: Dextrose, amino acids, and fat emulsion are added simultaneously while swirling and mixing. Additives are incorporated last.

PROCEDURES TO PREPARE RECONSTITUTED INJECTABLE AND NONINJECTABLE MEDICATIONS

- Reconstitution is the process of mixing a liquid and powder to form a suspension or solution.
- Solvent is the larger part of the solution.
- Solute is the agent or ingredient used with solvent.
- Solution is the solvent plus the solute.
- Measure solute and solvent (distilled water) to be used.
- Add solute to solvent in small portions; mix thoroughly.
- Check precipitation for solutions or changes in color.
- Add new expiration date to product bottle and affix a "SHAKE WELL" auxiliary label.

PROCEDURES TO PREPARE RADIOPHARMACEUTICALS

- Radiopharmaceuticals may be diagnostic or therapeutic; may be oral, IV, or inhaled.
- Individual must wear meter indicating the radioactive levels to which the individual is exposed.
- Quality-control tests are performed to ensure radiopharmaceutical is sterile, pyrogen-free, and pure.
- Proper handling of isotopes during preparation and disposal must be ensured.
- Radiopharmaceuticals are to be prepared in a vertical flow hood.
- Radiopharmaceuticals have strict packaging requirements, including the use of special shipping containers.
- Safety principles of time, distance, and shielding are observed.
- Special training must be completed if one is to work in a nuclear pharmacy.

PROCEDURES TO PREPARE ORAL DOSAGE FORMS

- Unit dose: Provides medication in the "final unit of use" form. Drug is contained in a small packet. Packet is made of thermal paper and foil laminate; other side is made of poly film material (Figure 1-7).
- Machines may be manually, semiautomatically, or automatically loaded.
- Single-drop machine: 60 packages/min; double-drop machine: 120 packages/min.

TPN ORDER SHEET

HOME HEALTH	DATE
PATIENT	ADDRESS

TPN FORMULA:

AMINO ACIDS: ☐ 5.5% ☐ 8.5% ☑ 10%	425	ml
☐ WITH STANDARD ELECTROLYTES		
DEXTROSE: ☐ 10% ☐ 20% ☐ 40% ☐ 50% ☑ 70%	357	ml
(check one)		
LIPIDS: ☐ 10% ☑ 20%	125	ml
FOR ALL-IN-ONE FORMULA		

FINAL VOLUME		ml
qsad STERILE WATER FOR INJECTION	400mL	1307

Patient Additives:

☐ MVC 9 + 3 10 ml Daily

☐ HUMULIN-R 10 u Daily

☐ FOLIC ACID _____ mg
_____ times weekly

☐ VITAMIN K _____ mg
_____ times weekly

☐ OTHER: MVI 12 1.5mL/daily

☐ OTHER: _____

Calcium Gluconate	0.465 mEq/ml	5	mEq
Magnesium Sulfate	4 mEq/ml	5	mEq
Potassium Acetate	2 mEq/ml		mEq
Potassium Chloride	2 mEq/ml		mEq
Potassium Phosphate	3 mM/ml	22	mM
Sodium Acetate	2 mEq/ml		mEq
Sodium Chloride	4 mEq/ml	35	mEq
Sodium Phosphate	3 mM/ml		mM
TRACE ELEMENTS CONCENTRATE	☐ 4 ☐ 5 ☐ 6		ml

Directions:

INFUSE: ☑ DAILY

☐ _____ TIMES WEEKLY

OTHER DIRECTIONS:
_____
_____
_____
_____
_____

Rate: ☐ CYCLIC INFUSION: OVER _____ HOURS (TAPER UP AND DOWN) ☐ CONTINUOUS INFUSION: AT _____ ml PER HOUR ☑ STANDARD RATE: AT 110 ml PER HOUR FOR 12 HOURS

LAB ORDERS:

☐ STANDARD LAB ORDERS
SMAC-20, CO2, Mg+2 TWICE WEEKLY
CBC WITH AUTO DIFF WEEKLY
UNTIL STABLE, THEN:
SMAC-20, CO2, Mg+2 WEEKLY
CBC WITH AUTO DIFF MONTHLY

☐ OTHER: _____
_____
_____

VALIDATION:

_____
DOCTOR'S SIGNATURE

Print Name: _____
Office Address: _____
Phone: _____

Fig. 1-6 Example of a total parenteral nutrition order. (Reprinted from Hopper T: *Mosby's pharmacy technician: principles and practice,* ed 2, St Louis, 2007, Saunders.)

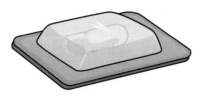

Fig. 1-7 A sample of a blister pack container. (Reprinted from Hopper T: *Mosby's pharmacy technician: principles and practice*, ed 2, St Louis, 2007, Saunders.)

- Machine drops drug into package, seals package, and prints medication information in one operation.

PROCEDURES TO COMPOUND STERILE NONINJECTABLE PRODUCTS

Factors to be considered in preparing ophthalmic products include the following:
- **Sterilization:** Can be accomplished by autoclave, filtration, gas, or radiation.
- **Clarity:** Free from foreign particles, which can be accomplished through filtration.
- **Stability:** Affected by chemical nature of the drug substance, pH, method of preparation, solution additives, and packaging.
- **Buffer and pH:** Should be formulated at a pH of 7.4, but this rarely occurs. The pH chosen should be optimum for stability.
- **Tonicity:** Refers to the osmotic pressure exerted by the salts. An isotonic solution should have tonicity equal to that of sodium chloride 0.9%.
- **Viscosity:** Agents are used to prolong contact time in the eye and enhance drug absorption and activity.

PROCEDURES TO COMPOUND NONSTERILE PRODUCTS

- **Blending:** An act of combining two substances
- **Comminution:** An act of reducing a substance to small, fine particles
- **Geometric dilution:** A technique used in mixing two ingredients of unequal quantities, where one begins with the smallest quantity and adds an equal quantity of the ingredient having the larger amount; process continues until all of the ingredients are used
- **Emulsifier:** A stabilizing agent in emulsions
- **Flocculating agent:** Electrolytes used in the preparation of suspensions

- **Levigation:** Trituration of a powder drug with a solvent, in which the drug is insoluble with the solvent
- **Mucilage:** A wet, slimy liquid formed as an initial step in the wet gum method
- **Pulverization by intervention:** Reducing the size of a particle in a solid with the aid of an additional material
- **Sifting:** A technique to either blend or combine powders
- **Spatulation:** Mixing powders using a spatula in a mortar, an ointment slab, or a plastic bag; process used when ingredients may liquefy on mixing; there is no reduction in particle size
- **Thickening agent:** An ingredient used in the preparation of a suspension to increase the viscosity of the suspension
- **Trituration:** A process of rubbing, grinding, or pulverizing a powder to create fine particles
- **Tumbling:** Combining powders in a bag and shaking it

WEIGHING PROCEDURES

- Unlock balance and make sure it is level. Relock balance before placing weights on it.
- Place weighing papers on pans of scale.
- Unlock scale and ensure that it is balanced.
- Place weights on right-hand pans using forceps.
- Place desired material on left-hand pans.
- Release the beam by unlocking balance.
- Lock balance before adding or removing additional powder.
- Unlock balance and check for equilibrium.
- After the appropriate quantity is on balance, close lid and have pharmacist verify weight.
- Remove ingredient and remove weight with forceps.

MEASURING USING A TORSION BALANCE

- Leave balance in a draft-free area (Figure 1-8).
- If balance has a level bubble, make sure the bubble is inside the bull's-eye and make adjustments using the leveling feet.
- Place weighing boat or a single piece of paper on the pan.
- When the balance has determined the final weight, press the tare bar to compensate for the weighing boat.
- As ingredients are added or removed, the digital display will show the weight.

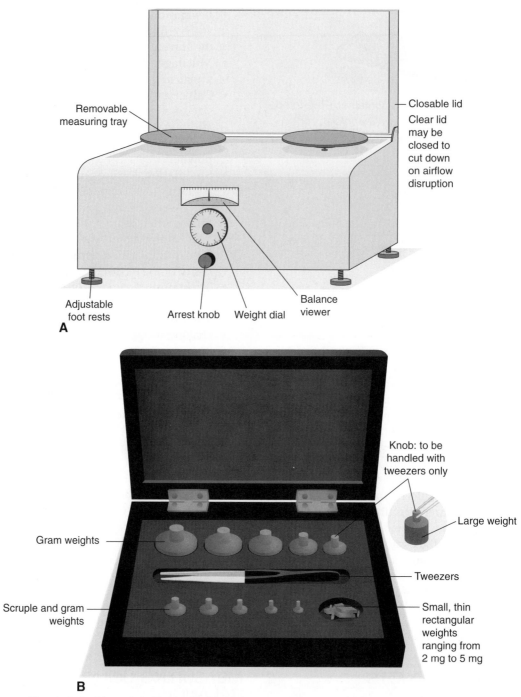

Fig. 1-8 A, Class A balance. **B,** Pharmaceutical weights. (Reprinted from Hopper T: *Mosby's pharmacy technician: principles and practice,* ed 2, St Louis, 2007, Saunders.)

PROCEDURES FOR MEASURING LIQUIDS

- Choose proper size graduate such that quantity to be measured is not less than 20% of the total volume of graduate (Figure 1-9).

- Pour liquid down the center of the graduate slowly, and watch the level of liquid rise to desired volume.
- Allow time for all liquid to fall in graduate before taking measurement.

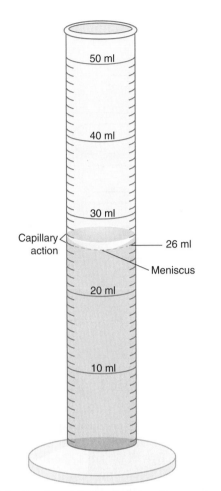

Fig. 1-9 A 50-mL graduate showing the meniscus and proper measurement of solutions. (Reprinted from Hopper T: *Mosby's pharmacy technician: principles and practice*, ed 2, St Louis, 2007, Saunders.)

- Measure level of liquid at eye level, and make observation at bottom of meniscus.
- Pour liquid into container and allow for liquid to be completely drained from the graduate.

PROCEDURES FOR FILLING CAPSULES

PUNCH METHOD

Triturate ingredients to the same particle size; mix using geometric dilution. Calculate enough ingredients for several extra capsules. Place powder on ointment slab, where depth of powder is approximately half the length of the capsule body. Hold capsule vertically and punch the open end into the powder until capsule is filled. Place cap on capsule, and weigh using an empty capsule as a counterweight. Add or

remove ingredient as needed. Hints: Remove exact number of capsules from box; wear finger cots to protect the fingers; roll capsules on a clean towel to remove traces of the drug on the outside; place completed capsules in either a glass or plastic vial; and store in a dry place to prevent them from absorbing moisture or becoming dry (Figure 1-10).

EMULSIONS

Contains two immiscible liquids, in which one liquid is dispersed throughout another liquid and is aided by a stabilizing agent. May either be oil-in-water (O/W) or water-in-oil (W/O).

Continental Method (Dry Gum Method)

The primary emulsion is formed from four parts oil, two parts water, and one part gum (emulsifier-acacia). With a Wedgwood or porcelain mortar, the gum and oil are levigated. Water is added and the trituration continues. After the primary emulsion is formed, additional ingredients may be added and are added up to the initial volume with the external phase.

Wet Gum Method

Primary emulsion is formed by triturating one part gum and two parts water to form a mucilage. Slowly add four parts oil and triturate slowly. Add additional ingredients.

Beaker Method

Water-soluble and oil-solute ingredients are mixed in separate containers. Both phases are heated to 70°C and are removed from heat. Internal phase is added to the external phase. Final product is cooled to room temperature but is continually stirred.

POWDERS

Powders are prepared through the use of trituration and geometric dilution.

LIQUID DRUG IN LIQUID VEHICLE

Measure quantities of each liquid in a graduated cylinder. Add drug to vehicle slowly, then shake and stir.

SOLID DRUG IN LIQUID VEHICLE

Weigh solid, and measure solvent. One must take into consideration the solubility of the drug and the solvent being used. Triturate drug if needed, and dissolve in solvent. May need to heat gently, stir, or shake gently.

NONAQUEOUS SOLUTIONS

Nonaqueous solutions contain solvents other than water and include elixirs, tinctures, spirits, fluid

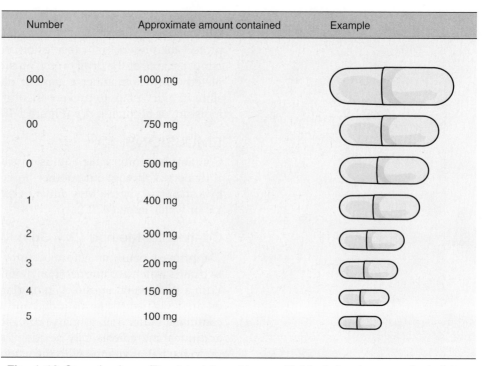

Number	Approximate amount contained	Example
000	1000 mg	
00	750 mg	
0	500 mg	
1	400 mg	
2	300 mg	
3	200 mg	
4	150 mg	
5	100 mg	

Fig. 1-10 Capsule sizes. (Reprinted from Hopper T: *Mosby's pharmacy technician: principles and practice,* ed 2, St Louis, 2007, Saunders.)

extracts, glycerates, collodions, liniments, and oleaginous solutions. Prepare by dissolving alcohol-soluble ingredients in alcohol and water-soluble ingredients in water. Add alcohol portion to aqueous portion and stir.

SUPPOSITORIES

Suppository bases may be oleaginous, water soluble, or hydrophilic.

Compression Mold

Mix the suppository base and drug ingredients. Force the mixture into a special compression mold.

Fusion Mold

Active ingredients are dispersed or dissolved in a melted base. Suppository base is melted at a low temperature, and the drug is dissolved in it. The base is poured and overfilled into a special suppository mold (metal, plastic, or rubber) and is left to harden. Excess material is removed from the top of the mold.

SUSPENSIONS

The solid drug to be suspended is weighed and is levigated in mortar and pestle with either alcohol or glycerin. A portion of the vehicle is added to mortar and is mixed with the levigated drug until a uniform consistency occurs. This portion of the drug is placed in the final container. The mortar and pestle are rinsed

with the balance of the vehicle and the suspension is added up to the final volume with the vehicle being used. A "SHAKE WELL" label should be affixed to the container. Flocculating and thickening agents may be used in the preparation of a suspension.

SYRUPS

Heat Method

Heat needs to be controlled; works fastest, but not all ingredients can be used with heat.

Without Heat Method

Must use a container that is twice the size of the final volume. The syrup needs to be shaken or stirred.

PROCEDURES TO PREPARE READY-TO-DISPENSE MULTIDOSE PACKAGES

PREPARING OINTMENTS

Ointments can be prepared on an ointment slab. Weigh quantities of each ingredient. Prepare by using geometric dilution and two spatulas to mix the ingredients. Transfer final product into ointment jar by using a spatula. Remove air pockets of ointment by using spatula. Spread evenly in container.

Ointment bases are chosen based on their characteristics to deliver a drug (Table 1-5).

TABLE **1-5** Property of Ointment Bases

PROPERTY	OLEAGINOUS BASE	ABSORPTION BASE	WATER-OIL EMULSION BASE	OIL-WATER EMULSION BASE	WATER-MISCIBLE BASE
Greasiness	Greasy	Greasy	Greasy	Nongreasy	Nongreasy
Occlusiveness	Yes	Yes	Sometimes	No	No
Spreadability	Difficult	Difficult	Moderate to easy	Easy	Moderate to easy
Washability	Nonwashable	Nonwashable	Nonwashable or poorly washable	Washable	Washable
Water content	Anhydrous	Anhydrous	Hydrous	Hydrous	Hydrous
Examples	White petrolatum	Aquaphor	Hydrous lanolin, Eucerin	Hydrophilic ointment	Polyethylene glycol (PEG)

ASEPTIC TECHNIQUES FOR TECHNICIANS

- No jewelry should be worn in the hood. This includes artificial nails because of microbial growth around or underneath.
- Long hair should be tied back away from the face.
- Hands must be washed after entering the IV area and before entering the laminar flow hood (Figure 1-11).
- Hands, wrists, and arms to the elbow should be washed with antimicrobial soap and hot water for at least 30 seconds and no more than 90 seconds.
- Gloves can be worn but should be washed down with 70% isopropyl alcohol after being put on.
- The surface of the hood should be washed down with 70% isopropyl alcohol using proper method (Figure 1-12).
- The hood must run at least 30 minutes before medications are placed inside.
- All vials and ports must be wiped down with alcohol. They should not be sprayed because the alcohol can make contact with the filter in the back of the hood, which breaks down the filter.
- Hands or any object within the hood cannot block the airflow at any time.
- Work at least 6 inches into the horizontal hood; keep pens and other objects out of the hood.
- All needles, syringes, vials, and other by-products must be disposed of in proper receptacles.
- No sneezing, talking, or coughing can be directed toward the airflow in a laminar flow hood.

INFECTION CONTROL PROCEDURES

UNIVERSAL PRECAUTIONS

- Universal precautions apply to all individuals in an institution who may come in contact with blood, other body fluids, or body substances.
- Latex gloves must be worn when there is a possibility the individual may come in contact with these substances.
- Hands must be washed after removing the latex gloves.
- Blood-soaked or contaminated materials must be disposed of in a wastebasket lined with a plastic bag.
- Specially trained individuals must be notified for cleanup or removal of contaminated waste.
- Contaminated materials such as syringes, needles, swabs, and catheters must be placed in red plastic containers labeled for disposal of biohazardous materials.
- A first-aid kit must be maintained and adequately stocked for use if an individual does come in contact with contaminated waste or body fluids. Items to be contained in the first-aid kit include adhesive bandages, alcohol, antiseptic or disinfectant, bleach, disposable latex gloves, disposable towels, medical tape, sterile gauze, and plastic bags for contaminated waste disposal.

REQUIREMENTS FOR HANDLING HAZARDOUS PRODUCTS AND DISPOSING OF HAZARDOUS WASTE

Sharps containers are used for the storage of used syringes, needles, ampules, and vials waiting for disposal. Needles should be clipped or snapped.

Other refuse, such as gloves, gowns, masks, and shoe and head coverings, should be placed in specially marked biohazard containers. Any clothing or linens that come in contact with body fluids need to be placed in these receptacles.

DOCUMENTATION REQUIREMENTS FOR CONTROLLED SUBSTANCES, INVESTIGATIONAL DRUGS, AND HAZARDOUS WASTE

- **DEA Form 224:** To register a pharmacy with the DEA to be able to stock controlled substances.
- **DEA Form 222:** To order Schedule II drugs.

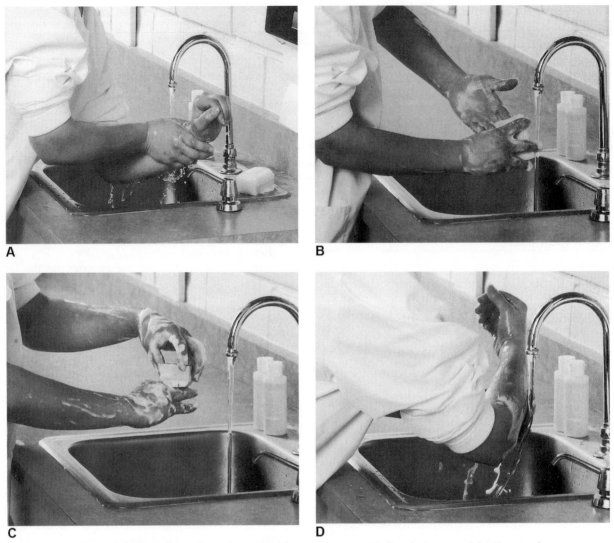

Fig. 1-11 A, Wet hands and arms with warm water. **B,** Scrub tops and bottoms of hands. **C,** Scrub between fingers and up to the elbows. **D,** Rinse arms and hands thoroughly. Foot pedals may be used rather than handles. (Reprinted from Hopper T: *Mosby's pharmacy technician: principles and practice,* ed 2, St Louis, 2007, Saunders.)

- **DEA Form 41:** To destroy outdated or unused controlled substances.
- **DEA Form 106:** To report theft of controlled substances.
- **Biennial Inventory:** Controlled Substances Act of 1970 requires that a pharmacy perform a biennial inventory (every 2 years) of all controlled substances in the pharmacy. An exact count must be performed on all Schedule II drugs, and an approximate count on Schedule III to V drugs.
- **Power of Attorney:** Authorizes a pharmacist to order Schedule II drugs.

Material Safety Data Sheet

Documentation that provides detailed information on the hazards of a particular substance. These hazards may be either physical or health related. Examples of substances with physical hazards are chemicals that are combustible, flammable, explosive, or corrosive. A health hazard may cause either acute or chronic effects in an individual who has been exposed. The manufacturer is responsible for providing the MSDS to the pharmacy, and the pharmacy is responsible for providing the MSDS to the purchaser.

Information Found on a Material Safety Data Sheet

- Identification of the substance or preparation: names and alternative names
- Composition of and information regarding the ingredients; includes uses

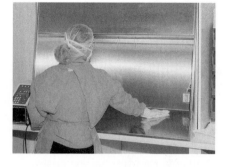

- It is important to be gowned up properly before cleaning the laminar flow hood. All items should be removed from the hood before cleaning.
- Moisten 4 × 4 inch gauze or other disposable cloth or gauze with 70% isopropyl alcohol and wet down the inside of the hood. This includes the sides and tabletop. Make sure you do not spray the HEPA filter at the back or the ceiling inside the hood.
- Then, starting from the top right-hand side of the hood, wipe down, across the surface, and up to the top of the left-hand side of the hood.
- Moving forward a few inches, repeat the motion in the opposite direction.
- The side-to-side, back-to-front motion must be done before using the hood each day. In addition, the hood should be cleaned periodically throughout the course of the day to ensure a sterile environment.

Fig. 1-12 Cleaning the horizontal hood. (Reprinted from Hopper T: *Mosby's pharmacy technician: principles and practice*, ed 2, St Louis, 2007, Saunders.)

- Hazards identification: toxicities identified
- First-aid measures: what to do if substance is inhaled, skin comes in contact with it, eye contact occurs, or substance is ingested
- Firefighting measures
- Accidental release measures
- Handling and storage
- Exposure control and personal protection
- Physical and chemical properties: includes form, color, pH, boiling point, melting point, vapor pressure, solubility, partition coefficient, flammable powder class, specific gravity, vapor density, dissociation constant
- Stability and reactivity
- Toxicologic information: inhalation, skin contact, eye contact, ingestion, long-term exposure
- Ecologic information: environmental fate and distribution, persistence and degradation, toxicity and effluent treatment
- Disposal considerations
- Transport information
- Regulatory information
- Other information

PHARMACY-RELATED SOFTWARE FOR DOCUMENTING THE DISPENSING OF PRESCRIPTIONS OR MEDICATION ORDERS

- Software is customized to meet the requirements of the pharmacy.
- Outpatient dispensing software is used to reduce errors, increase productivity, and perform inventory management.

- Inpatient dispensing software is used to reduce staff; software is accessible to medical staff and regulates controlled substances. Must interface with various other computer systems in the hospital. Hospitals using robotics possess the capability of scanning unit-dose labels and filling patients' orders.

CUSTOMER SERVICE PRINCIPLES

Customer satisfaction is the goal of customer service. Patients coming to a pharmacy do so because they are not feeling well or have a physical ailment. The customer must be treated in a positive manner. The pharmacist should be called to handle any difficult situations.

A technician working at the pharmacy counter or pharmacy window should listen carefully, make eye contact with the customer, repeat what the customer has said, and use positive language to emphasize what can be done rather than what cannot be done. If a pharmacy technician is using the telephone, he or she should maintain a pleasant and courteous manner, state the name of the pharmacy and his or her name, adhere to the standard procedures established by the pharmacy, and refer any questions requiring a pharmacist's judgment to the pharmacist.

COMMUNICATION TECHNIQUES

- Appearance
- Empathetic responses to the customer
- Listening
- Nonverbal communication

- Phone skills
- Verbal communication
- Writing skills

PATIENT CONFIDENTIALITY REQUIREMENTS

HIPAA requires that any personally identifiable information be protected as being confidential. Patients are allowed to access and request copies of their medical records. Health care providers and organizations must provide a written statement that states how medical information will be handled by a provider. Patients are entitled to a complete discussion of health care options from the health care provider. Patients may request that confidential communication is made in a manner that they feel is appropriate. Every organization must have a written privacy procedure. Training must be provided for all employees.

CASH-HANDLING PROCEDURES

The technician may be required to ring into the cash register both prescriptions and other purchases. Many cash registers feature scanners that enter the price into the cash register. If an error occurs, the transaction can be voided and entered manually. The pharmacy technician should accept and count the payment within the sight of the patient. The amount tendered should be entered into the cash register. The amount of change should be counted back to the customer, and the customer should be given a cash register receipt. The technician should thank the customer for the purchase.

Checks, debit cards, and credit cards are normally accepted at the pharmacy. Each of these different types of payment may require variations of this process. The pharmacy technician should follow the procedures established by the institution to process these forms of payment.

REIMBURSEMENT POLICIES AND PLANS

Average Wholesale Price (AWP) Applications

A form of reimbursement that follows the following formula:

$$AWP \pm percentage + dispensing\ fee$$

This form of reimbursement is the most commonly used and encourages a pharmacy to dispense generic medications because the percentage of return is greater for generics than for brand-name drugs.

- **AAC:** Actual acquisition cost; the price a pharmacy actually paid for a medication after receiving any discounts from either the manufacturer or the wholesaler. May be used instead of AWP.
- **MAC:** Maximum allowable cost; the maximum price an insurance company will pay for a generic medication.
- **Capitation fee:** A reimbursement system in which a pharmacy receives a fixed payment each month per patient, regardless of the number of prescriptions filled or the cost of the prescriptions filled. A practice commonly used by health maintenance organizations (HMOs).
- **Deductible:** A set amount that must be paid by the patient for each benefit period before the insurer will cover additional expenses.
- **Per diem:** A predetermined amount of money that is paid to an individual or institution for a daily service.

Copayments

- **Fixed:** The patient pays a fixed or set dollar amount.
- **Percentage:** The patient pays a fixed percentage of the total cost of the prescription.
- **Variable:** A different dollar amount is charged based on the type of drug dispensed. The variable copayment could be for a lifestyle drug, a nonformulary drug, or a medication that has a DAW2 code. A DAW2 indicates the prescriber has authorized the use of a generic medication but the patient has requested the brand-name medication.

Third-Party Plans

Health maintenance organization (HMO): The purpose is to keep the patient healthy; the plan is able to control costs by mandating generic usage. It is composed of a network of providers who are employed by the HMO or have signed contracts with the HMO to adhere to the conditions of the HMO. Expenses are not covered outside the network unless a referral has been made.

Preferred provider organization: A network of providers contracted by the insurer that offers the most flexibility to the patient. Costs outside the network may be partially reimbursed. They do not require that a physician within the network make referrals.

Point of sale: A network of providers under contract by the insurer. Patients are required to choose a primary care physician and are required to obtain a referral from the primary care physician for services outside the network.

Medicare: Federally funded program for individuals over the age of 65, disabled individuals younger than age 65, and patients with kidney failure.

Medicaid: A federally funded program administered by the states. States determine eligibility and services rendered. Prescription drug formularies are used, and not all drug products are covered.

Patient assistance programs: Special programs offered by pharmaceutical manufacturers for patients with specific needs who may be unable to afford their medication.

Workers' compensation: Federal and state laws require compensation for patients who have been accidentally injured on the job. Prescriptions for medications from the injury are billed either to the state bureau of workers' compensation or to the employer.

LEGAL REQUIREMENTS FOR PHARMACIST COUNSELING OF PATIENT OR PATIENT'S REPRESENTATIVE

An offer to counsel must be made to every patient, but the patient may refuse. Counseling may include name and description of medication; dosage form; dosage; route of administration; duration of drug therapy; action to take if a dose is missed; common adverse side effects; interactions and contraindications; self-monitoring for drug therapy; prescription refill information; proper storage of medication; and special directions.

CHAPTER 1 REVIEW QUESTIONS

1. What organization establishes standards of practice, addresses the quality of patient care and patient safety, and establishes standards for health care providers and home medical equipment and accredits the following: hospitals, home health care agencies, home infusion providers, long-term care pharmacies, and ambulatory infusion pharmacies?
   a. DEA
   b. EPA
   c. FDA
   d. TJC

2. What is Medicare?
   a. A federally funded program for drug addicts
   b. A federally funded program for elderly and disabled
   c. A federally funded program for the poor
   d. A federally funded program for injured victims of recalled medications

3. What is a deductible?
   a. Special programs offered by pharmaceutical manufacturers for patients with specific

   needs who may be unable to afford their medications
   b. A predetermined amount of money that is paid to an individual or institution for a daily service
   c. A set amount that must be paid by the patient for each benefit period before the insurer will cover additional expenses
   d. A fixed percentage, paid by the patient, of the total cost of the prescription

4. What is a Material Safety Data Sheet (MSDS)?
   a. Documentation that indicates the amount of each medication needed and lists the procedures to follow and labeling instructions
   b. Documentation that provides detailed information on the hazards of a particular substance
   c. Medication information sheet provided by the manufacturer that includes side effects, dosage forms, indications, and other important information
   d. A document provided to patients who are taking estrogens and progesterone

5. Where should one place used syringes?
   a. In a biohazard container
   b. In a cardboard box
   c. In a locked cabinet
   d. In a sharps container

6. Which of the following is not a universal precaution?
   a. Special handling of chemotherapy agents
   b. Using a sharps container to store used syringes and needles
   c. Wearing jewelry while preparing IV admixtures
   d. Wearing protective clothing while preparing IV admixtures

7. What is the process of mixing a liquid and powder to form a suspension or solution?
   a. Geometric dilution
   b. Levigation
   c. Reconstitution
   d. Trituration

8. Which of the following is not a characteristic of an absorption base?
   a. Anhydrous
   b. Difficult to spread
   c. Nongreasy
   d. Nonwashable

9. What type of order, used for specific classifications of medications, can be active for only a limited period of time, after which a new medication order is required to continue?
   a. Automatic stop order
   b. ASAP order
   c. PRN order
   d. STAT order

10. Which reference book provides information on drug prices?
    a. *Drug Topics Orange Book*
    b. *Drug Topics Red Book*
    c. *National Formulary*
    d. *USP*

11. What type of container is impervious to air under normal handling, shipment, storage, and distribution?
    a. Child-resistant
    b. Easy-open
    c. Hermetic
    d. Light-resistant

12. What classification of temperature is between 15°C and 30°C?
    a. Cold
    b. Cool
    c. Excessive heat
    d. Room temperature

13. What number is given by a manufacturer to identify a particular batch of medicine?
    a. Drug schedule
    b. UPC
    c. Lot number
    d. NDC number

14. Which piece of information is not required on a medication order label?
    a. Expiration date of medication
    b. Pharmacist or technician who processed the order
    c. Lot number of medication
    d. Trade or generic name of medication

15. Which of the following medications does not require that a patient package insert be given to the patient?
    a. Accutane
    b. ACE inhibitors
    c. Estrogens
    d. Oral contraceptives

16. If a pharmacy technician is using the continental (dry gum) method, what would he or she be compounding?
    a. Capsules
    b. Emulsions
    c. Suppositories
    d. Syrups

17. What should be used to clean the laminar flow hood?
    a. 70% rubbing alcohol
    b. 70% isopropyl alcohol
    c. 95% isopropyl alcohol
    d. 95% ethyl alcohol

18. What type of substance is composed of 50% dextrose, 20% fat, and 10% amino acid?
    a. Partial parenteral nutrition
    b. Peripheral parenteral nutrition
    c. Total parenteral nutrition
    d. Total peripheral nutrition

19. What technique is used in mixing two ingredients of unequal quantities?
    a. Blending
    b. Geometric dilution
    c. Levigation
    d. Spatulation

20. What type of agent increases the viscosity of a suspension?
    a. Emulsifier
    b. Flocculating agent
    c. Mucilage
    d. Thickening agent

21. What type of ointment base is Aquaphor?
    a. Absorption
    b. Oleaginous
    c. Oil-water emulsion base
    d. Water-oil emulsion base

22. What type of copayment is a predetermined amount of money to be paid for each prescription?
    a. Fixed
    b. Maximum allowable
    c. Percentage
    d. Variable

23. Which of the following is not found on an MSDS form?
    a. Accidental release measures
    b. Cost of the product

c. Exposure controls and personal protection
d. Handling and storage

24. Which of the following ointment bases is anhydrous?
    a. Absorption
    b. Water-oil emulsion base
    c. Oil-water base
    d. Water-miscible base

25. Who is responsible for providing a pharmacy with the MSDS?
    a. Drug manufacturer
    b. Drug wholesaler
    c. FDA
    d. EPA

26. How many times may a pharmacy transfer a controlled substance prescription of 30 tablets of Tylenol #3 with five refills indicated on the prescription?
    a. None
    b. One
    c. Three
    d. Five

27. What does a medication with an FDA therapeutic equivalence code "A" signify?
    a. Drug products that the FDA does not consider at this time to be therapeutically equivalent to other pharmaceutically equivalent products
    b. Drug products that are considered to be therapeutically equivalent to other pharmaceutically equivalent products
    c. Products meeting necessary bioequivalence requirements
    d. Products not presenting bioequivalence problems in conventional dosage forms

28. Which disease is characterized by an imbalance between oxygen supply and demand?
    a. Angina
    b. Hypertension
    c. MI
    d. Stroke

29. What type of a drug interaction occurs when one drug increases or prolongs the effect of another drug?
    a. Addition
    b. Antagonism
    c. Potentiation
    d. Synergism

30. What type of diabetes is caused by taking various medications?
    a. Gestational
    b. Type 1
    c. Type 2
    d. Secondary

31. What affective disorder is characterized by excessive phases of mania and depression?
    a. Bipolar disease
    b. Epilepsy
    c. Mania
    d. Schizophrenia

32. Which reference book provides monthly updates on FDA-approved medications, orphan drugs, and investigational drugs?
    a. *Drug Topics Red Book*
    b. *Drug Facts and Comparisons*
    c. *Physicians' Desk Reference*
    d. *Remington's Pharmaceutical Sciences*

33. Which of the following DEA numbers is incorrect for Dr. B. Yarhi?
    a. BY1234563
    b. BY5555555
    c. DBY1234563
    d. BY5555517

34. What type of syringe would be used to administer 0.5 mL of amoxicillin pediatric drops?
    a. Low-dose syringe
    b. Oral syringe
    c. Tuberculin syringe
    d. U-100 syringe

35. Which of the following screening or monitoring equipment is used to measure the vital capacity of an individual?
    a. Nebulizer
    b. Peak flow meter
    c. Pneumogram
    d. Sphygmomanometer

36. Which of the following pumps is used as a PCA?
    a. CADD Prizm PCS pump
    b. CADD-Plus pump
    c. CADD-TPN
    d. Elastometric balloon system

37. Which of the following pieces of equipment would be used by a diabetic?
    a. Glucometer
    b. Echocardiogram
    c. Electrocardiogram
    d. Syringe infusion system

38. Which of the following containers is a single-unit container intended for parenteral administration only?
    a. Tight container
    b. Single-unit container
    c. Single-dose container
    d. Unit-dose container

39. What dosage form can be prepared by the dry gum method, the wet gum method, or the beaker method?
    a. Capsules
    b. Emulsions
    c. Spirits
    d. Suspensions

40. Which dosage form can be prepared by the heat method?
    a. Elixir
    b. Suppository
    c. Syrup
    d. Tincture

41. Which dosage form can be prepared with either the compression mold or the fusion mold?
    a. Pills
    b. Suppositories
    c. Tablets
    d. Timed-released dosage forms

42. What type of an ointment base is white petrolatum?
    a. Absorption base
    b. Oleaginous
    c. Water-oil emulsion base
    d. Water-miscible base

43. Which of the following does not need to be placed in biohazard bag?
    a. Gloves
    b. Gowns
    c. Masks
    d. Needles

44. Which of the following is the price a pharmacy may pay for a medication after receiving a discount?
    a. AAC
    b. AWP
    c. Capitation
    d. MAC

45. Which of the following orders allows for a patient to receive a specific medication at a specific time each day in the hospital?
    a. ASAP orders
    b. Automatic orders
    c. PRN orders
    d. Standing orders

46. What temperature is considered a warm environment?
    a. Between 8° and 15°C
    b. Between 15° and 30°C
    c. Between 30° and 40°C
    d. Above 40°C

47. Which of the following is an automated dispensing device kept on the nursing unit?
    a. Baker Cells
    b. Omni Link Rx
    c. Pyxis Medstation
    d. Safety Pak

48. Which of the following is not required on a medication order label?
    a. Expiration date of medication
    b. Lot number of medication
    c. Medication number
    d. Name and location of patient

49. Which of the following is not found on a patient package insert?
    a. Description of medication
    b. Expiration date and lot number of medication
    c. Indications for medication
    d. Revisions of labeling

50. Which type of pharmacy processes, prepares, and distributes medication from one location?
    a. Centralized dispensing
    b. Decentralized dispensing
    c. Floor stock dispensing
    d. Satellite dispensing

ABBREVIATION QUESTIONS

1. Print the meaning of each abbreviation.
   a. ac
   b. amp
   c. bid
   d. cap
   e. emuls
   f. hs
   g. npo
   h. oint
   i. pc
   j. po
   k. pr
   l. q4h
   m. q6h
   n. q8h
   o. qd
   p. qid
   q. qod
   r. stat
   s. supp
   t. syr
   u. tab
   v. tid

2. Print the meaning of each abbreviation.
   a. tsp
   b. tbsp
   c. qt
   d. pt
   e. oz
   f. NS
   g. mL
   h. mg
   i. mEq
   j. mcg
   k. lb
   l. kg
   m. gr
   n. g
   o. gal
   p. fl oz
   q. DW
   r. D5W
   s. D5LR
   t. D20W
   u. D10W
   v. cc
   w. 1/2 NS

3. Print the meaning of each abbreviation.
   a. APhA
   b. ASAP
   c. AWP
   d. CMS
   e. DAW
   f. DEA
   g. EPA
   h. FDA
   i. GERD
   j. GPO
   k. HIPAA
   l. TJC
   m. MI
   n. NABP
   o. NF
   p. OSHA
   q. OTC
   r. P&T Committee
   s. PI
   t. U & C
   u. USP

4. Print the meaning of each abbreviation.
   a. 3TC
   b. APAP
   c. ASA
   d. AZT
   e. ddi
   f. D4T
   g. $FeSO_4$
   h. HCTZ
   i. INH
   j. KCl
   k. MOM
   l. NTG
   m. Pb
   n. PCN
   o. SMZ-TMP
   p. TCN

PRACTICE LAW QUESTIONS

1. What do the middle four numbers represent in an NDC number?
   a. Drug manufacturer
   b. Drug product
   c. Drug packaging
   d. None of the above

2. The pharmacist fails to place a prescription label on the medication container. Which law is being broken?
   a. Pure Food and Drug Act of 1906
   b. Food, Drug, and Cosmetic Act of 1938
   c. Durham-Humphrey Act of 1950
   d. Kefauver-Harris Act of 1962

3. An employee injures his back while lifting a carton of medication in the pharmacy. What law allows the employee to collect damages from the employer?
   a. Kefauver-Harris Act
   b. Occupational Safety and Health Act of 1970
   c. Omnibus Budget Reconciliation Act of 1987
   d. Poison Prevention Act of 1970

4. A patient requests that the pharmacist place his medication in an easy-open container. Which law allows the pharmacist to dispense the prescription in this manner?
   a. Kefauver-Harris Act
   b. Controlled Substances Act of 1970
   c. Occupational Safety and Health Act of 1970
   d. Poison Prevention Act of 1970

5. A pharmacist prepares a prescription with a mortar and pestle that have been contaminated by an antineoplastic agent and dispenses the prescription to a patient. Which law is he violating?
   a. Pure Food and Drug Act of 1906
   b. Food, Drug, and Cosmetic Act of 1938
   c. Durham-Humphrey Act of 1950
   d. Kefauver-Harris Act of 1962

6. Which law allows a pharmacist to accept a telephoned prescription from a physician's office?
   a. Pure Food and Drug Act of 1906
   b. Food, Drug, and Cosmetic Act of 1938
   c. Durham-Humphrey Act of 1950
   d. Kefauver-Harris Act of 1962

7. Which law allows a pharmacist to dispense nitroglycerin tablets in a non–child-resistant container?
   a. Durham-Humphrey Act
   b. Kefauver-Harris Act
   c. Controlled Substances Act
   d. Poison Control Act

8. Which law resulted in clearly distinguishing an over-the-counter medication from a prescription medication?
   a. Pure Food and Drug Act of 1906
   b. Food, Drug, and Cosmetic Act of 1938
   c. Durham-Humphrey Act of 1950
   d. Kefauver-Harris Act of 1962

9. Which law required that the federal legend appear on all prescriptions?
   a. Pure Food and Drug Act of 1906
   b. Food, Drug, and Cosmetic Act of 1938

   c. Durham-Humphrey Act of 1950
   d. Kefauver-Harris Act of 1962

10. For how long is a DEA Form 222 valid?
    a. 1 week
    b. 1 month
    c. 60 days
    d. 6 months

11. Which law requires that a manufacturer provide Material Safety Data Sheets (MSDSs) to a pharmacy for products that are combustible, are flammable, or can cause injury to an individual if he or she comes in contact with the substance?
    a. Kefauver-Harris Act of 1962
    b. Controlled Substances Act of 1970
    c. Occupational Safety and Health Act of 1970
    d. Poison Prevention Act of 1970

12. A pharmacist receives a prescription for 40 Percocet tablets, but the pharmacy has only 15 tablets in stock. The patient accepts the 15 tablets. How much time does the pharmacist have to provide the remaining 25 tablets?
    a. 24 hours
    b. 72 hours
    c. 96 hours
    d. 6 months

13. If a patient requests a partial filling of her Tylenol with Codeine #3 prescription, what can the pharmacist do for the patient?
    a. The pharmacist may provide the patient with the requested amount and places the remaining tablets in a bottle for the patient to pick up at a later date.
    b. The pharmacist may provide the patient with the requested amount and informs her that she must pick up the remaining quantity within 72 hours.
    c. The pharmacist may provide the patient with the requested amount and informs her that she must pick up the remaining quantity within 6 months of the date on which the prescription was filled.
    d. The pharmacist may provide the patient with the requested amount but can give her the balance only if there is a refill indicated on the prescription.

14. Which of the following is a correct DEA number for a Dr. Andrea J. Shedlock, who was Dr. Andrea Costello when she requested her DEA number before she was married?
    a. AC1234563

b. AS1234563
c. JC1234563
d. JS1234563

15. You are working for a chain pharmacy, and another member of the chain has run out of DEA Form 222s. They ask to borrow one of your DEA Form 222s. What would you do?
    a. Because you are members of the same pharmacy chain, you are allowed to let them use yours because you have the same DEA number.
    b. Give them one of your DEA Form 222s with the agreement that they will replace it after they receive their new ones.
    c. DEA Form 222s are for a specific pharmacy and can be used only by the pharmacy to which they were issued.
    d. Tell them to place an emergency order with the wholesaler and that you will provide them with a properly completed DEA Form 222 in 72 hours.

16. You receive a request from another pharmacy for 100 Percocet tablets. What do you do?
    a. You may loan them the requested 100 tablets of Percocet.
    b. You may sell them the 100 tablets of Percocet at the AWP.
    c. You may transfer to them the 100 tablets of Percocet through the use of a DEA Form 222.
    d. None of the above can be done.

17. What form is used to report the theft of controlled substances?
    a. DEA Form 41
    b. DEA Form 106
    c. DEA Form 222
    d. DEA Form 224

18. Which of the following is part of HIPAA?
    a. Allows a member of a plan to select any pharmacy for his or her pharmacy benefit as long as the pharmacy agrees to the terms and conditions of the plan
    b. Allows Rx to appear on a prescription instead of the federal legend
    c. Insurance reform
    d. Prohibits a prescription drug plan from requiring mail order prescription drug coverage without providing non–mail order coverage

19. Which organization oversees Medicare and Medicaid service?
    a. BOP
    b. CMS
    c. DEA
    d. TJC

20. Who reviews INDs?
    a. BOP
    b. DEA
    c. EPA
    d. FDA

21. Which law required opium to have a prescription?
    a. Comprehensive Drug Abuse Prevention and Control Act
    b. Federal Food and Drug Act
    c. Food, Drug, and Cosmetic Act
    d. Harrison Narcotic Act

22. Which law required that all narcotics be labeled "Warning: May Be Habit Forming"?
    a. Anabolic Steroid Control Act
    b. Comprehensive Drug Abuse Prevention and Control Act
    c. Harrison Narcotic Act
    d. Prescription Drug Marketing Act

23. Which law requires drug utilization evaluation to be performed on all prescriptions?
    a. Dietary Supplement Health and Education Act of 1994
    b. Omnibus Reconciliation Act of 1987
    c. Omnibus Reconciliation Act of 1990
    d. Prescription Drug Equity Law

24. Which law allowed pharmacists to take prescriptions over the telephone from a physician's office?
    a. Durham-Humphrey Act
    b. Food, Drug, and Cosmetic Act
    c. Kefauver-Harris Act
    d. Comprehensive Drug Abuse Prevention and Control Act

25. Which law established tax-free savings accounts?
    a. Freedom of Choice Law
    b. HIPAA
    c. Medicare Drug Improvement and Modernization Act of 2003
    d. Omnibus Budget Reconciliation Act of 1990

26. Which law stated that a resident's drug regimen must be free of unnecessary medications?
    a. Freedom of Choice Law
    b. HIPAA
    c. Omnibus Reconciliation Act of 1987
    d. Omnibus Reconciliation Act of 1990

27. Which law allows nasal inhalers to be dispensed without a child-resistant container?
    a. Americans with Disabilities Act
    b. Freedom of Choice Law
    c. Occupational Health and Safety Act of 1970
    d. Poison Control Act of 1970

28. Which law lowers the reimbursement rate for durable medical equipment?
    a. Drug Price Competition and Patent Term Restoration Act
    b. FDA Safe Medical Devices Act of 1990
    c. HIPAA
    d. Medicare Drug Improvement and Modernization Act of 2003

29. Which law prevents reimportation of medication into the United States other than by a manufacturer?
    a. Drug Listing Act of 1972
    b. Drug Price Competition and Patent Term Restoration Act of 1984
    c. Food, Drug, and Cosmetic Act
    d. Prescription Drug Marketing Act

30. Which agency oversees the practice of pharmacy?
    a. APhA
    b. DEA
    c. FDA
    d. State BOP

PHARMACOLOGY REVIEW QUESTIONS

1. Write the generic name for each of the following brand names.
    a. Premarin
    b. Lipitor
    c. Norvasc
    d. Lanoxin
    e. Zithromax
    f. Zocor
    g. Zestril
    h. Tenormin
    i. Xanax
    j. Cardizem
    k. Glucotrol
    l. Allegra
    m. Procardia
    n. Dilantin
    o. Wellbutrin
    p. Relafen
    q. Risperdal
    r. Serevent
    s. Zantac
    t. Plavix
    u. Azmacort
    v. Amaryl
    w. Phenergan
    x. Nolvadex
    y. Lasix
    z. Vasotec

2. Write the brand names for each of the following generic names.
    a. cephalexin
    b. fluoxetine
    c. paroxetine
    d. mupirocin
    e. acetaminophen + codeine
    f. propoxyphene N/APAP
    g. triamterene/HCTZ
    h. alendronate
    i. losartan
    j. fluconazole
    k. amitriptyline
    l. rosiglitazone
    m. esomeprazole
    n. olanzapine
    o. montelukast
    p. nefazodone
    q. tolterodine
    r. oxycodone
    s. acyclovir
    t. propranolol
    u. doxycycline
    v. nortriptyline
    w. etodolac
    x. clindamycin
    y. metronidazole
    z. naproxen

3. Which auxiliary labels should be affixed to a prescription container of the following medications?
    a. Vicodin
    b. Glucophage
    c. Coumadin
    d. Cipro
    e. Tetracycline
    f. Deltasone
    g. Biaxin
    h. Ambien
    i. Motrin

j. Depakote
k. Xalatan
l. Antivert
m. TobraDex
n. Proventil
o. Bactrim suspension
p. Augmentin
q. Benzamycin
r. Minocin
s. Amoxicillin suspension
t. Lotrisone cream
u. Feldene
v. Ritalin
w. Vicoprofen
x. Hydrochlorothiazide
y. Ultram
z. Humulin N

4. Identify the primary indication for which each brand of drug is used.
   a. Premarin
   b. Synthroid
   c. Lipitor
   d. Prilosec
   e. Vicodin
   f. Proventil
   g. Norvasc
   h. Amoxil
   i. Prozac
   j. Zoloft
   k. Glucophage
   l. Lanoxin
   m. Prempro
   n. Paxil
   o. Zithromax
   p. Zestril
   q. Zocor
   r. Prevacid
   s. Augmentin
   t. Celebrex
   u. Coumadin
   v. Vasotec
   w. Lasix
   x. Cipro
   y. Keflex
   z. Deltasone

5. Identify the primary indication for which each generic drug is used.
   a. pravastatin
   b. clarithromycin
   c. norgestimate–ethinyl estradiol
   d. acetaminophen-codeine
   e. atenolol
   f. cetirizine

g. zolpidem
h. alprazolam
i. tramadol
j. quinapril
k. diltiazem
l. glipizide
m. fexofenadine
n. triamterene-HCTZ
o. doxazosin
p. alendronate
q. benazepril
r. nifedipine
s. sildenafil citrate
t. ibuprofen
u. valproate
v. phenytoin
w. bupropion
x. gabapentin
y. losartan
z. fluconazole

6. To what drug classification does each drug belong?
   a. sulfasalazine
   b. erythromycin stearate
   c. doxycycline
   d. ranitidine
   e. ampicillin
   f. acyclovir
   g. lamivudine
   h. promethazine
   i. azelastine
   j. codeine
   k. carbamazepine
   l. albuterol
   m. beclomethasone
   n. diphenoxylate + atropine
   o. simethicone
   p. doxazosin
   q. quinidine
   r. amlodipine
   s. verapamil
   t. captopril
   u. hydrochlorothiazide
   v. lovastatin
   w. sumatriptan
   x. estradiol
   y. fluconazole
   z. terbinafine

7. To what drug classification does each drug belong?
   a. fluoxetine
   b. omeprazole
   c. cephalexin

d. pravastatin
e. celecoxib
f. sertraline
g. atenolol
h. furosemide
i. metformin
j. digoxin
k. sulfamethoxazole-trimethoprim
l. ibuprofen
m. rosiglitazone
n. salmeterol
o. cefprozil
p. quinapril
q. amitriptyline
r. lisinopril
s. imipramine
t. fluvastatin
u. ciprofloxacin
v. indomethacin
w. hydroxyzine HCl
x. carbamazepine
y. diltiazem
z. triamcinolone

8. To what drug classification does each drug belong?
    a. esomeprazole
    b. prednisone
    c. acetaminophen + codeine
    d. zolpidem
    e. alprazolam
    f. fexofenadine
    g. doxazosin
    h. citalopram
    i. naproxen
    j. oxycodone
    k. carvedilol
    l. etodolac
    m. piroxicam
    n. acetaminophen + hydrocodone
    o. levofloxacin
    p. enalapril
    q. lansoprazole
    r. acetaminophen + oxycodone
    s. tramadol
    t. clotrimazole
    u. nelfinavir
    v. butalbital/codeine/APAP
    w. ketoconazole
    x. clonidine
    y. nadolol
    z. doxycycline

9. Identify one indication for each of the following herbal agents.
    a. Aloe vera

b. Cascara sagrada
c. St. John's wort
d. Melatonin
e. Gingko
f. Glucosamine
g. Cranberry
h. Chondroitin
i. Goldenseal
j. Echinacea

PRACTICE MATH PROBLEMS

Conversions

1. How many lb are equal to 1 kg?

2. How many g are in 5.5 kg?

3. How many g are equal to 2500 mg?

4. How many mg are equal to 350 mcg?

5. How many cc equal 75 mL?

6. How many tsp equal 120 mL?

7. How many tbsp equal 6 tsp?

8. How many tsp equal 7.5 fl oz?

9. How many fl oz equal 1.5 cups?

10. How many qt equal 2 gal?

11. How many pt equal 6.5 qt?

12. How many mg equal 7.5 gr?

13. How many gr equal 2 g?

14. How many tsp equal 1 L?

15. How many gr equal 650 mg?

16. How many g equal 125 mg?

17. How many mcg equal 2.4 g?

18. How many tbsp equal 12 tsp?

19. How many fl oz equal 2.5 qt?

20. How many g equal 75 mg?

21. How many mL equal 2 gal?

22. How many gal equal 8 cups?

23. How many g equal 1 lb?

24. How many tbsp equal 6 fl oz?

25. How many tsp equal 2 fl oz?

Calculations

1. How many colchicine tablets each containing 600 mcg may be prepared from 30 g of colchicine?

2. The prescriber ordered atropine sulfate 0.2 mg SC q6h prn. What is the equivalent dose in micrograms?

3. The physician has ordered Coumadin 5 mg to be taken on Monday, Wednesday, and Friday. On Tuesday, Thursday, Saturday, and Sunday, the patient is to receive 2½ mg. How many milligrams will the patient take in 1 week?

4. The prescriber ordered 0.05 mg of Sandostatin PO, a hormone. How many micrograms are in this dose?

5. You have a 2-mL ampule of caffeine Na benzonatate containing gr viiss. If the physician orders gr v, how many milliliters will you dispense?

6. How many grams of reserpine would be required to make 25,000 tablets, each containing 250 mcg of reserpine?

7. How many milligrams are in one tablet of Nitrostat 1/150 gr?

8. How many grams of antipyrine should be used in preparing the following prescription?
Rx   Antipyrine 5%
Glycerin ad   60

9. A pediatric patient is to be given a 70-mg dose of Dilantin by administration of an oral suspension containing 50 mg of Dilantin per 5 mL. How many milliliters of the suspension must be administered?

10. A prefilled syringe of furosemide contains 20 mg of drug in 2 mL of solution. How many micrograms of drug would be administered by an injection of 0.5 mL of the solution?

11. The usual dose range of dimercapol is 2.5 mg to 5 mg/kg of body weight. What would be the dose range for a person weighing 165 lb?

12. How many chloramphenicol capsules each containing 250 mg of chloramphenicol are needed to provide 25 mg/kg/day of body weight for one week for a person weighing 154 lb?

13. Cyclosporine is an immunosuppressive agent administered before and after organ transplantation at a single dose of 15 mg/kg. How many milliliters of a 50-mL bottle containing 100 mg of cyclosporine per milliliter would be administered to a 140-lb kidney transplant patient?

14. How many milliliters of aminophylline injection containing 250 mg in each 10 mL should be used in filling a medication order calling for 15 mg of aminophylline?

15. The dose of a drug is 500 mcg/kg of body weight. How many milligrams should be given to a child weighing 55 lb?

16. The antiviral ophthalmic drug fomivirsen sodium (Vitravene) has been ordered by the physician, 330 mcg. The vial is labeled 6.6 mg/mL. How many milliliters contain the prescribed dose?

17. The physician ordered 0.725 mg of droperidol (Inapsine) IV stat. The vial reads 2.5 mg in 2 mL. Calculate the amount of drug you will administer to this patient in milliliters.

18. A patient is to receive a 100-mg dose of gentamicin. The medication is available in an 80-mg/mL vial. How many milliliters should the patient receive?

19. A drug has a concentration of 20 mg/mL. How many grams of the drug are in ½ L of the solution?

20. A dose of antacid is 1 tbsp. How many doses can be prepared from a pint bottle?

21. You are to prepare a dose of 300 mg and the tablets are available in 75-mg strength. How many tablets will the pharmacist need to dispense if the patient is to take 300 mg bid for 1 week?

22. What is the percent of a 1:25 (w/v) solution?

23. What is the percent of a 1:200 (w/w) ointment?

24. Convert 25°C to F.

25. Convert 65°F to C.

26. Convert 40°C to F

27. Convert 45°F to C.

28. The drug vial contains 1,000,000 units of penicillin G. The label directions state: Add 2.3 mL of sterile water to the vial, 1.2 mL = 500,000 units. How many milliliters equal 200,000 units?

29. A patient is to receive 25 units of the hormonal drug vasopressin (Pitressin) IM. If the label reads 50 units per 2 mL, how many milliliters will you administer to the patient?

30. The prescriber ordered 175,000 units of urokinase IVPB. The vial directions read: Add 4.2 mL to vial and each mL will contain 50,000 units. How many milliliters will you prepare?

31. The order is for K-Lor 60 mEq PO stat. Each packet contains 20 mEq. How many packets of K-Lor will you need?

32. A 20% KCl solution has a strength of 40 mEq/tbsp. How many milliliters need to be dispensed for the patient to receive 20 mEq?

33. If the dose of a drug is 150 mcg, how many doses are contained in 0.120 g?

34. If a physician prescribed cephalexin 250 mg qid for 10 days, how many milliliters of cephalexin oral suspension containing 250 mg/tsp should be dispensed?

35. A 25-lb child is to receive 4 mg of phenytoin per kg of body weight as an anticonvulsant. How many milliliters of pediatric phenytoin suspension containing 30 mg/5 mL should the child receive?

36. If a 3-year-old child weighing 33 lb accidentally ingested 20 81-mg aspirin tablets, how much aspirin did the child ingest on a milligram/kilogram basis?

37. The usual pediatric dose of cefazolin sodium is 25 mg/kg/day divided equally into three doses. What would be the single dose in milligrams for a child weighing 44 lb?

38. If a child is 4 years old and the adult dose of medication is 100 mg, how much medication should the child receive?

39. If a child is 36 months old and the adult dose is 250 mg, how much medication should the child receive?

40. If a child is 2½ years old and the adult dose is 100 mg, how many milligrams should the child receive?

41. If a child weighs 45 lb and the adult dose is 50 mg, how much medication should the child receive?

42. If a child weighs 50 lb and the adult dose is 1 tbsp, how many milliliters should the child receive?

43. If a child weighs 60 lb and the adult dose is 500 mg, how many milligrams should the child receive?

44. If a child weighs 15 kg and the adult dose is 75 mg, how many milligrams should the child receive?

45. If 125 mL of liquid weighs 95 g, what is its specific gravity?

46. A volume of fluid weighs 80 g and has a specific gravity of 1.05. What is its volume?

47. How many grams are in 100 mL of a liquid if its specific gravity is 1.25?

48. What is the specific gravity of a substance that weighs 60 g and occupies a volume of 75 mL?

49. How many grams of silver nitrate are needed to make 1 L of a 0.25% solution?

50. A pharmacist has received an order to prepare 1 lb of 5% (w/w) salicylic acid ointment. How much salicylic acid is needed to prepare this ointment?

51. How many grams of NaCl are in 250 mL of ½ NS (0.45%)?

52. How many grams are in 1 L of a 1:200 solution?

53. How many micrograms are in 1.0 mL of a 1:100 solution?

54. If a pharmacist adds 3 g of hydrocortisone to 120 g of a 5% hydrocortisone cream, what is the final percentage strength of hydrocortisone in the product?

55. How many 600-mg ibuprofen tablets will be needed to make 8 oz of a 15% ointment?

56. How many milliliters of a 3% (w/v) solution will be necessary to make 6 oz of a 1:200 solution?

57. A stock bottle of Lugol's solution contains 2 oz from the original pint bottle. The pharmacy technician is able to prepare four 8-oz bottles of a more dilute 4% solution. What was the original percentage strength of the Lugol's solution?

58. You receive an order for 125 mL of 4% acetic acid solution and you have in stock 75% acetic acid solution. How many milliliters of the 75% solution will you need?

59. If 100 mL of 25% (w/v) solution is diluted to 1 L, what will be the percentage strength (w/v)?

60. You are asked to prepare 80 mL of a 72% lidocaine solution and you have in stock a 75% solution. How many milliliters of the 75% solution will you use?

61. The formula for a buffer solution contains 1.24% (w/v) of boric acid. How many milliliters of a 10% (w/v) boric acid solution should be used to obtain the boric acid needed in preparing 1 gal of buffer solution?

62. How many grams of Eucerin should be added to 4 oz of a 10% ointment to make a 7% ointment?

63. You are asked to prepare 50 mL of a 1:100 rifampin suspension and you have in stock a 1:20 rifampin suspension. How many milliliters of the 1:20 suspension will you need?

64. You are asked to prepare 125 mL of a 1:8 nystatin suspension and you have in stock a 1:6 solution. How many milliliters of the 1:6 nystatin solution will you need?

65. You are asked to prepare 50 mL of a 1:3 folic acid solution and you have in stock a 1:2 solution. How many milliliters of the 1:2 solution will you use?

66. How many milliliters of a 1:50 (w/v) stock solution of a chemical should be used to prepare 2 L of a 1:4000 (w/v) solution?

67. How many milliliters of water should be added to 500 mL of a 1:2000 (w/v) solution to make a 1:5000 (w/v) solution?

68. How much water should be added to 1 quart of 70% isopropyl alcohol to prepare a 20% solution for soaking sponges?

69. How much metoclopramide 5 mg/mL is used to make 10 mL of 0.5 mg/mL solution?

70. Prepare 15 mL of cefazolin dilution 50 mg/mL from a stock of 1 g/5 mL. How many milliliters of the diluent and cefazolin will be needed?

71. Make 30 mL of a vitamin B_{12} dilution with a concentration of 100 mcg/mL from a stock solution of 1 mg/mL. How much B_{12} and diluent are needed?

72. You are asked to prepare 36 mL of a 1:4 Bactrim solution and you have in stock 30% solution. How many milliliters of the 30% solution will you use?

73. You are asked to prepare 52 mL of a 28% Flagyl solution and you have in stock 42 g/mL solution. How many milliliters of the 42 g/mL will you use?

74. How many milliliters of a ½% solution of gentian violet should be used in preparing 500 mL of a 1:100,000 solution?

75. How many milliliters of a 5% stock solution are needed to prepare 1 pint of a solution containing 100 mg of the chemical per liter?

76. How many milliliters of a 95% (v/v) alcohol should be used in preparing a pint of a 75% (v/v) solution?

77. In what proportions should alcohols of 95% and 50% strengths be mixed to prepare 250 mL of a 70% alcohol solution?

78. How many milliliters of a 1:2000 iodine solution and a 7.5% iodine solution are needed to make 120 mL of a 3.5% solution?

79. How many milliliters of a 2.5% (w/v) chlorpromazine hydrochloride injection and how many milliliters of a 0.9% (w/v) sodium chloride injection should be used to prepare 500 mL of a 1.25% (w/v) chlorpromazine hydrochloride injection?

80. How much 10% dextrose solution and 20% dextrose solution should be mixed to prepare 1 L of a 12.5% dextrose solution?

81. In what proportion should 5% and 1% hydrocortisone ointments be mixed to prepare a 2.5% ointment?

82. Prepare 300 mL of 7.5% dextrose using SWFI and D20W. How much of each is needed?

83. Prepare 500 mL of D12.5W. You have on hand D5W, D10W, and D20W. How much of which two solutions will you use?

84. How many grams of a 2.5% hydrocortisone cream should be mixed with 240 g of a 0.25% hydrocortisone cream to make a 1% cream?

85. What is the total volume that will be delivered if a patient receives normal saline solution at 25 mL/hr for 24 hr?

86. Calculate the flow rate to be used to infuse 1000 mL of NS over 8 hr if the set delivers 10 gtt/mL.

87. 1 L NS is to be administered over 24 hr. The administration set to be used has a DF of 15 gtt/mL. What is the rate of infusion in
   a. mL/hr?
   b. gtt/min?

88. 1500 mL TPN solution is given IV at 75 mL/hr using an administration set with a drop factor of 20 gtt/mL. If the infusion starts at 0900 hours, when will it end?

89. Medication: Solu-Cortef 250 mg

   Fluid volume: 250 mL
   Time of infusion: 4 hr
   How many mL/hr? How many mg/hr?

90. How many milliliters of IV fluid will a patient receive if infused at the rate of 120 mL/hr over 3½ hr?

91. What will be the rate in gtt/min if a patient receives 1 L of an IV fluid over an 8-hr period if the drop factor = 15 gtt/mL?

92. If 1000 mL at 20 drops/min is administered using a 15-drop set, what is the flow rate in milliliters per hour?

93. If 500 mL of an IV solution contains 0.1 g of a drug, at what flow rate in milliliters per minute should the solution be administered to provide 1 mg/min of the drug?

94. An initial heparin dose of not less than 150 units/kg of body weight has been recommended for open heart surgery. How many milliliters of an injection containing 5000 heparin units per milliliter should be administered to a 280-lb patient?

95. An IV piggyback of lincomycin containing 1 g of drug in 100 mL is to be infused over 1½ hours. The IV set is calibrated to deliver 15 gtt/mL. How many drops per minute will the patient receive?

96. An IV piggyback of pentamidine isethionate containing 300 mg of drug in 150 mL of D5W is to be infused over 2 hr. The IV set is calibrated to deliver 20 gtt/mL. How many drops per minute should be administered?

97. An IV piggyback of enalapril maleate containing 10 mg of drug in 50 mL of 0.9% sodium chloride injection is to be infused over 1 hour. The IV set is calibrated to deliver 15 gtt/mL. How many drops per minute should be administered?

98. A physician orders 3 L D5W to be administered over 24 hr. How many drops per minute will be delivered using an administration set calibrated to deliver 30 drops per milliliter?

99. What is the total overhead for a pharmacy that has the following expenses?

Pharmacist salary (2)	$90,000
Pharmacy technicians (3)	$30,000
Rent	$240,000
Pharmaceutical drugs	$2,850,000
Licenses	$545
Insurance	$2025
Electricity	$3625
Gas	$8525
Water	$895
Supplies	$1255
Software	$995

100. What is the gross profit for a drug that has an AWP of $59.99, has a dispensing cost of $3.75, and retails for $67.99?

101. What is the markup for a drug that costs $9.99, has a dispensing cost of $2.75, and retails for $13.99?

102. What is the markup rate for a drug that costs $19.99 and retails for $25.99?

103. What is the net profit for a drug that has an AAC of $99.99, has a dispensing cost of $4.25, and retails for $112.99?

104. The cost for a bottle of 100 test strips for a glucometer is $67.50. The overhead for the store is $3.50, and the store wants to make a net profit of $23.68. What should the selling price be?

105. How much will a pharmacy pay a wholesaler if the conditions are 2% net 30 if the invoice shows $1950.00?

106. What will the inventory turnover rate be for a pharmacy if the inventory value is $255,000 and the pharmacy has sales of $3 million?

107. How many inventory turns will a pharmacy experience if it has an initial inventory of $225,000 and a final inventory of $250,000 and sales totaling $2.6 million during the year?

108. Rx:

Hydrocodone bitartrate	0.2 g
Phenacetin	3.6 g
Aspirin	6.0 g
Caffeine	0.6 g
M ft	caps no 24
Sig	i cap tid prn pain

    a. How many milligrams of hydrocodone bitartrate would be contained in each capsule?
    b. What is the total weight, in milligrams, of the ingredients in each capsule?
    c. How many milligrams of caffeine would be taken daily?

109.

Carafate	400 mg/5 mL
Cherry syrup	40 mL
Sorbitol solution	40 mL
Flavor qs	
Purified water ad	125 mL
Sig: 5 mL tid	

    How many 1-g Carafate tablets should be used in preparing the prescription?

110. From the following formula for iodine topical solution, USP, calculate the number of grams of iodine needed to prepare 12 dozen 15-mL containers of the solution.

Iodine	20 g
Sodium iodide	24 g
Purified water ad	1000 mL

111. From the following formula, calculate the quantities to make 120 mL of benzyl benzoate lotion.

Benzyl benzoate	125 mL
Triethanolamine	2.5 mL
Oleic acid	10 mL
Purified water, to make 500 mL	

112. Each 5 mL of a pediatric cough syrup is to contain the following amounts of medications. Calculate the amount of each ingredient to prepare a gallon of the syrup.

Dextromethorphan hydrobromide	7.5 mg
Guaifenesin	100 mg
Flavored syrup, to make 5.0 mL	

113. The following is a formula for psoriasis ointment (*International Journal of Pharmaceutical Compounding* 2:305, 1998). Calculate, in grams, the quantity of each ingredient needed to make a pound of the ointment.

Coal tar	2.0 g
Precipitated sulfur	3.0 g
Salicylic acid	1.0 g
Lidex ointment	24.0 g
Aquabase	70.0 g

114. The following is a formula for 100 triple-estrogen capsules (*International Journal of Pharmaceutical Compounding* 1:187, 1997). Calculate the quantities of the first three ingredients in grams and the last two ingredients in kilograms required to prepare 2500 capsules.

Estriol	200 mg
Estrone	25 mg
Estradiol	25 mg
Polyethylene glycol	145,020 g
Polyethylene glycol	335,020 g

Maintaining Medication and Inventory Control Systems

PHARMACEUTICAL INDUSTRY PROCEDURES FOR OBTAINING PHARMACEUTICALS

- **Group purchasing organization:** Negotiates prices for hospitals and institutions but does not make the actual purchase for institution.
- **Purchase from drug manufacturers:** Allows pharmacies to purchase in bulk, resulting in a savings for the company. Wholesalers may not always stock specific medications because of storage conditions, expense, or low demand.
- **Purchase from wholesalers:** Stocks medications from all manufacturers. Pharmacies are able to purchase when they need a product, rather than far in advance. Wholesalers may provide special services to the pharmacy, such as emergency deliveries, automated ordering systems, or automated purchasing systems.
- **Government:** Requires pharmacies to use Drug Enforcement Agency (DEA) Form 222 to purchase Schedule II drugs.

PURCHASING POLICIES, PROCEDURES, AND PRACTICES

- **Just-in-time ordering:** Ordering a product before running out; the product is shipped to the pharmacy immediately. The pharmacy will normally receive it the same day or the next business day. A method to keep an inventory low and maximize profit.
- **Point of sale:** Item is deducted from inventory as it is dispensed and in many situations is automatically reordered.
- **Purchase order:** A form that is used to order drugs and supplies from a wholesaler. Information found on a purchase order includes the following:
  - Name and address of the institution
  - Shipping address
  - Date the order was placed
  - Vendor's name and address
  - Purchase order number—a tracking number used to identify a purchase order
  - Ordering department's name and location
  - Expected date of delivery
  - Shipping terms
  - Account name or billing designation
  - Description of items ordered
  - Quantity of items ordered
  - Unit price
  - Extended price
  - Total price of the order
  - Buyer's name and phone number

DOSAGE FORMS

A dosage form is a system or device for delivering a drug to a biologic system.

SOLIDS

Advantages of Solid Dosage Forms

- Easy to package, transport, store, and dispense
- Convenient for self-medication
- Lack smell or taste
- Extremely stable for products that are not stable in liquid form
- Predivided dosage form
- Suited for sustained- or delayed-release medications

Examples of Solid Dosage Forms

- **Tablets:** Prepared either by compressing or by molding. The dosage form is accurate, compact, portable, and easy to administer. May come in various shapes; may be scored (able to be broken in halves or quarters). The most common types of marketable tablets include standard compressed, enteric coated, sugar-coated, film-coated, sublingual or buccal, multiple compressed, chewable, sustained-action, and delayed-action tablets.
- **Capsules:** A drug is contained in a shell of gelatin (either soft or hard) that dissolves in 10 to 20 minutes. Drug may be in either a solid or a liquid form. Shape of dosage form may be spheric or ovoid. Capacity of capsule may vary up to 1 g. Can be produced manually by using the punch method.
- **Effervescent salts:** Granules or powders; when dissolved in water, they effervesce and release carbon dioxide.
- **Implants or pellets:** Dosage forms that are placed under the skin through injection and are effective for a long period.
- **Lozenges, troches, or pastilles:** Solid dosage forms with flavoring that dissolve in the mouth.
- **Pellets:** Small cylinders that are implanted subcutaneously for continuous absorption.
- **Plasters:** Medicated or nonmedicated preparations that adhere to the skin by a backing material.
- **Powders:** Finely ground substances that can be administered internally or externally. Chief disadvantages are their taste and that they are not stable when exposed to the atmosphere. May be dispensed in a bulk form, in a multidose form, or as a divided dose such as a powder paper.
- **Suppositories:** Solid dosage forms to be inserted in body orifices, such as the rectum, vagina, or urethra. May work either locally or systemically. Mechanism of action is either through melting or dissolving and release of medication over time. Not all products are available as a suppository.

Major disadvantages of a suppository are that it may be easily expelled from the body and that absorption of medication into the body can be erratic.

Oral Sustained-Release Dosage Forms

- Constant release
- Continuous action
- Continuous release
- Controlled action
- Controlled release
- Delayed absorption
- Delayed action
- Depot
- Extended action
- Extended release
- Gradual release
- Long acting
- Long lasting
- Long-term release
- Programmed release
- Prolonged action
- Prolonged release
- Protracted release
- Repeat action
- Repository
- Slow acting
- Sustained action
- Sustained release
- Sustained-release depot
- Timed disintegration
- Timed release

LIQUIDS

Advantages of Liquids

- Effective more quickly than a solid dosage form because the drug is already dissolved in a liquid.
- Easier to swallow than a solid dosage form for many patients.
- Drugs may be available only in liquid form owing to convenience of administration.
- Uniformity and flexibility of dosage form.
- Certain medications may cause gastrointestinal distress if administered in a solid dosage form.

Disadvantages of Liquids

- Deterioration and loss of potency occur more quickly than in a solid dosage form.
- May require special sweetening or flavoring to be palatable.
- Incompatibilities of dissolved substances.
- May require preservatives to prevent bacteria or mold from developing.

- Inaccurate measuring of a dose for a patient may occur.
- Bulkier to carry than solid dosage forms.
- Interactions may develop from changes in solubility.

SOLUTIONS

Solutions contain a solute that is dissolved in a solvent. They may be aqueous, alcoholic, or hydroalcoholic.

- **Aromatic waters:** Solutions of water-containing oils that have a smell and are volatile.
- **Collodion:** Topical dosage form that contains pyroxylin and is dissolved in alcohol and ether.
- **Elixir:** A clear, sweetened, flavored hydroalcoholic solution, containing water and alcohol, that may or may not be medicated.
- **Enema:** A solution administered rectally for either cleansing or drug administration.
- **Extract:** A process by which active ingredients are removed from their source through the application of solvents.
- **Douche:** An irrigating or bathing solution.
- **Isotonic (Iso-osmotic):** Having the same tone or osmolarity of another substance. There is no loss or gain of water by the cell. Dilution of an isotonic solution may affect the composition of solution. An example is an ophthalmic solution.
- **Liniments:** Either alcoholic or oleaginous solutions or emulsions that are applied through rubbing.
- **Spirits:** Alcoholic or hydroalcoholic solutions containing volatile aromatic ingredients.
- **Syrups:** Aqueous solutions containing sucrose or sucrose substitutes.
- **Tinctures:** Alcoholic or hydroalcoholic solutions of pure chemicals or extracts.

DISPERSIONS

A dispersion consists of a solute dispersed through a dispersing vehicle.

- **Suspension:** A two-phase system in which solid particles are dispersed in a liquid vehicle. A suspension may be oral, topical, or injectable. Suspended material should not settle rapidly and should pour freely. Topical solutions should be fluid enough to spread over the affected area, but should not run off the surface of application. They dry quickly. They provide a protective film and have an acceptable color and odor.
- **Emulsion:** One liquid is dispersed in another liquid; may be water in oil (w/o) or oil in water (o/w). Emulsions are stabilized through the use of an emulsifying agent. Oral emulsions are o/w preparations; topical emulsions may be either o/w (washable and nonstaining) or w/o. An o/w emulsion will become diluted with water, but a w/o emulsion will not.
- **Lotion:** A liquid for topical application that contains insoluble solids or liquids.
- **Gel:** A two-phase system containing an extremely fine solid particle that, when mixed, has a semisolid form. It is very difficult to distinguish between the two phases.
- **Ointment:** A semisolid dosage form for topical application. Anhydrous ointments absorb water but are insoluble in water and are not water washable. Oleaginous ointments are insoluble in water, do not contain or absorb water, and are not water washable.
- **Pastes:** Similar to ointments but contain more solid materials.
- **Creams:** Topically applied o/w emulsions.

INHALANTS

Inhalants are gases, vapors, solutions, or suspensions intended to be inhaled either orally or intranasally.

- **Aerosol:** A spray in a pressurized container that contains a propellant, an inert liquid, or gas under pressure meant to carry the active ingredient to its location of application. Particles may be either a fine solid or a liquid. Aerosols are used for administration into body cavities. They are convenient and easy to apply.
- **Spray:** A dosage form that consists of a container with a valve assembly that, when activated, will emit a dispersion of liquid, solid, or gaseous material.

TRANSDERMAL PRODUCTS

Transdermal products provide systemic therapy for acute or chronic conditions that do not involve the skin. A transdermal product delivers a controlled dose of medication through the skin and is absorbed directly into the bloodstream. It is a convenient system that results in improved patient compliance, accurate drug dosage, and regulation of drug concentration.

FORMULARY OR APPROVED STOCK LIST

- **Formulary:** A list of drugs that are approved for use in an institution such as a hospital or whose cost will be reimbursed by a third-party carrier to a pharmacy. Formulary systems include open formulary (all pharmaceutical products carried), closed formulary (limited number of products of each drug classification covered), or restricted formulary (a hybrid of both open and closed formularies). Formularies may define policies, procedures, and guidelines established by the medical staff regarding a medication's usage. Formularies are revised yearly and a process must be in place for revisions.

- **Pharmacy and therapeutics (P&T) committee:** A committee composed of pharmacists, physicians, nurses, pharmacy buyers, and accountants who develop a formulary for a hospital. The most effective therapeutic agents are chosen for an institution. A formulary may contain a generic and name-brand name index, dosage forms and strengths, formulations, packaging and sizes available, dosage guidelines, approved abbreviations for the institution, policies on investigational medications, electrolyte content of large-volume parenterals, and lists of available nutritional and sugar-free products.
- **Third-party (managed care) provider:** A provider that may develop a formulary for its members regarding products covered for reimbursement. They are referred to as *pharmacy benefit providers.*

PAR AND REORDER LEVELS AND DRUG USAGE

- **PAR value (periodic automatic replacement):** The amount of drug that is automatically reordered. In automatic reordering systems, when a drug falls below a predetermined quantity, it is automatically reordered.
- **Minimum and maximum:** A predetermined number that states the minimum and maximum amount of medication to be kept on a shelf. The smaller the range, the more accurate the quantity to be stocked. This system eliminates guesswork from the individual ordering the medication. The system is based on historical data for an institution and current trends.

INVENTORY RECEIVING PROCESS

1. Verify incoming merchandise (drug, dosage form, strength, package size, number of units, and expiration date) against packing slip or invoice.
2. Any merchandise requiring special storage, such as refrigeration, should promptly be verified and placed in proper conditions to avoid damage or loss of potency.
3. Sign and date invoice.
4. Forward documentation to accounts payable.
5. Place merchandise on shelf, and rotate product by placing product with shortest dating in front and longest dating behind it.

6. Retain appropriate paperwork in the pharmacy as outlined in the Controlled Substances Act, Occupational Safety and Health Administration (OSHA) requirements, or the institution's policy and procedure manual.

BIOAVAILABILITY STANDARDS AND GENERIC SUBSTITUTES

- **Bioavailability of pharmaceutical products:** A measurement of both the rate of absorption and the total amount of drug that reaches the general circulation from an administered dosage form. Dissolution of the pharmaceutical product affects the absorption of the drug, which is also affected by properties of the drug and the dosage form. All generic drugs must contain the same active ingredients as the original brand indications; meet the same batch requirements for identity, strength, purity, and quality; and yield similar blood absorption and urinary excretion curves as the active ingredient.
- **Therapeutic equivalent:** A drug product that, when administered in the same amount, will provide the same therapeutic effect and pharmacokinetic characteristics as another drug with which it is compared.
- **Therapeutic substitution:** The substitution of a new drug product with another that differs in composition but is considered to have the same or very similar pharmacologic and therapeutic activity.

REGULATORY REQUIREMENTS REGARDING RECORD KEEPING FOR REPACKAGED, RECALLED, AND REFUNDED PRODUCTS

REPACKAGING

- **Labeling:** The labeling must contain the following information:
  - Generic name of the drug
  - Strength
  - Dosage form
  - Manufacturer's name and lot number
  - Expiration date after repackaging
- **Repackaging log:** The log contains documentation required for repackaging medication and must be signed by the pharmacist.
  - Date of repackaging
  - Name of drug
  - Dosage form
  - Drug manufacturer

Item	Description
Date	The date that the drug is made, which includes day, month, and year
Drug	Drug name, usually by generic name then brand name if indicated on log sheet
Dosage form	Tablet, capsule, spansule, troche, liquid, etc
Manufacturer	Manufacturer of the drug, usually abbreviated
Manufacturer's lot number	Control number located on the side of the label or on the bottom of the bottle
Manufacturer's expiration date	Located with the lot number; remember that if the date indicates only the month, the drug is good through the end of the month
Pharmacy lot number	Each item repackaged in the pharmacy is given a number consecutive to the previously made batch
Pharmacy expiration date	Calculate the new expiration date, which is 6 months or 1/4 of the time of the manufacturer's expiration date, whichever is less
Technician	Must initial the logbook entry
Pharmacist	Each item made must be checked off by a pharmacist

The information on the label of the unit dose item is much less than what is required in the logbook, but it is just as important. The following sample lists the components necessary on a typical unit dose label:

Name of drug
    Generic name
    Trade name (trade name commonly given for the easy identification of the proper medication)

Strength
Dosage form
Pharmacy lot number
Pharmacy expiration date

Fig. 2-1 Example of a record log sheet used for documentation.

- Manufacturer's expiration date and lot number
- Pharmacy lot number
- Expiration date assigned by the pharmacy
- Quantity of drug repackaged
- Pharmacy technician's initials (if a pharmacy technician participated in the repackaging)
- Licensed pharmacist's initials
- **Expiration date of repackaged drugs:** Federal law mandates that the expiration date cannot exceed 6 months and cannot exceed 25% of the remaining time on the manufacturer's original expiration date on the bulk container (Figure 2-1).

RECALLED MEDICATIONS

- Pharmacy notified by manufacturer or wholesaler by mail or fax.
- Pharmacy determines if recalled medication is currently in stock.
- Pharmacy contacts patients who may have received medication. If a customer has the recalled product, the medication should be returned to the pharmacy for refund or substitution.
- Recalled medication returned to manufacturer for credit.
- Reorder medication that has been recalled. Notify physician of recalled medication; inquire if the physician wishes to change the medication order, especially if product may not be available for a long period.

REFUNDED PRODUCTS

- **Unit dose:** May be redispensed if not tampered with or beyond use date.
- **Multidose vial:** Cannot be redispensed in many states. A pharmacy technician must be aware of state pharmacy regulations on this issue. Many states are examining this issue.

POLICIES, PROCEDURES, AND PRACTICES FOR INVENTORY SYSTEMS

Inventory management: Focuses on the procurement, drug storage and inventory control, repackaging and label considerations, distribution systems, and recapture and disposal of used and unused pharmaceutical products.

PURPOSE OF INVENTORY MANAGEMENT

- Provide an adequate stock of pharmaceuticals and supplies
- Reduce unexpected stock-outs and temporary shortages, which may affect patient care
- Reduce carrying cost (financial investment) in drug products
- Minimize costs associated with placing orders to the wholesaler
- Minimize time spent on purchasing functions
- Minimize capital charge on average inventory
- Minimize shrinkage, breakage, and obsolescence of inventory
- Reduce purchasing dollars spent by selecting products with the best price

INVENTORY PRACTICES

- **Cost analysis:** Examination of all costs associated with the purchase of a product, which may include acquisition costs, storage costs, costs associated with preparing and packaging a product, and costs involved in getting the final product to the patient.
- **Formulary:** A basis for the dispensing of medications purchased and prescribed in a hospital or reimbursed under a managed care program. A formulary may be either an open or a closed formulary.
- **Group purchasing organizations:** Organization responsible for negotiating discounted drug prices for hospitals or other institutions with drug manufacturers. They develop contracts with pharmaceutical companies. They do not purchase the medications for the institution. It is the responsibility of the institution to make its purchases.
- **Just-in-time ordering:** A strategy of ordering a product just before it is used. This process minimizes tying up funds for long periods and reduces the cost associated with inventory management.
- **Prime vendor agreement:** An agreement between a pharmacy and a wholesaler in which the pharmacy agrees to purchase the majority of its products from that wholesaler in return for other considerations.
- **Therapeutic interchange:** A substitution of one medication for another medication that is not generically equivalent but has the same therapeutic effect.
- **Want list:** A list of items that are in short supply and need to be ordered or reordered from a vendor.

TABLE 2-1 ABC Analysis

ABC ITEM RANK	TOTAL ANNUAL % OF COSTS	% OF PRODUCTS
A	80%	20%
B	15%	15%
C	5%	65%
Total	100%	100%

INVENTORY MANAGEMENT STRATEGIES

- **80/20 rule:** Eighty percent of a pharmacy's drug costs are derived from 20% of the pharmaceuticals carried. Focuses on inventory control of the top 20% of the items carried.
- **80/20 report (velocity report):** A detailed summary of purchasing history based on the 80/20 rule, designating those medications that account for 80% of the drug costs for that period of time.
- **ABC analysis:** A method to identify and define inventory items based on their usage. Products are ranked based on their purchase history and dollar amount of total annual costs. Focuses efforts based on the products that will have the greatest inventory turnover rate (Table 2-1).
- **Compliance report:** A report summarizing all items that were not purchased on bid.
- **Inventory turnover rate:** A tool to evaluate inventory dollars. Can be calculated using the following formula: Total annual purchases/Inventory value. A greater number of inventory turns indicates greater financial well-being for an institution. Twelve inventory turns per year is considered very good for a pharmacy.
- **Minimum/maximum:** An inventory ordering system that identifies a predetermined order of quantity (PAR value) and maximum order point of medications. The min/max system ensures that a firm maintains an adequate quantity on its shelves without incurring additional costs from purchasing from a wholesaler or outside vendor.

PRODUCTS USED IN PACKAGING AND REPACKAGING

- Child-resistant caps are required on all prescriptions unless the patient or physician requests easy-open containers. If the patient requests an easy-open container, the patient must sign on the back of the prescription. Easy-open containers may be used in the following situations: patients are being administered medication in institutions;

multiple sizes of same product are available and package is marked as not being child resistant (such as over-the-counter [OTC] medications); and certain medications, such as nitroglycerin.

- Packaging is light resistant to prevent ultraviolet rays from breaking down the compound.

RISK MANAGEMENT OPPORTUNITIES

- **Dress code:** Persons involved in the preparation of sterile products should scrub their hands with an appropriate antibacterial agent for a predetermined time and dry them with paper towels. Procedure should be repeated if possible contamination occurs. Jewelry should not be worn during aseptic technique because of the possibility of contamination. Makeup should not be worn because of the particulate nature of the substance. Clean, particulate-free clothing should be worn. The pharmacy technician should be familiar with USP <797>.
- **Personal protective equipment:** Used to place a barrier between the employee and specific substances. Includes latex gloves, masks, goggles, face shields, gowns, laboratory coats, shoe coverings, and head coverings.
- **Needle recapping:** Never recap used needles using both hands or perform any other technique that involves directing the point of the needle toward the body. Use a one-handed "scoop" technique or a mechanical device designed for holding the needle sheath. Do not remove used needles from disposable syringes by hand, and do not bend, break, or manipulate the needles by hand.
- **Use of sharps container:** Used disposable syringes are to be placed in the sharp containers (a thick red plastic container) in an area close to where sharps are being used.

FOOD AND DRUG ADMINISTRATION CLASSIFICATIONS OF RECALLS

- **Class I:** Reasonable probability that use of the product will cause or lead to serious adverse health events or death.
- **Class II:** Probability exists that use of the product will cause adverse health events that are temporary or medically reversible.
- **Class III:** Use of product will probably not cause an adverse health event.

SYSTEMS TO IDENTIFY AND RETURN EXPIRED AND UNSALEABLE PRODUCTS

- Policies are established by each pharmacy regarding the process of pulling medications that will expire within a given period.
- A system must be in place in all practices of pharmacy to check for expired medications. Expired medications must be kept away from in-date medications.
- Contracts with wholesalers and manufacturers will determine if products may be returned for partial or full credit. Proper inventory management skills may eliminate the necessity of returns to the manufacturer if a product is being properly rotated.
- Cytotoxic medications are destroyed with biohazardous waste goods.
- The DEA must be notified through the issue of Form 41 for expired controlled substances before destruction may occur. A copy of Form 41 must be maintained for a minimum of 2 years after the destruction of controlled substances at the pharmacy site. The destruction of medications must follow all local, state, and federal guidelines involving environmental issues, such as burning, flushing, or rinsing.
- Reconstituted or compounded drugs are not returnable to the manufacturer. Other examples of nonreturnable items include partially used bottles of medication.
- Unused unit-dose medications may be redispensed after medication has been checked for integrity.

RULES AND REGULATIONS FOR THE REMOVAL AND DISPOSAL OF PRODUCTS

- Medication should never be dispensed to a patient if it has passed its expiration date or will expire before the patient is able to complete the current course of therapy. Multidose containers cannot be redispensed to another patient (refer to state regulations for direction on this issue); unit-dose medications can be redispensed to other patients.
- Controlled substances can be returned only by institutions having a DEA number. For example, long-term facilities cannot return controlled substances to pharmacies because long-term care facilities do not have a DEA number.
- Every pharmacy technician in a particular pharmacy should be aware of the pharmacy's

disposition procedures. Depending on the vendor or wholesaler, some will accept outdated medication for credit.

- If medication is to be destroyed, the pharmacy technician needs to be familiar with the procedures of the institution regarding outdated products.
- A DEA Form 41 is a triplicate form that needs to be completed at least 2 weeks before the scheduled destruction of controlled substances. The destruction must be done in the presence of another individual. The required copies of DEA Form 41 are submitted to the DEA.

LEGAL AND REGULATORY REQUIREMENTS AND PROFESSIONAL STANDARDS GOVERNING OPERATIONS OF PHARMACIES

Compounding: "The preparation, mixing, assembling, packaging, or labeling of a drug or device (1) as the result of a practitioner's prescription drug order or initiative based on the practitioner-patient-pharmacist relationship, or (2) for the purpose of or as an incident to research, teaching, or chemical analysis and not for sale or dispensing. Compounding also includes the preparation of drugs or devices in anticipation of prescription drug orders based on routine, regularly observed prescribing patterns" (*United States Pharmacopeia*).

Manufacturing: "The production, preparation, propagation, conversion, or processing of a drug or device either directly or indirectly by extraction from substances of natural origin or independently by means of chemical or biological synthesis and includes any packaging or repackaging of the substance(s) or labeling of its container, and the promotion and marketing of such drugs or devices. Manufacturing also includes the preparation and promotion of commercially available products from bulk compounds for resale by pharmacies, practitioners, or other persons" (*United States Pharmacopeia*).

Prepackaging

- **Unit-dose system:** A system that provides a medication in its final "unit of use." Unit-dose packaging machines may be manual, semiautomatic, or automatic. May be a single-drop (60 packages/min) or double-drop (120 packages/min) system.
- **Modified unit-dose system:** A drug distribution system that combines unit-dose medications, which are blister-packaged onto a multiple-dose

card instead of being placed in a box. Synonymous with *punch cards, bingo cards,* or *blister cards.*

- **Blended unit-dose system:** Combines a unit-dose system with a non–unit-dose system. May be a multiple-medication package or a modular cassette. Multiple-medication package has all the medication, which is administered at the same time. Modular cassette is a combination cassette or drawer exchange system.

LEGAL AND REGULATORY REQUIREMENTS AND PROFESSIONAL STANDARDS FOR PREPARING, LABELING, DISPENSING, DISTRIBUTING, AND ADMINISTERING MEDICATIONS

- The DEA is responsible for enforcing the Controlled Substances Act.
- The FDA is accountable for ensuring that medications and food are pure, safe, and effective. It can issue drug recalls.
- State Boards of Pharmacy ensure that specific standards are met for the licensing of pharmacists, permits are issued for pharmacies, and requirements are met regarding pharmacy technicians.
- The Joint Commission requires unit-dose dispensing and pharmacy-based intravenous (IV) additive programs. Bulk packaging and floor stock have been eliminated because of safety and contamination issues.
- The United States Pharmacopeia sets requirements for labeling of medications, whether they are in a multidose vial or unit-dose container, an IV admixture, or a compound.
- The Bureau of Alcohol, Tobacco, Firearms and Explosives (ATF) oversees the use and taxing of alcohol in hospitals and other institutions.

REQUIRED INFORMATION FOR ALL PRESCRIPTIONS

- Prescriber information:
  - Name of physician
  - Office address of physician—includes street number, street name (office or suite number if applicable), city, state, zip code
- Date prescription was written
- Patient information:
  - Patient's name
  - Patient's home address—includes number, street, city, state, zip code

- Inscription:
  - Name of medication: may be either brand or generic
  - Strength of medication (if applicable)
  - Quantity of medication to be dispensed
- Subscription: instructions to the pharmacist
- Physician's signature: must be in ink; stamped signatures are illegal

REQUIRED INFORMATION ON MEDICATION ORDERS

- Prescriber's information
- Date of order
- Patient information—room number, bed number, and ID number assigned to patient
- Name, strength, and dosage form of medication
- When to be administered (specific time of day)
- Duration of therapy
- Prescriber's signature

MEDICATION DISTRIBUTION AND CONTROL SYSTEM REQUIREMENTS FOR THE USE OF MEDICATIONS IN VARIOUS PRACTICE SETTINGS

INPATIENT SETTINGS

- Automation is being used to regulate and track controlled substances.
- Bar-coded labels are used as part of automation to reduce errors and to streamline the medication process. Will improve the quality of patient care.
- Computerized dispensing systems are being used because of the need to have medication available 24 hours per day.
- A "code blue" in a hospital signifies that a patient is in a life-threatening situation such as the stopping of a patient's heart or a cessation of breathing. Crash carts are located on the floors of a hospital, are stocked with the necessary medications and equipment for a code blue situation, and are used to stabilize a patient.
- Robotics is being used to scan unit-dose medication and fill patients' medication cassettes.
- Scanning patient identification bracelets ensures patients are receiving the proper medication.

OUTPATIENT SETTINGS

- Automated dispensing machines such as Baker Cells (McKesson Corp., San Francisco, Calif.) and Pyxis systems (Cardinal Health, Dublin, Ohio) are being used to improve efficiency.
- Scanning of prescription orders and imaging are being used.

REPACKAGING, STORAGE REQUIREMENTS, AND DOCUMENTATION FOR FINISHED DOSAGE FORMS PREPARED IN ANTICIPATION OF PRESCRIPTIONS OR MEDICATION ORDERS

- Storage of all medications is based on environmental considerations, security issues, and safety requirements.
- Environmental consideration involves proper temperature, ventilation, humidity, light, and sanitation. Standards for storage are found in the United States Pharmacopeia and National Formulary under the "General Notices and Requirements" section.
- Faxed prescriptions must not be dispensed until the original prescription is presented to the pharmacy. Exceptions exist for emergency prescriptions for Schedule II medications and Schedule II medications in long-term care facilities.
- Master formula must be maintained for any pharmacy engaging in extemporaneous compounding.
- Repackaging log must be maintained in any pharmacy that prepares or repackages medication.

POLICIES, PROCEDURES, AND PRACTICES REGARDING STORAGE AND HANDLING OF HAZARDOUS MATERIALS AND WASTE

The Material Safety Data Sheet (MSDS) provides detailed information on the hazards associated with a particular substance. A hazardous chemical is one that poses a threat to health or safety. A list of hazardous drugs can be found in a patient product insert, in the *Physicians' Desk Reference,* and in *American Hospital Formulary Service Drug Information.* These drugs are considered to be hazardous in their final dosage form, especially if they are crushed or broken. The manufacturer provides an MSDS to the pharmacy, and the pharmacy must provide it to long-term care facilities.

MEDICATION DISTRIBUTION AND CONTROL SYSTEM REQUIREMENTS FOR CONTROLLED SUBSTANCES, INVESTIGATIONAL DRUGS, AND HAZARDOUS MATERIALS AND WASTE

CONTROLLED SUBSTANCES

Schedule II medications must be kept in a locked safe in the pharmacy. Schedule III to V medications may be dispersed throughout the pharmacy. Refrigerated Schedule II substances must be kept in a locked refrigerator with no other medications. Controlled substances on a nursing floor must be in a locked cart.

Controlled substance administration record: Assists in the accountability of controlled substances in a nursing unit. Controlled substance forms allow a nurse to verify counts of a controlled substance at the change of a shift. Counts must be witnessed by the incoming nurse. A controlled substance usage form monitors receipt, administration, and disposal of individual controlled substances. A separate form is used to account for the amount of controlled substances a patient is taking.

Medication delivery record: Documents receipt of medication on a nursing floor from the pharmacy. Records are checked against records in the pharmacy.

Medication administration record: Documents medication dispensed to a patient.

INVESTIGATIONAL DRUGS

Under the Federal Food, Drug, and Cosmetic Act, a medication must obtain premarketing approval from the government before use. A hospital pharmacy is responsible for the distribution and control of investigational drugs, including procurement, storage, inventory management, packaging, labeling, distribution, and disposition of unused drugs. The pharmacy must provide clinical services such as patient education, staff in-service training, monitoring, and reporting of adverse reactions. The pharmacy is involved with research activities, such as participating in the preparation or review of research proposals and protocols, assisting in data collection, and analysis. The pharmacy may undertake clinical study management by providing reports to the sponsor.

HAZARDOUS MATERIALS AND WASTE

The Occupational Safety and Health Act requires that all employees be aware of the hazards of chemicals to which they are exposed. The Hazard Communication Standard is based on the belief that all employees have both a need and a right to be informed of the hazards and identities of the chemicals to which they will be exposed. Every institution handling hazardous chemicals must have a written hazard communication program, and it must receive an MSDS from the manufacturer, importer, or distributor for each hazardous chemical in the workplace.

QUALITY ASSURANCE POLICIES, PROCEDURES, AND PRACTICES FOR MEDICATION AND INVENTORY CONTROL SYSTEMS

GUIDE TO PREVENTING PRESCRIPTION ERRORS

The following simple procedures will help avoid errors in the pharmacy:

- Always keep the prescription and the label together during the fill process.
- Know the common look-alike and sound-alike drugs, and keep them stored in different areas of the pharmacy so they will not be easily mistaken (Table 2-2).
- Always question illegible handwriting.
- Be aware of insulin mistakes. Insulin brands should be clearly separated from one another. Educate patients to always verify their insulin purchase.
- Clear stock bottles no longer needed away from the work area in a timely fashion. Keep only what is needed for immediate use in the work area.
- Keep dangerous or high-alert medications in a separate storage area of the pharmacy.
- Make sure prescriptions and orders include the correctly spelled drug name, strength, appropriate dosing, quantity or duration of therapy, dosage form, and route. Missing information should be obtained from the prescriber.
- Question ambiguous orders.
- Question the prescription order that uses abbreviations you are not familiar with or that are uncommon. Avoid using abbreviations that have more than one meaning, and verify the meaning of these abbreviations with the prescriber.
- The label should always be compared with the original prescription by at least two people. If an error occurs at this stage, the refills may be filled incorrectly as well (Table 2-3).
- Use the metric system. A leading zero should always be present in decimal values less than 1. Remember that an error of this nature will mean a dosage error of at least tenfold.

What Can the Technician Do to Reduce Errors?

- Do a mental check on dosage appropriateness.
- Keep your work area free of clutter.
- Observe and report pertinent OTC purchases.
- Triple-check your work.
- Verify your own data entry before processing.

TABLE **2-2** Common Look-Alike and Sound-Alike Medications

Accupril	Accutane	Fioricet	Fiorinal
acetazolamide	acetohexamide	Flomax	Volmax
AcipHex	Accupril, Aricept	flurbiprofen	fenoprofen
Actos	Actonel	folinic acid	folic acid
albuterol	atenolol	Gantrisin	Gantanol
Aldomet	Aldoril	glipizide	glyburide
Alkeran	Leukeran, Myleran	glyburide	Glucotrol
alprazolam	lorazepam	Hycodan	Hycomine
Amaryl	Reminyl	hydralazine	hydroxyzine
Ambien	Amen	hydrocodone	hydrocortisone
amiloride	amlodipine	Hydrogesic	hydroxyzine
amiodarone	amrinone	hydromorphone	morphine
amitriptyline	nortriptyline	Hydropres	Diupres
Apresazide	Apresoline	Hytone	Vytone
Arlidin	Aralen	imipramine	Norpramin
Artane	Altace	Inderal	Inderide, Isordil
asparaginase	pegaspargase	Indocin	Minocin
Atarax	Ativan	K-Phos	Neutra-Phos-K
atenolol	timolol	Lamictal	Lamisil, Ludiomil
Atrovent	Alupent	Lanoxin	Lasix
Avandia	Coumadin, Prandin	Lantus	Lente insulin
Bacitracin	Bactroban	Lioresal	lisinopril
Benylin	Ventolin	Lithostat	Lithobid, Lithotabs
Brevital	Brevibloc	Lodine	Codeine
Bumex	Buprenex	Lopid	Lorabid
bupropion	buspirone	lovastatin	Lotensin
Cafergot	Carafate	Ludiomil	Lomotil
calciferol	calcitriol	Medrol	Haldol
Cardene	Cardizem	metolazone	methotrexate, metoclopramide
Cataflam	Catapres	metoprolol	misoprostol
Catapres	Combipres	metoprolol	metoclopramide
cefotaxime	cefoxitin	Monopril	minoxidil
Cerebryx	Celebrex, Celera	nelfinavir	nevirapine
chlorpromazine	prochlorperazine, promethazine	nicardipine	nifedipine
Clinoril	Clozaril	Norlutate	Norlutin
clomipramine	Clomiphene	Noroxin	Neurontin
clonidine	Klonopin	Norvasc	Navane
Combivir	Combivent	Norvir	Retrovir
Cozaar	Zocor	Ocufen	Ocuflox
cyclobenzaprine	cyproheptadine	Orinase	Ornade
cyclophosphamide	cyclosporine	paroxetine	Paclitaxel
cyclosporine	cycloserine	Paxil	Paclitaxel, Taxol
Cytovene	Cytosar	penicillamine	penicillin
Cytoxan	Cytotec, Cytosar	Percocet	Percodan
Darvocet-N	Darvon-N	pindolol	Parlodel
daunorubicin	doxorubicin	Pravachol	Prevacid, propranolol
desipramine	diphenhydramine	prednisolone	prednisone
DiaBeta	Zebeta	Prilosec	Prozac
digitoxin	digoxin	Prinivil	Prilosec, Proventil
diphenhydramine	dimenhydrinate	Procanbid	Procan SR
dopamine	dobutamine	Provera	Premarin
Edecrin	Eulexin	Prozac	Proscar
enalapril	Anafranil, Eldepryl	quinidine	clonidine, Quinamm
Eryc	Ery-Tab	quinine	quinidine
etidronate	etretinate, etomidate	Regroton	Hygroton
E-Vista	Evista	Reminyl	Robinul
Femara	Femhrt	Retrovir	ritonavir

Continued

TABLE **2-2** Common Look-Alike and Sound-Alike Medications—Cont'd

Rifamate	rifampin	Ultram	Ultrase
rimantadine	flutamide	Vancenase	Vanceril
Roxicodone	Roxicet	Vasosulf	Velosef
Sarafem	Serophene	Versed	Vistaril
Seroquel	Serzone	Xanax	Zantac
Stadol	Haldol	Xenical	Xeloda
sulfadiazine	sulfasalazine	Zantac	Zyrtec
Tegretol	Tequin	Zebeta	DiaBeta
terazosin	temazepam	Zinacef	Zithromax
terbinafine	terfenadine	Zocor	Zoloft
terbutaline	tolbutamide	Zofran	Zantac
Ticlid	Tequin	Zosyn	Zofran
tolazamide	tolbutamide	Zovirax	Zyvox
torsemide	furosemide	Zyrtec	Zyprexa
trifluoperazine	trihexyphenidyl	Zyvox	Vioxx
Trimox	Diamox		

TABLE **2-3** Common Abbreviation Errors

ABBREVIATION	MEANING	MISINTERPRETATION
ac	Before meals	After meals
ad	Right ear	Right eye
ARA-A	Vidarabine	Cytarabine
As	Left ear	Left eye
AU	Both ears	Both eyes
AZT	Zidovudine	Azathioprine
CPZ	Compazine	Chlorpromazine
D/C	Discontinue	Discharge
	Discharge	Discontinue
HCl	Hydrochloride salt	Potassium chloride
HCT	Hydrocortisone	Hydrochlorothiazide
HCTZ	Hydrochlorothiazide	Hydrocortisone
IU	International units	Intravenous
MTX	Methotrexate	Mitoxantrone
Nitro Drip	Nitroglycerin infusion	Sodium nitroprusside infusion
od or OD	Right eye	Right ear
os	Left eye	Left ear
ou	Each (both) eye(s)	Each (both) ear(s)
Per os	Orally	Left eye
qd or QD	Each or every day	Four times a day
qhs	At bedtime	Every hour
qod or QOD	Every other day	Every day or every other day
SC	Subcutaneous	Sublingual
sub q	Subcutaneous	Subcutaneous every
TAC	Triamcinolone	Tetracaine
TIW	Three times a week	Three times a day
x3d	For 3 days	For three doses

What Can the Pharmacist Do to Reduce Errors?

- Check prescriptions in a timely manner.
- Document all clarifications on orders.
- Encourage OTC and herbal remedy documentation.
- Initial checked prescriptions.
- Use the USP-ISMP (Institute for Safe Medication Practices) Medication Error Reporting Form to inform manufacturers of errors caused by commercial packaging and labeling.
- Visually check the product in the bottle.

What Can the Pharmacy Do to Reduce Errors?

- Automate and bar code all fill procedures.
- Encourage physicians to use common terminology and abbreviations.
- Maintain a safe work area.
- Provide adequate computer applications and hardware.
- Provide adequate storage areas.

By the year 2010 the E-Health Initiative is to be implemented; it will require all prescriptions and medication orders to be submitted electronically. This will alleviate many of the legibility problems associated with handwritten prescriptions.

CHAPTER 2 REVIEW QUESTIONS

1. What is the purpose of a group purchasing organization for a hospital pharmacy?
   a. Negotiate prices with drug manufacturers
   b. Negotiate prices with a local drug wholesaler
   c. Purchase drugs from a drug manufacturer for the hospital
   d. Purchase drugs from a local drug wholesaler

2. Which of the following is not an advantage of a solid dosage form?
   a. Convenient for self-medication
   b. Easier to swallow than other dosage forms
   c. Easy to package and dispense
   d. Lacks taste or smell

3. Which dosage form is contained in a gelatin shell?
   a. Capsule
   b. Effervescent salts
   c. Pastilles
   d. Suppositories

4. Which dosage form may be prepared by either compressing or molding?
   a. Capsule
   b. Pellet
   c. Plaster
   d. Tablet

5. Which dosage form releases carbon dioxide when it is dissolved in water?
   a. Effervescent salts
   b. Plasters
   c. Powders
   d. Troches

6. Which of the following is not a disadvantage of liquid?
   a. Deterioration and loss of potency occur quickly
   b. Easier to swallow than solid dosage forms
   c. Interactions develop owing to changes in solubility
   d. Requires sweetening and flavoring to be palatable

7. Which type of solution is a clear, sweetened, flavored hydroalcoholic containing water and alcohol?
   a. An aromatic water
   b. An elixir
   c. A suspension
   d. A syrup

8. What type of dispersion is either water in oil or oil in water?
   a. An emulsion
   b. A gel
   c. A lotion
   d. An ointment

9. Which of the following is not required on the label of a repackaged medication?
   a. Date of repackaging
   b. Generic name of the medication
   c. Manufacturer's name and lot number
   d. Expiration date after repackaging

10. Which of the following information is not required on a repackaging log?
    a. Date of repackaging
    b. Expiration date after repackaging
    c. Pharmacist's initials
    d. Quantity of drug repackaged

11. Which regulatory agency may issue a drug recall?
    a. BOP
    b. DEA
    c. FDA
    d. TJC

12. What type of unit-dose system may be referred to as a "punch card" or "bingo card"?
    a. Blended unit-dose system
    b. Modified unit-dose system
    c. Modular cassette unit-dose system
    d. Multiple-medication package unit-dose system

13. What type of agreement is made between a pharmacy and a wholesaler in which the pharmacy agrees to purchase the majority of its product from that wholesaler?
    a. Prime purchaser agreement
    b. Prime vendor agreement
    c. Purchase order
    d. Velocity agreement

14. Which of the following dosage forms is an aqueous solution containing sucrose or sucrose substitute?
    a. Elixir
    b. Spirit
    c. Syrup
    d. Tincture

15. Which of the following dosage forms is not an example of dispersion?
    a. Gel
    b. Liniment
    c. Lotion
    d. Suspension

16. Which of the following dosage forms is not an example of a solution?
    a. Elixir
    b. Emulsion
    c. Enema
    d. Syrup

17. Which of the following dosage forms is not an example of a sustained-release dosage form?
    a. Controlled action
    b. Depot
    c. Pastille
    d. Repository

18. Which type of solution is a topical dosage form containing pyroxylin and is dissolved in alcohol and ether?
    a. Collodion
    b. Extract
    c. Liniment
    d. Spirit

19. How many phases are in a suspension?
    a. Two
    b. Three
    c. Four
    d. Five

20. Which type of dispersion is similar to an ointment but contains more solid materials?
    a. Cream
    b. Gel
    c. Lotion
    d. Paste

21. Which committee develops a formulary for an institution?
    a. BOP
    b. FDA
    c. TJC
    d. P&T

22. What is the maximum amount of time that can be assigned to a repackaged drug?
    a. 3 months
    b. 6 months
    c. 9 months
    d. 12 months

23. What is the subscription on a prescription?
    a. Any special instructions or directions to the pharmacist
    b. Directions to be typed on the prescription label
    c. Name, strength, and quantity of medication
    d. The Rx symbol

24. What types of substances require an MSDS?
    a. Hazardous drugs and chemicals
    b. Investigational drugs
    c. Intravenous admixtures
    d. OTC drugs

25. What type of products must be isotonic?
    a. External medications
    b. Ophthalmic products
    c. Oral inhalation products
    d. Otic preparations

26. Which of the following must be done if a patient requests an easy-open container?
    a. Verify with the physician that the dispensing of a medication in an easy-open container is permitted.
    b. Verify that there are no children younger than 12 years living with the patient.
    c. Verify that the patient has ipecac at home in case of a potential overdose.
    d. Have the patient sign the back of the prescription, indicating that he has requested an easy-open container.

27. Which of the following pieces of information is not needed on a patient's prescription?
    a. Patient's name
    b. Patient's ID number
    c. Name of the medication
    d. Directions for use

28. Which of the following forms is required to be completed in the destruction of noncontrolled substances?
    a. DEA Form 41
    b. DEA Form 106
    c. DEA Form 222
    d. No form is required

29. Which of the following is not an environmental factor affecting the storage of medications?
    a. Heat
    b. Humidity
    c. Light
    d. Security requirements

30. Which of the following is not a dispersion?
    a. Cream
    b. Gel
    c. Solution
    d. Suspension

31. Which of the following is not a delayed-release dosage form?
    a. Controlled release
    b. Repository
    c. Sublingual tablet
    d. Time release

32. Which of the following is not a solid dosage form?
    a. Pill
    b. Suppository
    c. Tablet
    d. All are solid dosage forms

33. Which federal agency is responsible for hazardous waste and materials?
    a. DEA
    b. FDA
    c. ISMP
    d. OSHA

34. What type of drug recall is associated with irreversible damage or death to an individual?
    a. Class I
    b. Class II
    c. Class III
    d. Class IV

35. When must an MSDS be provided to the patient?
    a. When dispensing a controlled substance
    b. When dispensing a hazardous substance
    c. When dispensing an investigational drug
    d. On request from the patient

Participating in the Administration and Management of Pharmacy Practice

THE PRACTICE SETTING'S MISSION, GOALS, AND OBJECTIVES; ORGANIZATIONAL STRUCTURE; AND POLICIES AND PROCEDURES

- **Mission statement:** States the purpose and goals of an organization.
- **Organizational structure:** Shows the chain of command in an organization. Examples of organizational structure include matrix and product line. Matrix emphasizes overlapping of responsibility among departments and common areas of decision making. Product line is organized along a common product or service being offered.
- **Policy:** A definite course or method of action; a plan establishing goals and objectives.
- **Procedure:** Process of accomplishing a task to ensure efficiency and consistency; a step-by-step method to accomplish a policy.

Policies and procedures are found in all types of pharmacy practice. They are required by professional and regulatory agencies, such as the American Society of Health-System Pharmacists (ASHP), the American Pharmacists Association, and The Joint Commission (TJC). Policies and procedures provide standards for the operation of a pharmacy. The policy and procedure manual can be used as a reference book and can promote safety in the workplace.

LINES OF COMMUNICATION THROUGHOUT THE ORGANIZATION

- Face-to-face meetings
- Telephone
- Voice mail
- E-mail
- Memorandums (written letters)

PRINCIPLES OF RESOURCE ALLOCATION

- **Cross-training (cross-functional):** Bringing together persons from different functions to work on a common task; designed to help improve lateral communication. They have the ability to solve problems based on "total systems thinking." They have the ability to work well based on better information and speed of transmitting the information.
- **Multiskilling:** Team members are trained in skills to perform more than one job.
- **Scheduling:** Productivity reports can be used to show the peak times of the day when prescription processing is heaviest and when prescriptions are being picked up by customers. The staff should be scheduled based on these times.
- **Self-managing teams:** Teams that are empowered to make decisions about planning, doing, and evaluating their daily work.

- **Virtual groups:** Convene and operate with members linked together electronically by computers.
- **Workflow:** An organized way of performing a task. It is efficient in nature and it is a repeatable, defined set of activities.

PRODUCTIVITY, EFFICIENCY, AND CUSTOMER SATISFACTION MEASURES

- **Customer service:** Follow-up survey with customers. Use of focus groups to gauge opinions of customers, comparing customer service in one location or organization with that in another.
- **Efficiency:** Inventory turnover rates, reduction in prescription errors per shift. Compliance reports from vendors. Average waiting time per prescription.
- **Productivity:** Prescriptions filled per pharmacist per hour. Absenteeism and tardiness reports through payroll.

WRITTEN, ORAL, AND ELECTRONIC COMMUNICATION SYSTEMS

- **Organizational communication:** Process by which information is exchanged in an organizational setting.
- **Channel richness:** The capacity of a channel to convey information effectively. In the following list the channels are shown in decreasing order of channel richness:
  - Face-to-face: most effective
  - Telephone
  - E-mail
  - Written memos
  - Letters
  - Posted notices
  - Bulletins: least effective
- **Formal channels:** Follow the chain of command or hierarchy in an organization.
- **Informal channels:** Do not follow chain of command; allow for the transfer of information through networks and acquaintances.

REQUIRED OPERATIONAL LICENSES AND CERTIFICATES

All pharmacists must have licenses on site (which may include continuing education documentation):
  - Business license
  - Drug Enforcement Agency (DEA) Form 222 to order Schedule II medications

- DEA Form 224 to order controlled substances
- DEA Form 41 to destroy controlled substances
- TJC accreditation is highly recommended for hospitals and long-term care facilities, such as nursing homes
- Permits collection of taxes if any products are sold and tax is to be collected
- Pharmacist in charge must have appropriate documentation to order Schedule II medications, such as the "power of attorney"

ROLES AND RESPONSIBILITIES OF PHARMACISTS, PHARMACY TECHNICIANS, AND OTHER PHARMACY EMPLOYEES

The primary duty of a pharmacy technician is to assist the pharmacist. Pharmacy technicians provide technical assistance in the pharmacy but are not involved in judgmental duties. The following sections list duties associated with community, institutional (e.g., hospital), and managed care pharmacy technicians.

RESPONSIBILITIES OF COMMUNITY TECHNICIANS

- Help patients who are dropping off or picking up prescription orders
- Enter prescription orders into the computer
- Create a profile of the patient's health and insurance information in the computer, or update the patient's profile
- Assist the pharmacist, under direct supervision, in the practice of pharmacy, in accordance with local, state, federal, and company regulations
- Communicate with insurance carriers to obtain payment for prescription claims
- At point of sale, verify that customer receives correct prescription(s)
- Complete weekly distribution center medication orders, place orders on shelves, and verify all associated paperwork
- Assist the pharmacist with filling and labeling prescriptions
- Prepare the pharmacy inventory
- Screen telephone calls for the pharmacist
- Communicate with prescribers and their agents to obtain refill authorization
- Compound oral solutions, ointments, and creams
- Prepackage bulk medications
- Maintain an awareness of developments in the community and the pharmaceutical field that relate to job responsibilities, and integrate them into own practices

- Assist in training new employees
- Assist other pharmacy technicians
- Assist pharmacist in scheduling and maintaining workflow
- Maintain knowledge of loss-prevention techniques

RESPONSIBILITIES OF INSTITUTIONAL TECHNICIANS

- Rotate through all work areas of the pharmacy
- Transport medications, drug-delivery devices, and other pharmacy equipment from the pharmacy to nursing units and clinics
- Pick up copies of physician orders, automated medication administration records, and unused medications from the nursing units and return them to the pharmacy
- Fill patient medication cassettes
- Prepare medications and supplies for dispensing, including the following:
  - Prepacking bulk medications, compounding ointments, creams, oral solutions, and other medications
  - Preparing chemotherapeutic agents
  - Compounding total parenteral nutrition (TPN) solutions
  - Compounding large-volume intravenous (IV) mixtures
  - Packaging and preparing drugs being used in clinical investigations
  - Preparing prescriptions for outpatients
  - Checking continuous unit-dose medications
  - Controlling and auditing narcotics and stock substances
- Assist pharmacists with entering medication orders into the computer system
- Prepare inventories, order drugs and supplies from the storeroom, receive drugs, and stock shelves in various pharmacy locations
- Screen telephone calls
- Perform monthly nursing unit inspections, maintain workload records, and collect quality assurance data
- Assist in training new employees
- Assist other pharmacy technicians
- Coordinate insurance billing, including third-party prescriptions
- Deliver unit dose to automated dispensing technology
- Triage telephone and window inquiries

RESPONSIBILITIES OF MANAGED CARE TECHNICIANS

- Under the supervision of a pharmacist, perform daily handling of ongoing pharmacy benefit telephone calls from members, pharmacy providers, and physicians
- Troubleshoot third-party prescription claims questions with an understanding of online rejections and plan parameters
- Develop and maintain an electronic service log of all telephone calls with complete follow-up history
- Develop a trending report on the aforementioned service calls with an eye toward forecasting possible trends in pharmacy service
- Provide as-needed telephone and administrative support for the department

LEGAL AND REGULATORY REQUIREMENTS FOR PERSONNEL, FACILITIES, EQUIPMENT, AND SUPPLIES

- **Drug storage:** All Schedule II forms must be stored in a locked safe (either combination or key lock); Schedule III to V medications may be dispersed throughout the pharmacy with the other medications; refrigerated medication must be stored in a refrigerator.
- **Equipment:** Required equipment in all pharmacies includes a Class A balance, pharmacy weights; equipment for reconstitution such as graduated cylinders, various mortars and pestles for mixing, spatulas, and stirring rods. Laminar airflow hoods are required for preparing IV preparations and chemotherapy agents.
- **Facilities:** State Boards of Pharmacy require a minimum amount of counter space in a pharmacy, an alarm system to be activated when the pharmacy is not open, separate refrigerators for refrigerated medications and controlled substances (must be lockable), a safe for Schedule II medications, and a sink with hot and cold water. The pharmacy must be kept clean and uncluttered.
- **Personnel:** Pharmacists must be licensed by the State Board of Pharmacy for the state in which they practice. Pharmacists must maintain their licensure by meeting specific requirements established by the Board of Pharmacy, which include continuing education. Pharmacy technicians must follow state regulations set by the Board, which may include registering with the Board of Pharmacy, becoming certified either by the Pharmacy Technician Certification Board or the state, and maintaining their certification, which may include continuing education. Some states require that a pharmacy technician be licensed by the Board of Pharmacy.

- **Prescription storage:** Prescriptions, biennial inventories, invoices, and Forms 222 and 41 must be readily retrievable (able to be produced within 72 hours of the request). Prescriptions may be filed either by separating the Schedule II, Schedule III to V, and noncontrolled prescriptions or by filing the Schedule II to V prescriptions separately from prescriptions for nonscheduled drugs.

PROFESSIONAL LIBRARY

All pharmacies must have a professional library. Required resources include the Federal Controlled Substances Act, United States Pharmacopeia (USP) and National Formulary (NF), and other texts (statutes) required by the State Board of Pharmacy. Examples of reference books that may be found in a pharmacy library include the following:

- *American Drug Index 2002*, St. Louis, Mo, 2002, Facts and Comparisons.

  This standard reference work contains more than 20,000 entries on drugs and drug products, including alphabetically listed drug names, cross-indexing, phonetic pronunciations, brand names, manufacturers, generic or chemical names, composition and strength, pharmaceutical forms available, package size, use, and common abbreviations. It also contains a listing of orphan drugs. The work is available in hardbound and CD-ROM editions. *www.factsandcomparisons.com*

- *American Hospital Formulary Service Drug Information 2002*, Bethesda, Md, 2002, American Society of Health-System Pharmacists.

  The complete text of roughly 1400 monographs covering about 50,000 commercially available and experimental drugs, including information on uses, interactions, pharmacokinetics, dosage, and administration. *www.ashp.org*

- Ansel HC, Allen LV, Popovich NG: *Pharmaceutical Dosage Forms and Drug Delivery Systems*, ed 7, Baltimore, 1999, Williams & Wilkins.

  A superb survey of contemporary dosage forms and delivery systems. *www.lww.com*

- *Drug Facts and Comparisons*, St. Louis, Mo, 2002, Facts and Comparisons.

  This comprehensive source of information about 16,000 prescription and 6000 over-the-counter (OTC) drugs contains monographs about individual drugs and groups of related drugs; product listings in table format providing information on dosage forms and strength, distributor names, costs, package sizes, product identification codes, flavors, colors, and distribution status; and information on therapeutic uses, interactions, and adverse reactions. The publication includes an index of manufacturers and distributors and controlled-substance regulations. This reference work is available in hardbound form, on CD-ROM, or in a loose-leaf form that is updated monthly. *www.factsandcomparisons.com*

- *Drug Information Fulltext (DIF)*, Norwood, Mass, Silverplatter.

  A searchable computer database combining two publications: the *American Hospital Formulary Service Drug Information* and the *Handbook on Injectable Drugs*. This database is available on hard disk, CD-ROM, or the Internet. *www.silverplatter.com*

- *Drug Interaction Facts*, St. Louis, Mo, 2002, Facts and Comparisons.

  This reference, available as a hardbound book, CD-ROM, or loose-leaf book that is updated quarterly, provides comprehensive information on potential interactions that can be reviewed by drug class, generic drug name, or trade name. Provides information on drug-drug and drug-food interactions. *www.factsandcomparisons.com*

- Food and Drug Administration (FDA): *Approved Drug Products with Therapeutic Equivalence Evaluations*, Washington, DC, U.S. Government Printing Office.

  Revised annually, with monthly updates, this source lists drug products approved for use in the United States. Also known as the *Orange Book* because of its orange-colored cover, it is available online at *www.fda.gov/cder/ob/default.htm*.

- Fudyuma J: *What Do I Take? A Consumer's Guide to Nonprescription Drugs*, New York, 1997, HarperCollins.

  A simple-to-read guide to OTC drugs.

- *Goodman and Gilman's the Pharmacological Basis of Therapeutics*, ed 10, New York, 2002, McGraw-Hill.

  An authoritative text on pharmacology and therapeutics containing 67 articles by leading experts in the field. This text provides information for pharmacists to help them answer clinical questions about how drugs work under different conditions in the body. *www.pbg.mcgraw-hill.com*

- *Index Nominum*, Geneva, 1995, Swiss Pharmaceutical Society.

  A compilation of synonyms, formulas, and therapeutic classes of more than 7000 drugs and 28,000 proprietary preparations from 27 countries. Available in text and CD-ROM formats.

- *The International Pharmacopeia*, ed 3, New York, 1994, World Health Organization.

  Recommended production methods and specifications for drugs, in four volumes. *www.who.ch*

- Koda-Kimble M, Young LY: *Applied Therapeutics: The Clinical Use of Drugs*, ed 6, Vancouver, Wash, 1995, Applied Therapeutics.

- *MedCoach CD-ROM* (Windows NT and Macintosh), Rockville, Md., 1997, United States Pharmacopeial Convention.

   A database of information for patients containing more than 6000 generic and brand-name drug products, OTC drugs, nutritional and home infusion items, test devices, and infant formulas. Provides information for patients on proper drug use and preparation, drug and food interactions, side effects and adverse effects, therapeutic contraindications, and product storage. Information is tailored to particular patients' needs (e.g., pediatric, male or female, geriatric). Subscription includes quarterly updates. *www.usp.org*

- *Orange Book*. See Food and Drug Administration.

- *Patient Drug Facts, 1996: Professionals Guide to Patient Drug Facts,* St. Louis, Mo, 1996, Facts and Comparisons.

   Comprehensive guide to patient counseling about drugs, available in loose-leaf format for verbal patient counseling and in PC format (on disk) for creation of patient handouts. *www. factsandcomparisons.com*

- *Physicians' Desk Reference (PDR),* ed 63, Oradell, NJ, 2009, Medical Economics.

   Available in hardbound and CD-ROM form, with two supplements published twice a year, this standard reference work contains information from package inserts for more than 4000 prescription drugs, as well as information on 250 drug manufacturers. *www.medec.com*

- Stringer JL: *Basic Concepts in Pharmacology: A Student's Survival Guide,* ed 2, New York, 2001, McGraw-Hill.

   Survey of basic pharmacologic concepts for students. *www.pbg.mcgraw-hill.com*

- *United States Pharmacopeia,* 23rd rev, and the *National Formulary,* ed 20, Rockville, Md, 2001, United States Pharmacopeial Convention.

   Combined compendium of monographs setting official national standards for drug substances and dosage forms *(United States Pharmacopeia)* and standards for pharmaceutical ingredients *(National Formulary).* Available in book or CD-ROM form and in English- and Spanish-language editions. *www.usp.org*

- *USP Dictionary of USAN and International Drug Names,* Rockville, Md, 2001, United States Pharmacopeial Convention.

   An authoritative guide to drug names, including chemical names, brand names, manufacturers, molecular formulas, therapeutic uses, and chemical structures. *www.usp.org*

- Benitz WE, Tatro DS: *The Pediatric Drug Handbook,* ed 3, St. Louis, Mo, 1995, Mosby.

   Information on drugs, dosage forms, and administration for pediatric patients. *www.mosby.com*

- Davies DM: *Textbook of Adverse Drug Reactions,* ed 5, New York, 1999, Oxford University Press.

   A standard textbook on the subject. *www. oup-usa.org*

- *Goldfrank's Toxicologic Emergencies,* ed 6, New York, 1998, Appleton & Lange.

   Information on treating toxicologic emergencies. The medical titles of Appleton & Lange are distributed by McGraw-Hill and may be found at that Web site. *www.pbg.mcgraw-hill.com*

- *Handbook of Nonprescription Drugs,* 2 vols, ed 11, Washington, DC, 1996-1997, American Pharmaceutical Association.

   A reference work on OTC medications. *www. aphanet.org*

- Hunt ML Jr: *Training Manual for Intravenous Admixture Personnel,* ed 5, Chicago, 1995, Bonus Books.

   A manual for training people to create parenteral preparations. *www.bonus-books.com*

- *The King Guide to Parenteral Admixtures, 2001 Edition,* Napa, Calif, 2001, King Guide Publications.

   Available in four loose-leaf volumes, on microfiche, and on CD-ROM, the *King Guide* provides 350 monographs on compatibility and stability information critical to determining the advisability of preparing admixtures of drugs for parenteral administration. The guide is updated quarterly. *www.kingguide.com*

- Nahata MC, Hipple TF: *Pediatric Drug Formulations,* ed 3, Cincinnati, 1997, Harvey Whitney.

   Information on formulation and compounding of drugs for pediatric patients. *hwb@eos.net*

- *Poisindex System,* Englewood, Colo, Micromedex.

   A computerized poison information system. *www.mdx.com*

- Remington: The Science and Practice of Pharmacology, ed 20, Philadelphia, 2000, Lippincott.

   The compounding "bible" of the pharmacy profession.

- Stoklosa MJ, Ansel HC: *Pharmaceutical Calculations,* ed 11, Baltimore, Md, 2001, Williams & Wilkins.

   A clear, concise, thorough introduction to pharmaceutical mathematics. *www.lww.com*

- Trissel LA: *Handbook on Injectable Drugs, with Supplement,* ed 11, Bethesda, Md, 2000, American Society of Health-System Pharmacists.

   Provides information on stability and compatibility of injectable drug products, including formulations, concentrations, and pH values. *www. ashp.org*

- *Understanding and Preventing Errors in Medication Orders and Prescription Writing,* Bethesda, Md, 1998, United States Pharmacopeial Convention.

An education resource consisting of lecture materials, videotapes, and 35-mm slides describing medication errors that arise from poorly written orders and prescriptions, using examples of actual reports received through the USP Medication Errors Reporting Program. Contains recommendations for preventing errors. *www.usp.org* (search within USP Educational Programs)

PROFESSIONAL STANDARDS

TJC requires the following:
- Unit-dose systems are preferred over floor stock inventories in hospitals and long-term care facilities.
- Internal and external products must be kept in separate locations in a pharmacy to prevent an error from occurring.
- The dispensing of professional samples to patients is discouraged because of the potential for the samples to be out of date before being administered to patients and because use of the samples may cause a bias toward the purchase of a medication.
- IV admixtures are prepared in a pharmacy using aseptic technique and a laminar flow hood.

The state, TJC, and the State Boards of Pharmacy require that the pharmacy receive the physician's prescription or a copy of the original prescription when filling medication orders.

QUALITY IMPROVEMENT STANDARDS AND GUIDELINES

- Encouraging pharmacies to report errors and find causes for the error without fear of punishment
- Establishing the maximum number of prescriptions a pharmacist may fill during a shift
- Improving lighting in a pharmacy
- Improving workflow in a pharmacy
- Limiting the number of hours a pharmacist or technician may work in a given pay period
- Limiting the number of pharmacy technicians a pharmacist may supervise during a shift
- Requiring certification of technicians (30 states have required that technicians be certified and registered with the state board of pharmacy to assist a pharmacist)

STATE BOARD OF PHARMACY REGULATIONS

Every pharmacy technician must be familiar with regulations governing the practice of pharmacy in his or her respective state by the state board of pharmacy.

These regulations may include registering with the state board of pharmacy, maintaining certification status, and completing continuing education requirements. All pharmacy technicians must obey all state statutes in addition to federal statutes. A complete listing of all state board of pharmacy information is found in Appendix K.

STORAGE REQUIREMENTS AND EXPIRATION DATES FOR EQUIPMENT AND SUPPLIES

- Cardiopulmonary resuscitation training and certification may be required of all employees. Each employee is responsible for maintaining his or her certification.
- Employees should know the location of and how to use the automated external defibrillator kit.
- Fire extinguishers must be certified on a yearly basis. Personnel should know the location of fire extinguishers in a facility.
- First-aid kits need to be periodically checked to ensure contents have not expired.
- Pharmacy balances require certification by the Department of Taxation on a yearly basis.
- Laminar flow hoods need to be certified every 6 months unless the HEPA filter becomes damaged, which will require certification.
- Medications must be checked periodically to ensure they are in date. Medications that are out of date must be separated from other medications to ensure patient safety.
- Recalled medications must be separated from all usable medications.

STORAGE AND HANDLING REQUIREMENTS FOR HAZARDOUS SUBSTANCES

- **Chemotherapeutic agents** and cytotoxic materials must be prepared in a biologic safety cabinet or vertical flow hood and placed in bags identifying them as such. The preparer should wear a gown, goggles, and two pairs of gloves to protect him or her from possible contamination. A 4 × 4 inch piece of gauze should be kept inside the hood in case of a spill. A preparer should know the location of the cleanup kit. Refer to Occupational Safety and Health Administration (OSHA) guidelines regarding the storage and handling of chemotherapeutic agents.
- **Hazardous substances** include syringes, needles, and toxic medications. Used needles and syringes should be placed in a red plastic sharps container to be autoclaved and disposed of. Toxic substances

(e.g., chemotherapeutic agents) should be placed in a red biohazard bag to be picked up by the appropriate authorities for destruction. Refer to OSHA guidelines regarding the storage and handling of hazardous substances.

- **Radiopharmaceuticals:** A pharmacy must be designed to protect employees from radiation exposure; prevent radioactive contamination of pharmacy work areas and equipment; ensure proper ventilation of the pharmacy; provide for the safe disposal of radioactive waste; limit access into the pharmacy; and ensure security of the pharmacy. Refer to Nuclear Regulatory Agency for the storage and handling of all radiopharmaceuticals.

A nuclear pharmacy has designated rooms to perform the following specific functions:

- Breakdown room: area where empty or used radiopharmaceuticals are returned and dismantled for reuse
- Order entry area: area in which prescription orders for radiopharmaceuticals are entered
- Compounding area: compounding or dispensing area
- Quality-control area: quality assurance tests are performed before delivery
- Packaging area: finished product is packaged for delivery
- Storage and disposal area: storage area for radioactive waste
- Requires special equipment: fume box, glove box, dose calibrator, Geiger-Müller counter, dosimeter, lead-lined refrigerator and freezer, lead-lined storage boxes, autoclave, heating equipment, testing equipment, centrifuge, lead barrier shield, stainless steel sink, shower, and respirator

The U.S. Department of Transportation (DOT) regulates the shipment of hazardous materials under the Hazardous Materials Transportation Act of 1994. Radioactive materials are considered hazardous materials. DOT has set regulations regarding packaging, labeling, and transporting of radioactive materials.

The shipping container (metal) for transporting radioactive material must be able to maintain the integrity of the product during shipping. The container must be specifically labeled based on the activity of the radioactive material: Radioactive White I, Radioactive Yellow II, and Radioactive Yellow III, which contains the highest concentration of radiation. The container must have a "Caution: Radioactive" label with the name of the nucleotide, the quantity, the date, and the time.

Shipping papers must be inside the shipping container and include the following information: name of nucleotide, quantity, form, label category, emergency response telephone number, information regarding emergency personnel, and pharmacy name. The driver carries a copy of the shipping papers. A placard must be on the vehicle if it is carrying Radioactive Yellow III material. Shipped material must be braced inside the transportation vehicle.

PROCEDURES FOR THE TREATMENT OF EXPOSURE TO HAZARDOUS SUBSTANCES

- Chemotherapy spill kits should be used for the cleanup of accidental spills of antineoplastic agents. These kits include waste disposal bags, respirator, latex gloves, heavy utility gloves, eyeglasses, gowns, shoe covers, toweling, and sealable bags.
- The technician should know the location of the Material Safety Data Sheets and should follow the directions on them for a particular item. After completion of the cleanup, an incident report should be filed with the supervisor.
- If a hazardous substance comes in contact with the skin, it must be washed immediately with soap and water for at least 5 minutes. If a substance comes in contact with the eyes, they should be rinsed for 15 minutes. This can be done at the eyewash station.

SECURITY SYSTEMS FOR THE PROTECTION OF EMPLOYEES, CUSTOMERS, AND PROPERTY

- All pharmacies are required to have a workable alarm service when the pharmacy is closed.
- Closed-circuit televisions and hold-up alarm buttons may be installed in pharmacies, but such installation is at the discretion of the institution.
- Each facility (organization) will have established policies and procedures to ensure the safety of staff, customers, and property.
- Facilities may provide lockers for employees' belongings in a secure area.
- Keys may be required to be signed out from a security location to gain access to a pharmacy.
- Motion detectors must be installed and in working condition.
- Only licensed pharmacists may dispense a prescription and supervise a pharmacy technician.
- Only pharmacists or designated employees will have access to keys to open or close the pharmacy.
- Security requirements that restrict access to medications to "authorized personnel only" are in place because of legal and institutional standards and standards of practice.

- Volatile substances must be stored in an area that is properly ventilated and has been designed to prevent explosion.
- Touchpads and scannable means of identification may be used for an employee to gain access to a particular area.

LAMINAR FLOW HOOD MAINTENANCE REQUIREMENTS

1. The blower of the laminar airflow hood should be kept on at all times. If it is shut down, then it must be in operation for at least 30 minutes before use.
2. The hood is wiped down with 70% isopropyl alcohol beginning with the bar, followed by the sides, and continuing from the area closest to the filter, working outward and wiping from the top edge of the side to the bottom.
3. The bench is cleaned last by beginning from the back of the bench and wiping from side to side and moving outward.
4. The laminar flow hood should be cleaned at the beginning of every shift and whenever a spill occurs. Sanitizing agents should not be sprayed because the HEPA filter may become damp and develop a hole.
5. The flow hood needs to be certified every 6 months or whenever the HEPA filter becomes wet.

The pharmacy technician should be familiar with USP <797> as it applies to the preparation of sterile products.

SANITATION REQUIREMENTS

- Counting trays should be cleaned with alcohol after every use to prevent cross-contamination from occurring, which might result in an allergic reaction in another patient. A separate counting tray should be used for chemotherapeutic agents only.
- Proper hand-washing techniques include washing the hands and arms with hot water and Betadine; scrubbing both the top and bottom of the hands; scrubbing between the fingers up to the elbow; and rinsing arms and hands thoroughly.
- Every pharmacy must have running hot and cold water. A mild detergent may be used to clean instruments used in extemporaneous compounding; 70% isopropyl alcohol should be used to clean all countertops in the pharmacy. All pharmacy equipment should be kept clean and in good condition.
- Microorganisms can be introduced into the laminar flow hood by jewelry, cosmetics, coughing or sneezing (if a mask is not worn), or loose facial hair.
- The laminar flow hood should provide an ISO Class 5 clean environment, and the work surface should be cleaned with 70% isopropyl alcohol. The prefilter and the HEPA filter need to be maintained such that particles greater than 3 microns cannot enter the sterile area.
- Radiation may be used in hospitals to sterilize supplies, vitamins, antibiotics, syringes, and needles.

EQUIPMENT CALIBRATION AND MAINTENANCE PROCEDURES

- Automated compounding and repackaging equipment must be calibrated before each use.
- A buffer room must be at least a Class 100,000 clean room but may be a Class 10,000 clean room.
- **ISO Class 5 (formerly known as a Class 100 Area):** An area in which there are no more than 100 particles 0.5 micron or larger per cubic foot of air.
- **ISO Class 7 (formerly known as a Class 10,000 Area):** An area in which there are no more than 10,000 particles 0.5 micron or larger per cubic foot of air.
- **ISO Class 9 (formerly known as a Class 100,000 Area):** An area in which there are no more than 100,000 particles 0.5 micron or larger per cubic foot of air.
- **Class A balance:** Can accurately weigh 120 mg to 15 g.
- **Class B balance:** Can weigh 650 mg to 120 g. Prescription balances should be placed on a level counter away from customer traffic. Before weighing, place equal size glassine papers on the pans of the balance and "zero out" or level until indicator on the balance shows both pans are of even weight. This procedure needs to be done before each weighing.
- **Graduates.** Refer to Figure 3-1.
- **TC** (to contain): Volume measured on the scale is equal to the volume of liquid inside the graduate.
- **TD** (to deliver): Allows one to measure the amount of liquid needed by considering the residual amount of liquid that is left inside the graduate once the liquid is poured out.
- A HEPA filter is monitored by introducing aerosolized Emery 3004 into the plenum of the laminar flow hood while monitoring the penetration of the Emery 3004 on the downstream side of the HEPA filter. No more than 0.01% of the upstream concentration may be detected downstream from the HEPA filter.
- Laminar flow hoods must be turned on for a minimum of 30 minutes before being used. The

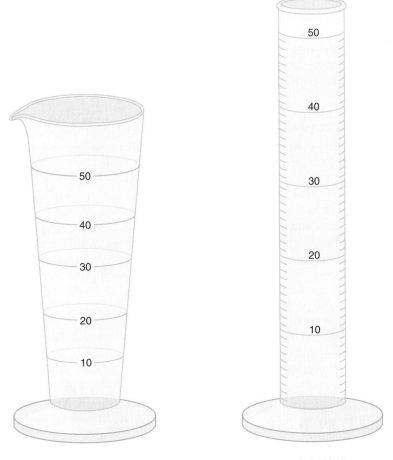

Conical   Cylindrical

Fig. 3-1 Graduated cylinders for liquid measurement. (From Hopper T: *Mosby's pharmacy technician: principles and practice*, ed 2, St Louis, 2007, Saunders.)

velocity of air from the HEPA filter is measured using a volumeter. Average air velocity is 90 linear feet per minute ±20%.

- Pharmacy balances (scales) need to be evaluated on a yearly basis by the Department of Taxation for accuracy.
- Pharmacy weights need to be calibrated once per year.

SUPPLY PROCUREMENT PROCEDURES

- Procurement includes drug selection, source selection, cost analysis, group purchasing, prime vendor relationships, purchasing procedures, record keeping, and receiving control.
- Drug selection includes a cost analysis (cost per dose, cost per day, or cost per treatment). Cost-benefit analysis examines the perceived benefit versus the cost of the medication.

- Source selection is deciding whether a generic or brand-name drug is to be purchased. It examines the therapeutic equivalency of the products. Examination of the reputation of the drug manufacturer and knowledge of drug analysis data are taken into consideration. Consideration of product is affected by the *ASHP Guidelines for Selecting Pharmaceutical Manufacturers and Suppliers.*
- Cost analysis is an examination of acquisition and storage costs and the costs associated with the time required to prepare or package a drug.
- Group purchasing organizations allow hospitals to purchase medications at a lower cost based on volume. These organizations negotiate prices but do not make purchases for an institution. The ability to purchase contract items is known as a "bid" or "contract compliance."
- A primary or prime vendor is one source, a wholesaler, from which as many products as possible are purchased. When choosing a primary vendor, one

should consider the following: delivery rate of items, 24-hour emergency service, computer system for ordering drugs from the vendor, electronic order entry devices, bar-coded shelf labels, competitive pricing, purchasing history reports (80/20 and compliance reports), pricing updates, and drug recalls.

- Purchasing procedures include negotiating discounts and establishing payment schedules, terms of payment, prepayment policies, nonperformance penalties, and returned and damaged goods policies.
- Records must be maintained to meet government regulations, standards of practice requirements, accreditation standards, policies, and management information requirements. Records may include purchase orders that authorize the purchase of a product.
- Receiving procedures include shipments, invoices, and purchase orders that must be reconciled by item. Quantity and strength of each item must be checked; prices on invoice should correspond to price that has been negotiated; and discrepancies must be addressed promptly with the pharmacist and the vendor.

TECHNOLOGY USED IN THE PREPARATION, DELIVERY, AND ADMINISTRATION OF MEDICATION

- **Accusource monitoring system (Baxter, Deerfield, Ill.):** Automated TPN compounder with total nutrient admixture.
- **Baker cells (McKesson Corp., San Francisco, Calif.):** An example of an automated counting and filling device. Each cell contains a particular medication. The desired quantity is entered, and the Baker cell counts the desired quantity for the pharmacist.
- **Bar code scanners:** The Food and Drug Administration has proposed that bar codes be placed on all human drugs and biologicals, which will result in an improvement in both patient and medication safety. The potential for errors will be greatly reduced because the right patient will be receiving the right drug and dose at the right time through the right route.
- **Enteral pump:** A special pump to infuse enteral substances into the stomach.
- **Gravity infusion system:** A stationary infusion system using a minibag that is regulated by the patient.
- **Homerus (Cardinal Health, Dublin, Ohio):** Centralized robotic unit-dose dispensing device. Has

the ability to individually package medications from bulk and deliver bar-coded medications to 24-hour patient-specific bins and return medication to bins on discharge of patient.

- **Infusion control devices**
  - Nonmechanical rate controller (dial calibrated gravity flow regulator, such as Dial-a-Flow [Zoeller Pump Co., Louisville, Ky.])
  - Nonmechanical external pump (elastometric balloon system—a stationary infusion system controlled by the use of a special tube; examples include Intermate [Baxter], ReadyMed [Cardinal Health], MedFlo II [MPS Acacia, Brea, Calif.], and Homepump Eclipse [I-FLOW Corporation, Lake Forest, Calif.])
  - Spring-controlled pump such as the SideKick (I-FLOW Corporation)
- **Mechanical peristaltic pumps** deliver a controlled amount of medication at a controlled rate, such as the CADD line of products (Deltec, St. Paul, Minn.).
  - CADD-Plus—An ambulatory-specific therapy pump used to infuse antibiotics.
  - CADD-Prizm PCS Pump—An ambulatory-specific therapy infusion pump. Patient-controlled analgesia (PCA) used to infuse analgesics.
  - CADD-TPN—An ambulatory-specific infusion pump used in the infusion of TPN.
- **Mechanical piston pump:** Similar to mechanical peristaltic pump, except that it is controlled by a piston that is electromagnetically operated by a battery; the advantage of the system is miniaturization. An example is the Lifecare Omni-Flow 4000 (Abbott Laboratories, Abbott Park, Ill.).
- **Implantable pumps:** Implanted under the skin with a catheter entering a vein. Examples include the SynchroMed (Medtronic, Minneapolis, Minn.) and Infusaid (Shiley Infusaid, Norwood, Mass.).
- **Physician order entry system** results in a reduction of medical errors by having complete and accurate information, accurate dose calculation, and appropriate clinical decision support.
- **Mobile robots** that travel through a hospital to the various nursing units delivering medication.
- **Pyxis** (Cardinal Health) is an automated point-of-use storage system for making floor stock items available to nursing staff. Servers are connected to a Pyxis server and link hospital billing and information systems together.
- **Syringe infusion system** is a stationary infusion system requiring the use of a special syringe.

PURPOSE AND FUNCTION OF PHARMACY EQUIPMENT

EXTEMPORANEOUS COMPOUNDING EQUIPMENT

- **Beakers:** May be either glass or plastic and are used to estimate and mix solutions.
- **Class A (III) balance:** Required in all pharmacies. Used to weigh small quantities of weight. Has a sensitivity requirement of 6 mg.
- **Counter balance (bulk balance):** Two-pan balance used to weigh quantities up to 5 kg. Sensitivity of 100 mg.
- **Digital balances:** Sensitive to a tenth of a milligram and are used to replace Class A balances.
- **Compounding slab (ointment slab):** Used for mixing compounds.
- **Filter paper:** Can be used to weigh or filter a solution.
- **Forceps:** Used to pick up prescription weights. Forceps are used to ensure that oil is not deposited on the weight, which would affect it.
- **Funnels:** Used to filter or pour liquids.
- **Glass stirring rods:** Used to stir solutions and suspensions.
- **Glycine paper:** Used under substances to be weighed.
- **Graduates:** Used to measure liquids. There are two types of graduates: conical and cylindric (most accurate method to measure a volume). Graduates will either be "TD" or "TC." "TD" means the volume delivered is the exact amount desired and the residual remaining solution is in addition to the volume measured. "TC" will hold the desired volume but, when transferred, a residual remains, making the amount measured inaccurate.
- **Master formula sheet (pharmacy compounding log):** Lists the ingredients and their quantities and the procedures to follow in the preparation (Figure 3-2).
- **Mortar and pestle:** Used to mix ingredients. Glass is used for mixing liquids and semisolid dosage forms. Wedgwood is used in the trituration of crystals, granules, and powders. Porcelain is similar to Wedgwood and is more commonly used in the blending of powders (Figure 3-3).
- **Pharmaceutical weights:** Brass weights measured in both metric and apothecary systems. They should never be touched by the hand, should be stored in a clean state, and should be calibrated once per year.
- **Pipettes:** Used to measure volumes less than 1.5 mL.
- **Sink:** Used to wash and clean equipment and hands.
- **Spatula:** Rubber (used for corrosive ingredients), plastic, or steel. Hard rubber is used in the

Ranitidine suspension			
Formulation ingredients	15 mg/ml		
Ingredients	150 mg tablets	#6	
Simple syrup		30 ml	
Distilled water		qs to 60 ml	
Compounding procedure	1. Pulverize tabs in mortar		
	2. Levigate with a small amount of distilled water to disintegrate the film-coating fragments		
	3. Add, by geometric proportion, the syrup and levigate until a uniform mixture is obtained		
	4. Transfer the contents of the mortar to a conical graduate		
	5. Qs ad to 60 ml with distilled water		
	6. Pour into an amber bottle and shake vigorously		
Auxiliary labels	**Shake well**		
	Protect from light		
Stability	1 week at 20 to 30 degrees Celsius		

Fig. 3-2 A recipe book for formula cards. (From Hopper T: *Mosby's pharmacy technician: principles and practice,* ed 2, St Louis, 2007, Saunders.)

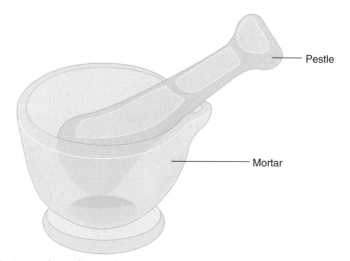

Fig. 3-3 Mortar and pestle used to crush solids. (From Hopper T: *Mosby's pharmacy technician: principles and practice,* ed 2, St Louis, 2007, Saunders.)

compounding of ingredients that react with metal. Stainless steel is most commonly used because of its flexibility and ability to remove materials from a mortar.

INTRAVENOUS ADMIXTURES

- **70% isopropyl alcohol:** Used to clean laminar air hood surfaces.
- **Administration sets:** Disposable, sterile tubing that connects the IV solution to the injection site.
- **Alcohol pads:** Used to clean the ports on an IV bag, the rubber stopper of a vial, or an area of the skin before an injection.
- **Ambulatory pumps:** A small, lightweight, portable pump worn by a patient. May be either therapy-specific or used for multiple therapies.
- **Ampule breaker:** A device used to break the neck of an ampule. May range from 1 to 50 mL.
- **Ampules:** Elongated glass container in which the neck is broken off.
- **Catheters:** Devices that are inserted into veins for direct access to the vascular system. May be either peripheral venous catheters or central venous catheters.
- **Clamps:** Adjust the rate and shutting down of the flow. Types of clamps include slide clamps, screw clamps, and roller clamps.
- **Depth filter:** A filter that works by trapping particles as solution moves through channels.
- **Drip chamber:** A hollow chamber where drops of an IV solution accumulate. The purpose of the drip chamber is to prevent air bubbles from entering the tubing.

- **Filters:** Used to remove particulate material and microorganisms from solution. Can be attached to the end of a syringe, the end of the administration kit, or the end of the needle.
- **Filter needles:** Needles that include a filter that prevents glass from entering the final solution when one draws from an ampule.
- **Filter straws:** Used for pulling medication from ampules.
- **Final filters:** A filter used before a solution enters a patient's body.
- **Flexible bag:** Plastic container that may hold volumes ranging from 50 to 3000 mL.
- **Heparin lock:** A short piece of tubing attached to a needle or catheter when the tubing is filled with heparin to prevent potential clotting.
- **Infusion pumps:** Regulate the flow of medication into a patient. May either be stationary or ambulatory.
- **Laminar flow hoods**
  - **Type A hoods:** Recirculate a portion of the air (after it first passes through a HEPA filter) within the hood, and exhaust a portion of this air back into the parenteral room.
  - **Type B1 hoods:** Exhaust most of the contaminated air through a duct to the outside atmosphere. This air passes through a HEPA filter.
  - **Type B2 hoods:** Exhaust all of the contaminated air to the outside atmosphere after it passes through a HEPA filter. Air is not recirculated within the hood or returned to the parenteral room atmosphere.

- **Type B3 hoods:** Use recycled air within the hood. All exhaust air is discharged to the outside atmosphere. A Type A hood may be converted to a Type B3 hood.
- **Large-volume parenterals (LVPs):** Parenterals with a volume greater than 100 mL.
- **Male and female adapters:** Available in a universal size. Fit a syringe on each end and are used in the mixing of the two contents.
- **Membrane filters:** Consist of small pores that retain particles that are larger than the pores. Membrane filters may be placed between syringe and needle before a medication is introduced into an LVP or a small-volume parenteral (SVP).
- **Minibags:** Contain volumes between 50 and 100 mL.
- **Multidose vial:** Contains a preservative to prevent bacterial contamination and allows for multiple doses of variable amounts. Rubber closure reseals after syringe is withdrawn from it.
- **Needles:** Composed of a hub and a shaft and are designated by two numbers (gauge and length). The gauge measures the diameter of the needle bore; the larger the gauge, the smaller the bore. The length of the needle is measured in inches.
- **Needle adapter:** A needle or catheter may be attached to it.
- **Piggyback:** A small-volume solution added to an LVP.
- **Roll clamp:** Allows for variable flow rates.
- **Single-dose vial:** Does not contain a preservative and must be discarded after one use.
- **Small-volume parenterals:** Packaged products that are either directly administered to the patient or added to another parenteral. Contain a volume of 100 mL or less.
- **Spike:** A rigid, sharpened plastic piece that is inserted into the IV bag.
- **Syringe:** Components of a syringe include plunger, plunger flange, barrel, and tip (Figure 3-4).
- **Syringe caps:** A sterile cap used to prevent contamination of syringes during the transportation out of the pharmacy.
- **Syringes needles:** Components include hub, shaft, bevel, lumen, and point (Figure 3-5).
- **Transfer needles:** Specially designed needles that look like two needles attached together at the hub. Are used to transfer sterile solutions from one vial directly into another without the use of a syringe.
- **Tubing for pumps:** Tubing is specific for manufacturer's machine.
- **Tubing transfer sets:** Blood transfer sets; used to transfer contents of large containers into empty containers.
- **Vials:** Glass or plastic containers with rubber stoppers. Single-dose vials do not contain a preservative, whereas multidose vials do.
- **Solutions used:**
  - ¼ NS—one-fourth normal saline (0.225% sodium chloride)
  - ½ NS—one-half normal saline (0.45% sodium chloride)
  - D10W—10% dextrose in water
  - D5NS—5% dextrose in normal saline (0.9% solution)
  - D5W—5% dextrose in water
  - LR—Lactated Ringer's solution

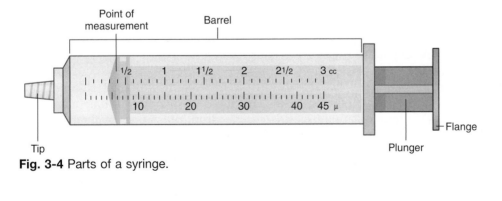

Fig. 3-4 Parts of a syringe.

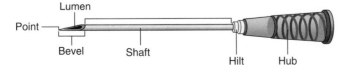

Fig. 3-5 Parts of a needle.

- NS—normal saline solution (0.9%)
- SW—sterile water

TYPES OF WATER

- **Purified water USP:** not intended for parenteral administration; used in the reconstitution of oral products
- **Water for injection USP:** is not sterile and cannot be used in aseptic compounding of sterile products
- **Sterile water for injection USP:** has been sterilized but has no antimicrobial agents; can be used in parenteral solutions
- **Bacteriostatic water for injection USP:** sterile water with antimicrobial agents that can be used for injection
- **Water for injection USP:** not sterile; has no antimicrobial agents and cannot be used for aseptic compounding
- **Sterile water for irrigation USP:** has been sterilized but contains no antimicrobial agents; used as an irrigating solution

DOCUMENTATION REQUIREMENTS FOR ROUTINE SANITATION, MAINTENANCE, AND EQUIPMENT CALIBRATION

- **Balances:** Must be certified yearly by the state Department of Taxation.
- **Laminar hoods and HEPA filters:** Need to be certified a minimum of every 6 months or when the HEPA filter is wetted or the laminar flow hood is moved. Validation is documented evidence that provides a high degree of assurance that the process will produce a product with predetermined specifications.

AMERICANS WITH DISABILITIES ACT REQUIREMENTS

The Americans with Disabilities Act (ADA) is a federal civil rights law that prohibits discrimination against people with disabilities in everyday activities, such as buying an item at the store, going to the movies, enjoying a meal at a local restaurant, exercising at the health club, or having a car serviced at a local garage.

To meet the goals of the ADA, the law established requirements for businesses of all sizes. These requirements went into effect on January 26, 1992. Businesses that serve the public must modify policies and practices that discriminate against people with disabilities; comply with accessible design standards when constructing or altering facilities; remove barriers in existing facilities where readily achievable; and provide auxiliary aids and services when needed to ensure effective communication with people who have hearing, vision, or speech impairments. All businesses, even those that do not serve the public, must comply with accessible design standards when constructing or altering facilities.

MANUAL AND COMPUTER-BASED SYSTEMS FOR STORING, RETRIEVING, AND USING PHARMACY-RELATED INFORMATION

MANUAL PROCESSING OF MEDICATION ORDERS

- Medication order is written in patient chart.
- Copy of medication order is removed from chart.
- Order is picked up at nursing station, faxed, or tubed to the pharmacy.
- Medication order is entered into the pharmacy computer system.
- Pharmacist reviews and verifies medication order.
- Medication order is filled by technician and checked by pharmacist.
- Patient-specific medication is manually delivered or tubed to nursing unit.

AUTOMATIC PROCESSING OF MEDICATION ORDERS

- Physician or physician's representative enters medication order directly into hospital computer service, which communicates order to pharmacy.
- Pharmacist reviews and verifies order.
- Registered nurse retrieves medication from point-of-use automated medication station.
- Pharmacy technician fills inventory as medication supplies fall below PAR (periodic automatic replacement) levels.

Drug Interactions

The Omnibus Budget Reconciliation Act of 1990 (OBRA 90) requires that all pharmacists perform a drug utilization evaluation (DUE) during the processing of prescriptions. The DUE will alert the pharmacist of any potential drug interactions or contraindication a patient may experience while taking a prescribed medication.

Patient Profiles

Patient profiles are required to be maintained by a pharmacy as a result of OBRA 90. Information to be collected includes personal information such as name, home address, home telephone number, and patient's birthday; billing information such as insurance carrier (plan and group number); disease states of the patient; and drug allergies of the patient.

Label Generation

Labels are generated on successful adjudication of an insurance claim or if the patient is a cash customer.

SECURITY PROCEDURES RELATED TO DATA INTEGRITY, SECURITY, AND CONFIDENTIALITY

The second part of the Health Insurance Portability and Accountability Act was enacted in April 2005 and requires that pharmacies have established appropriate safeguards to prevent a patient's information from becoming compromised by an outside source.

KNOWLEDGE OF DOWNTIME EMERGENCY POLICIES AND PROCEDURES

A pharmacy technician should be familiar with procedures to be followed when a system is down. These procedures may include filling prescriptions manually and entering the information into the computer system when the system returns to normal. The pharmacy technician should know how to bill prescriptions during an emergency.

BACKUP AND ARCHIVING PROCEDURES FOR STORED DATA AND DOCUMENTATION

Computer systems need to be backed up at regularly scheduled times (possibly daily) to prevent loss of data if the system goes down for any reason.

Defragmentation of computer files reorganizes files that have been stored on a computer.

LEGAL REQUIREMENTS REGARDING ARCHIVING

Federal law requires that the following documents be maintained for a minimum of 2 years and be readily retrievable (able to be produced within 72 hours of inquiry):

- DEA Forms 41, 106, 222, and 224
- All prescriptions for controlled substances
- All controlled-substance invoices
- All initial narcotic inventories, biennial inventories, and change of pharmacist inventories
- All exempt narcotic and poison sales records

If a particular state requires retention of these records for longer than 2 years, a pharmacy must adhere to whichever is the more stringent of the two regulations.

HEALTH CARE REIMBURSEMENT SYSTEMS

Acute care: Does not allow pharmacy to make a profit. Pharmacy-related expenses are incorporated into the per diem hospital charge.

Ambulatory care parenteral therapy: The Centers for Medicare and Medicaid Services has created a list of health insurance continuation program codes for drugs in this setting. Reimbursable costs are also included. Other fees include a professional fee component and a facility fee.

Cognitive services: These services include prescriptive authority by the pharmacist, administration of medications by the pharmacist, patient assessment and treatment, pharmacist intervention with prescribers and other health care providers, patient education, and patient reassessment and monitoring. Reimbursement is based on prior years' data.

Community care: Cost of medication plus a dispensing fee for dispensing, monitoring, and record keeping.

Disease state management services: Health Care Financing Administration 1500 form may be used for billing of these services.

Long-term care: Per diem reimbursement (predetermined daily rate) that is based on prior medication costs of the facility. Formulary control is important. Regulatory agencies have developed lists of medications they have deemed unnecessary based on excessive adverse effects or poor outcomes obtained.

BILLING AND ACCOUNTING POLICIES AND PROCEDURES

Allowances: A deduction is given from the purchase price by the seller to the purchaser.

Average cost method: An inventory costing method that uses the weighted average unit cost to allocate the costs of goods available for sale to inventory and cost of goods sold.

Consigned goods: Goods held for sale by one party (the consignee), although ownership of the goods is retained by another party.

Cost of goods available for sale: The sum of the beginning merchandise inventory and the cost of goods purchased.

Cost of goods purchased: The sum of the net purchases and freight charges associated with a product.

Cost of goods sold: The total cost of merchandise sold during the period, determined by subtracting ending inventory from the cost of goods available for sale.

Credit terms: Terms that specify the amount of cash discount and the time period during which it is offered. They indicate the length of time in which the purchaser is expected to pay the full invoice price. An example includes 2/10, where a 2% discount can be taken off the invoice price less any returns or allowances, if the invoice is paid within 10 days of the invoice date.

Current replacement cost: The current cost to replace an inventory item.

Days in inventory: Measure of the average number of days the inventory is held; calculated as 365 divided by inventory turnover rate.

Depreciation: A process of allocating to expense the cost of a plant asset over its useful life in a rational and systematic manner. It is not a process of asset valuation. Depreciation takes into account the cost (all expenditures necessary to acquire the asset and make it ready for intended use); the useful life (estimate of the expected life based on need for repair, service life, and vulnerability to obsolescence); and the salvage value (an estimate of the asset's value at the end of its useful life). Can be computed by either the straight-line, declining-balance, or units-of-activity method.

First in, first out: An inventory costing method that assumes the cost at the earliest purchase of goods is the first to be recognized as the cost of the goods sold.

FOB (free on board) destination: Freight terms indicating that the goods are placed free on board at the buyer's place of business and the seller pays the freight cost; goods belong to the seller while in transit.

FOB shipping point: Freight terms indicating that the goods are placed free on board the carrier by the seller; the buyer pays the freight cost; goods belong to the buyer while in transit.

Gross profit (gross margin): Excess of net sales over the cost of goods sold.

Gross profit rate: Gross profit expressed as a percentage by dividing the amount of gross profit by net sales.

Inventory turnover rate: A ratio that measures the number of times on average the inventory sold during the period; computed by dividing cost of goods sold by the average inventory during the period.

Last in, first out: An inventory costing method that assumes that the costs of the latest units purchased are the first to be allocated to cost of goods sold.

Lower of cost or market basis: A basis whereby inventory is slated at the lower of cost or market (current replacement cost).

Net profit: Sales minus cost of goods minus expenses.

Net purchases: Purchases less purchase returns and allowances and purchase discounts.

Net sales: Sales less sales returns and allowances and sales discounts.

Periodic inventory system: An inventory system in which costs are allocated to ending inventories and cost of goods sold at the end of the period. Cost of goods is computed at the end of the period by subtracting the ending inventory (costs are assigned to a physical count of items on hand) from the cost of goods available for sale.

Purchase discount: A cash discount claimed by a buyer for prompt payment of a balance due.

Purchase invoice: A document that supports each credit purchase.

Sales discounts: A reduction given by a seller for prompt payment of a credit sale.

Specific identification method: An actual physical flow costing method in which items still in inventory are specifically costed to arrive at the total cost of the ending inventory.

Weighted average unit cost: Average cost that is weighted by the number of units purchased at each unit cost.

INFORMATION SOURCES USED TO OBTAIN DATA IN A QUALITY IMPROVEMENT SYSTEM

Controlled-substance form: Allows a nursing staff to verify controlled substances at each change of shift of nurses. Monitors receipt, administration, and disposal of a controlled substance.

Medication administration record (MAR): Documents medication administered to a patient. It includes the drug, dose, route of administration, frequency of administration, and administration times. The MAR lists the patient's allergies and diagnoses. It is used every time a medication is administered.

Medication delivery record: Provides accountability for medication distribution between the pharmacy and hospital or long-term care facility. It lists the medication found in a particular delivery.

Patient profile: A patient profile may be either a hardcopy or a computerized list of a patient's prescriptions (medications) and other information. A patient profile will identify the patient by name, Social Security number, birth date, and gender. It provides billing information, such as insurance (group number, patient's identification, patient's relationship to the cardholder [spouse, dependent]). A patient profile contains a patient's medical history that includes current conditions, known allergies, and adverse reactions. It provides a listing of medications, whether legend or OTC, that have been filled for the patient, including dates, quantities, directions for use, and physician's name. It may list whether the patient requests easy-open containers or use of generic medications if authorized by the physician.

Physician order sheet: List of all of the physician's orders for a patient, including both drug and nondrug orders. Nondrug orders may include allergies, diagnoses, diet orders, directives, laboratory orders, and orders for ancillary services, such as physical therapy, occupational therapy, respiratory therapy, or speech therapy.

Resident monitoring form: Documents behavior of a patient and any precipitating factors, drug and nondrug intervention, outcomes, and adverse reactions.

Treatment administration record: Documents external treatments given to a patient in a hospital or long-term care facility.

PROCEDURES TO DOCUMENT OCCURRENCES SUCH AS MEDICATION ERRORS, ADVERSE EFFECTS, AND PRODUCT INTEGRITY

The following agencies track medication errors:

- **AHRQ:** Agency for Healthcare Research and Quality
- **AMA:** American Medical Association
- **ASHP:** American Society of Health-System Pharmacists
- **CDER:** Center for Drug Evaluation and Research
- **FDA:** Food and Drug Administration; MedWatch is a voluntary program reporting adverse health events and medical problems
- **TJC:** The Joint Commission
- **USP:** Medmarx is a national, Internet-accessible database used by hospitals and health care systems to track and trend adverse drug reactions and medication errors.
- **FDA and the Centers for Disease Control and Prevention:** Vaccine Adverse Event Reporting System is a postmarketing safety surveillance program that collects information about adverse events that occur after the administration of U.S.-licensed vaccines.

STAFF TRAINING TECHNIQUES

Training: A set of activities that provides the opportunity to acquire and improve job-related skills. Should include both technical skills (e.g., computer and systems technology) and nontechnical skills (e.g., diversity and sexual harassment).

On-the-job training: Involves job instruction while performing the job in the actual workplace.

Apprenticeship: Learning a trade from an experienced worker.

Internship: A form of on-the-job training for which the intern may or may not be paid.

Job rotation: Provides a wide range of experience in different kinds of jobs in a firm. May include mentoring.

Off-the-job training: Involves lectures, videos, and simulations.

EMPLOYEE PERFORMANCE EVALUATION TECHNIQUES

Performance appraisal: A process of systematically evaluating performance and providing feedback on which performance adjustments can be made. Performance appraisals define specific job criteria against which performance will be measured, measure past job performance accurately, justify rewards given to individuals and groups, and define the developmental experiences employees need to enhance their performance in the current job and to prepare for future responsibilities.

Activity measures: A rating system based on an evaluator's observation and rating.

Ranking: A comparative technique of performance appraisal that involves rank ordering of each individual from best to worst on each performance dimension.

Paired comparison: A comparative method of performance appraisal whereby each person is directly compared with every other person.

Forced distribution: A method of performance appraisal that uses a small number of performance categories, such as "very good," "good," "adequate," and "very poor" and forces a certain proportion of people into each.

Graphic rating scales: A scale that lists a variety of dimensions thought to be related to high performance outcomes in a given job and that the individual is expected to exhibit.

Critical incident diary: A method of performance appraisal that records incidents of unusual success or failure in a given performance aspect.

Behaviorally anchored rating scales: A performance appraisal approach that describes observable job behaviors, each of which is evaluated to determine good versus bad performance.

Management by objective: A process of joint goal setting between a supervisor and a subordinate.

360 evaluations: A comprehensive approach that uses self-ratings, customer ratings, and others outside the workforce.

EMPLOYEE PERFORMANCE FEEDBACK TECHNIQUES

Feedback is the process through which the receiver communicates with the sender by returning another message. Suggestions for giving constructive feedback include the following:

- Give feedback directly and in a spirit of mutual trust.
- Be specific.
- Give feedback when receiver is most ready to accept it.
- Be accurate; check validity with others.
- Focus on things the receiver can control.
- Limit how much the receiver gets at one time.

CHAPTER 3 REVIEW QUESTIONS

1. Which type of mortar and pestle is used to mix liquids?
   a. Glass
   b. Porcelain
   c. Wedgwood
   d. None of the above

2. Who is responsible for the transportation of hazardous materials?
   a. Department of Transportation (DOT)
   b. Environmental Protection Agency (EPA)
   c. Food and Drug Administration (FDA)
   d. The Joint Commission (TJC)

3. How often must HEPA filters be certified?
   a. Every 3 months
   b. Every 6 months
   c. Every year
   d. Every 2 years

4. Which of the following symbols indicates the highest level of radiation?
   a. Radioactive White I
   b. Radioactive Yellow II
   c. Radioactive Yellow III
   d. Radioactive Orange IV

5. How often must laminar flow hoods be certified?
   a. Every 3 months
   b. Every 6 months
   c. Every year
   d. Every 2 years

6. Which reference book is a compendium of monographs setting official national standards for drug substances, dosage forms, and standards for pharmaceutical ingredients?
   a. *Approved Drug Products with Therapeutic Equivalence Evaluations*
   b. *Drug Facts and Comparisons*
   c. *PDR*
   d. *USP-NF*

7. What is the sensitivity of a Class A balance?
   a. 5 mg
   b. 6 mg
   c. 10 mg
   d. 20 mg

8. What type of spatula should be used in measuring corrosive ingredients?
   a. Plastic
   b. Rubber
   c. Steel
   d. All the above

9. What type of alcohol should be used to clean a laminar flow hood?
   a. 70% Isopropyl alcohol
   b. 70% Methyl alcohol
   c. 70% Rubbing alcohol
   d. All the above

10. What is the name of the opening of a needle?
    a. Bevel
    b. Hilt
    c. Lumen
    d. Shaft

11. What type of environment should a laminar flow hood provide?
    a. ISO 5, formerly known as a Class 100 area
    b. ISO 6, formerly known as a Class 1000 area
    c. ISO 7, formerly known as a Class 10,000 area
    d. ISO 8, formerly known as a Class 100,000 area

12. What is used to measure volumes less than 1.5 mL?
    a. 5-mL conical graduate
    b. 5-mL cylindric graduate

c. Pipette
d. Syringe

13. How are disease management services reimbursed?
    a. Capitation
    b. Cost of service cost to monitor cost for record keeping
    c. Fee-cost spread
    d. HCFS 1500 form

14. Who is responsible for pharmaceuticals in transit if they are designated as "FOB destination"?
    a. Buyer
    b. Drug manufacturer
    c. Drug wholesaler
    d. Seller

15. Which of the following is not a duty of an institutional pharmacy technician?
    a. Compound parenteral medications
    b. Enter prescription orders into the computer
    c. Fill patient medication cassettes
    d. Transport medications throughout the institution

16. Which of the following is not true regarding TJC's policies regarding the pharmacy in an institution?
    a. External and internal products should not be stocked next to each other, to avoid errors.
    b. IV admixtures are prepared in a pharmacy using aseptic technique and a laminar flow hood.
    c. Professional samples should be dispensed as soon as the pharmacy receives them to prevent them from going out of date.
    d. Unit doses are preferred over a traditional vial system.

17. What type of balance can weigh objects between 650 mg and 120 g?
    a. Class A
    b. Class B
    c. Electronic
    d. Triple-beam

18. How long should the blower be on for a laminar airflow hood?
    a. 10 minutes
    b. 15 minutes
    c. 20 minutes
    d. 30 minutes

19. What type of laminar flow hood can be converted to a Type B3 hood?
    a. Type A hood
    b. Type A1 hood
    c. Type B1 hood
    d. Type B2 hood

20. How often does a pharmacy balance need to be certified?
    a. Every 3 months
    b. Every 6 months
    c. Every 9 months
    d. Every 12 months

21. Where is a finished radiopharmaceutical product stored?
    a. Breakdown room
    b. Compounding area
    c. Packaging area
    d. Storage and disposal area

22. Which is the most effective method of communication?
    a. E-mail
    b. Face to face
    c. Memos
    d. Telephone

23. Which of the following does TJC not certify?
    a. Hospitals
    b. Long-term care facilities
    c. Nursing homes
    d. Retail pharmacies

24. What type of balance must a pharmacy have?
    a. Class A
    b. Class B
    c. Electronic
    d. Triple-beam

25. What is the air velocity of a laminar flow hood?
    a. 70 linear feet/min (±20%)
    b. 80 linear feet/min (±20%)
    c. 90 linear feet/min (±20%)
    d. 100 linear feet/min (±20%)

Chapter 4

Practice Examinations

PRACTICE EXAMINATION I

Select the response that best answers the question.

1. Drugs in which classification should not be taken with potassium-sparing diuretics?
   a. ACE inhibitors
   b. Beta-blockers
   c. Calcium channel blockers
   d. Nitrates

2. Which interpretation of the following instructions is correct? 30 mL MOM PO ac and hs prn
   a. Take one teaspoonful of Milk of Magnesia by mouth before meals and at bedtime as needed.
   b. Take one tablespoonful of Milk of Magnesia by mouth after meals and at bedtime as needed.
   c. Take 1 oz of Milk of Magnesia by mouth after meals and at bedtime as needed.
   d. Take 1 oz of Milk of Magnesia by mouth before meals and at bedtime as needed.

3. A pharmacy technician receives a prescription to make 4 oz of a 10% solution and has a 25% stock solution on hand. How much diluent will be added to fill this prescription?
   a. 7.2 mL
   b. 48 mL
   c. 72 mL
   d. 300 mL

4. What type of solution has greater osmolarity than blood?
   a. Hypertonic
   b. Hypotonic
   c. Isotonic
   d. Pyrogenic

5. Which of the following dosage forms is not a solid dosage form?
   a. Capsule
   b. Elixir
   c. Plaster
   d. Powder

6. A 180-lb man is to receive 1.75 mg of tobramycin per kilogram per day. The pharmacy technician is to prepare the tobramycin in 100 mL of D5W, and it is to be given three times per day. The drug is available in a 40-mg/mL vial and is to be administered over 30 min. How much medication will the patient receive each day?
   a. 48 mg
   b. 96 mg
   c. 143 mg
   d. 315 mg

7. Which of the following drugs is not a beta-blocker?
   a. Atenolol
   b. Metoprolol
   c. Nifedipine
   d. Propranolol

8. Which of the following terms does not mean a "proprietary" drug?
   a. Brand
   b. Generic
   c. Patented
   d. Trade

9. If a patient is hypokalemic, the patient has which of the following?
   a. Low sodium
   b. High sodium
   c. Low potassium
   d. High potassium

10. What is not found in a total nutrient admixture?
    a. Amino acid
    b. Dextrose
    c. Lipids
    d. Protein

11. What does UTI stand for?
    a. Undiagnosed treatment inconclusive
    b. Upper respiratory infection
    c. Urethral tract infection
    d. Urinary tract infection

12. Which of the following is not a required text in a pharmacy?
    a. A copy of the Controlled Substance Act
    b. *USP-NF*
    c. *Drug Facts and Comparisons*
    d. All are required references

13. How many teaspoon doses are in a pint of elixir?
    a. 24
    b. 48
    c. 72
    d. 96

14. Which of the following is not an advantage of a plastic bag IV parenteral system?
    a. The plastic bag is light and cheap to transport.
    b. The plastic bag takes less room for storage and disposal.
    c. The quantity remaining in the bag is easy to read.
    d. All the above.

15. What does FDA refer to?
    a. Food and Drug Abuse
    b. Food and Drug Administration
    c. Food and Drug Association
    d. Free Drug Assistance

16. Drugs in which classification may yield side effects such as dry eyes, dry mouth, or difficult urination or defecation?
    a. Alpha-blockers
    b. Anticholinergics
    c. Beta-blockers
    d. Cephalosporins

17. Which vitamin will increase the blood coagulation of a patient taking Coumadin?
    a. Vitamin B_1
    b. Vitamin B_6
    c. Vitamin C
    d. Vitamin K

18. Which of the following must appear on a unit-dose product label?
    a. Dose strength of the medication
    b. Expiration date of the medication
    c. Medication name
    d. All the above

19. How many day(s) will 40 tablets last if the patient is taking the medication "ii bid"?
    a. 1 day
    b. 5 days
    c. 10 days
    d. 20 days

20. A potassium chloride solution has a concentration of 1.5 mEq/mL. How many milliliters contain 30 mEq?
    a. 0.05 mL
    b. 15 mL
    c. 20 mL
    d. 45 mL

21. What is the maximum number of refills allowed for a Schedule IV drug?
    a. None
    b. One
    c. Five
    d. Unlimited

22. How many days will the following prescription last?
    Ampicillin 250 mg #40
    1 cap PO qid
    Ref × ii
    a. 4
    b. 10
    c. 20
    d. 30

23. How many times a day would a patient take a medication if it was "q6h"?
    a. 3
    b. 4
    c. 6
    d. 8

24. How many milliliters are in 1 pint?
    a. 120 mL
    b. 240 mL
    c. 480 mL
    d. 960 mL

25. Which organ would be affected if the root word *nephro* was indicated?
    a. Ear
    b. Heart
    c. Kidney
    d. Liver

26. Which of the following would require a potassium supplement?
    a. Aldactone
    b. Dyazide
    c. Dyrenium
    d. Lasix

27. Which of the following drugs would be administered to a patient if he or she had received an overdose of heparin?
    a. Aspirin
    b. Phytonadione
    c. Protamine sulfate
    d. Warfarin

28. How many units of heparin are in 50 mL of 100,000 units/L?
    a. 50 units
    b. 500 units
    c. 5000 units
    d. 50,000 units

29. What does the term "od" mean?
    a. Right ear
    b. Right eye
    c. Left ear
    d. Left eye

30. You have received the following prescription for Robitussin A-C: "1 tsp qid for 10 days." How much would you dispense?
    a. 50 mL
    b. 100 mL
    c. 150 mL
    d. 200 mL

31. What is the generic name for Lodine?
    a. Diclofenac
    b. Etodolac
    c. Naproxen
    d. Oxaprozin

32. Which of the following signs or symptoms may indicate digoxin toxicity?
    a. Arrhythmias
    b. Auditory disturbances
    c. Fever
    d. Hypotension

33. An intravenous solution containing 20,000 units of heparin in 500 mL of a 0.45% sodium chloride solution is to be infused at a rate of 1000 units/hr. How many drops per minute should be infused to deliver the desired dose if the intravenous set is calibrated at a rate of 15 gtt/mL?
    a. 0.42 gtt/min
    b. 6 gtt/min
    c. 16 gtt/min
    d. 32 gtt/min

34. Which of the following is a federal program for patients older than 65 years or with certain diseases?
    a. ADC
    b. Medicaid
    c. Medicare
    d. Workers' Compensation

35. How much medication should a 70-lb child receive if the adult dose is 250 mg?
    a. 70 mg
    b. 79 mg
    c. 116 mg
    d. 1458 mg

36. What does the word root *derm* mean?
    a. Brain
    b. Skin
    c. Skull
    d. Tooth

37. Which of the following ratings indicates that the drug is contraindicated in pregnancy?
    a. A
    b. B
    c. C
    d. X

38. What is the meaning of the Latin abbreviation *Rx* on a prescription?
    a. Insigna
    b. Sig
    c. Take this drug
    d. Write on label

39. What term refers to the amount of money a patient must pay in a given period before the third-party insurer will make a payment?
    a. AWP + dispensing fee
    b. Capitation
    c. Copayment
    d. Deductible

40. How often must an inventory of controlled substances be taken?
    a. Weekly
    b. Monthly
    c. Yearly
    d. Every 2 years

41. The following prescription is presented to the pharmacy:

    Hctz 50 mg #30
    i tab PO qod c OJ

    How many days will the prescription last the patient?
    a. 15 days
    b. 30 days
    c. 45 days
    d. 60 days

42. What system does tuberculosis affect?
    a. Cardiovascular
    b. Digestive
    c. Endocrine
    d. Respiratory

43. Which of the following drugs does not require blood work from a patient?
    a. Lithium
    b. Phenytoin
    c. Sulfasalazine
    d. Warfarin

44. Where would meperidine be stored in the pharmacy?
    a. In the refrigerator
    b. In the pharmacy safe
    c. With the "fast movers"
    d. With the pills and tablets

45. What is the maximum number of refills allowed on Accutane prescriptions?
    a. None
    b. One
    c. Six
    d. 12

46. A pharmacy technician is preparing heparin 25,000 units in 500 mL of D5W. What concentration should be on the label?
    a. 50 units/mL
    b. 75 units/mL
    c. 100 units/mL
    d. 125 units/mL

47. Where should an otic product be placed?
    a. In the ear
    b. In the eye
    c. In the rectum
    d. Under the tongue

48. What is the minimum amount of time that a patient must wait before purchasing another bottle of an exempt narcotic?
    a. 24 hr
    b. 48 hr
    c. 72 hr
    d. 96 hr

49. Which of the following drugs is not available as an OTC product?
    a. Ibuprofen
    b. Naproxen sodium
    c. Ranitidine
    d. Tramadol

50. How is insulin administered?
    a. ID
    b. IM
    c. PO
    d. SC

51. Which of the following is the strongest dose?
    a. NTG 1/100 gr
    b. NTG 1/150 gr
    c. NTG 1/200 gr
    d. NTG 1/400 gr

52. What is the meaning of the abbreviation "qs ad"?
    a. A sufficient quantity for the left ear
    b. A sufficient quantity for the right ear
    c. A sufficient quantity for the right eye
    d. A sufficient quantity to make up to

53. Which of the following antidepressants may be used to treat bedwetting in small children?
    a. Amitriptyline
    b. Desipramine
    c. Doxepin
    d. Imipramine

54. What auxiliary label should be affixed to a prescription of ibuprofen?
    a. Avoid sunlight
    b. For external use
    c. Take on an empty stomach
    d. Take with food

55. Which of the following antifungal agents is not available as an OTC product?
    a. Clotrimazole
    b. Itraconazole
    c. Miconazole
    d. Terbinafine

56. Which of the following may be used to treat sleep disorders?
    a. Chromium picolinate
    b. Ginseng
    c. Glucosamine
    d. Melatonin

57. Which of the following is not a task completed by pharmacy technicians?
    a. Counseling patients
    b. Performing inventory management tasks
    c. Ordering medications
    d. Refilling prescriptions

58. Which drug law stated that all drugs must be pure, safe, and effective?
    a. FDCA 1938
    b. Durham-Humphrey Amendment
    c. Kefauver-Harris Amendment
    d. Poison Prevention Act of 1970

59. Which of the following should be used in lifting pharmacy weights to be placed on a balance?
    a. Filter paper
    b. Forceps
    c. Latex gloves
    d. Weighing papers

60. What is the correct interpretation of the following prescription: 1 tsp PCN 250 mg PO qid for 10 days?
    a. Take one tablespoonful of penicillin 250 mg by mouth four times a day for 10 days.
    b. Take one teaspoonful of penicillin 250 mg by mouth every other day for 10 days.
    c. Take one teaspoonful of penicillin G 250 mg by mouth four times a day for 10 days.
    d. Take one teaspoonful of penicillin 250 mg by mouth four times a day for 10 days.

61. What does the word root *cardio* mean?
    a. Heart
    b. Lungs
    c. Skin
    d. Stomach

62. What is the meaning of "DAW2" in billing a prescription to an insurance carrier?
    a. Brand dispensed as a generic
    b. Physician approved the use of a generic drug
    c. Physician approved the use of a generic drug; the patient requested brand name
    d. Physician requested brand name

63. How much 1% boric acid solution and 5% boric acid solution are needed to make 30 mL of 3% boric acid solution?
    a. 5%: 20 mL; 1%: 10 mL
    b. 5%: 5 mL; 1%: 15 mL
    c. 5%: 10 mL; 1%: 20 mL
    d. 5%: 5 mL; 1%: 25 mL

64. Which of the following natural supplements might be used to treat depression?
    a. Chamomile
    b. Ginger
    c. Ginkgo
    d. St. John's wort

65. Which of the following drugs is not a proton pump inhibitor?
    a. Esomeprazole
    b. Itraconazole
    c. Lansoprazole
    d. Pantoprazole

66. Which reference book is a compilation of package inserts?
    a. *Drug Topics Red Book*
    b. *Facts and Comparisons*
    c. *Physicians' Desk Reference*
    d. *USP DI*

67. How much medication should a 9-year-old child receive if the adult dose is 50 mg?
    a. 19.4 mg
    b. 21.4 mg
    c. 24.4 mg
    d. 26.4 mg

68. How old must a person be to purchase an exempt narcotic?
    a. 12 years
    b. 16 years
    c. 18 years
    d. 21 years

69. Which of the following drugs is not an antifungal agent?
    a. Fluconazole
    b. Miconazole
    c. Nystatin
    d. Sulfisoxazole

70. What is the meaning of URI?
    a. Upper respiratory infection
    b. Urethral and rectal infection
    c. Urine receptacle infection
    d. Upper respiratory influenza

71. Which of the following would not be used in the preparation of intravenous medications?
    a. Ampules
    b. Class A prescription balance
    c. Laminar flow hood
    d. Syringes

72. Which term encompasses the absorption, distribution, metabolism, and elimination of a drug?
    a. Pharmacokinetics
    b. Pharmacognosy
    c. Pharmacology
    d. Pharmacopeia

73. A pharmacy technician receives a medication order that requires him to add 40 units of insulin to an intravenous solution. How many milliliters will he need?
    a. 0.3 mL
    b. 0.4 mL
    c. 0.5 mL
    d. 0.6 mL

74. How much codeine is contained in one tablet of Tylenol #3?
    a. ¼ gr
    b. ½ gr
    c. ¾ gr
    d. 1 gr

75. Which instrument should be used to measure a volume less than 1.0 mL?
    a. Beaker
    b. Conical graduate
    c. Cylindric graduate
    d. Pipette

76. What standards must be followed during extemporaneous compounding?
    a. DEA
    b. FDA
    c. GMP
    d. OBRA 90

77. What term describes the willingness of the patient to take a drug in the amounts and on schedule as prescribed?
    a. Compliance
    b. Ease of administration
    c. First-pass effect
    d. Second-pass effect

78. What is the generic name for Glucophage?
    a. Glipizide
    b. Glyburide
    c. Metformin
    d. Pioglitazone

79. What is the generic name for Zithromax?
    a. Azithromycin
    b. Clarithromycin
    c. Minocycline
    d. Ofloxacin

80. Which of the following auxiliary labels should be placed on a prescription container of antianxiety, antidepressant, or anticonvulsant medication?
    a. Avoid dairy products
    b. May cause drowsiness
    c. Refrigerate
    d. Shake well

81. Which dosage form is described as "solid particles dispersed in liquid vehicle"?
    a. Emulsions
    b. Gel
    c. Lotion
    d. Suspensions

82. If a patient is to receive 5 mg/kg of a drug, how much should a 176-lb patient receive?
    a. 40 mg
    b. 193.6 mg
    c. 1936 mg
    d. 0.4 g

83. Which of the following interpretations of "ii gtt bid os" is correct?
    a. Instill two drops in right ear twice per day.
    b. Instill two drops in left ear twice per day.
    c. Instill two drops in right eye twice per day.
    d. Instill two drops in left eye twice per day.

84. Which of the following is not an effect of narcotics?
    a. Analgesia
    b. CNS stimulation
    c. Euphoria
    d. Sedation

85. How many 150-mg clindamycin capsules are required to compound a prescription reading "clindamycin 2%, propylene glycol 5%, isopropyl alcohol qs ad 480 mL"?
    a. 10
    b. 64
    c. 96
    d. 112

86. You have received a prescription for amoxicillin 500 mg PO. The patient is unable to chew or swallow capsules or tablets. How many milliliters should be given in each dose if the concentration is 125 mg/5 mL?
    a. 5 mL
    b. 10 mL
    c. 15 mL
    d. 20 mL

87. A pharmacy is reimbursed by an insurance company for AWP + $3.25 per prescription. If the AWP for 100 tablets is $120.00, how much will the pharmacy be reimbursed for a prescription of 30 tablets?
    a. $36.00
    b. $39.25
    c. $120.00
    d. $123.25

88. How many milliliters of water should be mixed with 1200 mL of 65% (v/v) to make a 45% (v/v) solution?
    a. 533 mL
    b. 667 mL
    c. 830 mL
    d. 1733 mL

89. If 500 mL of D5W is to be infused over 6 hours and the drop factor is 15 gtt/mL, what will the rate in gtt/min be?
    a. 1 gtt/min
    b. 2 gtt/min
    c. 10 gtt/min
    d. 20 gtt/min

90. How much time does a pharmacist have to complete the partial filling of a Schedule II prescription?
    a. 24 hours
    b. 48 hours
    c. 72 hours
    d. 96 hours

91. Which of the following could be used to prepare an ointment if another technician is using the ointment slab?
    a. A graduate
    b. A mortar
    c. Parchment paper
    d. Weighing paper

92. Which of the following duties may the pharmacy technician not perform?
    a. Labeling medication doses, preparing intravenous admixtures, and maintaining the cleanliness of the laminar flow hood
    b. Maintaining patient records, filling and dispensing routine orders for stock supplies, and preparing routine compounding
    c. Prepackaging drugs in single dose or unit of use, maintaining inventories of drug supplies, and completing insurance forms
    d. Providing clinical counseling, providing clinical information to medical staff, and providing patient medical history data to requestors

93. What is the most common route of administration?
    a. Inhalation
    b. Inunction
    c. Oral
    d. Rectal

94. Which route of administration should be used in taking nitroglycerin?
    a. Buccal
    b. Oral
    c. Rectal
    d. Sublingual

95. Which of the following is not true with regard to ordering Schedule II drugs?
    a. Form 222 is a triplicate form.
    b. Form 222 must be kept in a secure location.
    c. If an error is made on a Form 222, one can cross it out and initial it.
    d. A maximum of 10 different drugs can be ordered on one form.

96. What is the basic reimbursement formula for pharmacies?
    a. Copayment
    b. Drug cost × standard markup rate
    c. Drug cost + dispensing fee
    d. Drug cost + dispensing fee − deductible

97. How much dextrose does 1 L of D10W contain?
    a. 10 mg
    b. 100 mg
    c. 1 g
    d. 100 g

98. Which classification of drug recall occurs if the patient experiences a reversible side effect?
    a. Class I
    b. Class II
    c. Class III
    d. Class IV

99. A pharmacy bases its retail prices on AWP plus a professional fee as follows:

Fee	AWP
$2.25	$25.00 or less
$3.25	$25.01-$50.00
$10.00	$50.01-$75.00
$20.00	$75.01 or more

    A prescription is presented that reads "Sig: 2 tabs bid × 25 days." If the AWP of this drug is $321.66 for 500 tablets, what will be the retail price of the prescription?
    a. $66.53
    b. $70.20
    c. $74.33
    d. $85.25

100. Which of the following is not an automated dispensing system?
     a. TJC
     b. Pyxis
     c. Robot-Rx
     d. SureMed

PRACTICE EXAMINATION II

Select the response that best answers the question.

1. Which auxiliary label should be affixed to a container of tetracycline?
   a. Avoid sunlight
   b. Take 1 hr before or 2 hr after taking dairy products or antacids
   c. Take all medication
   d. All the above

2. Five pints of diluted hydrochloric acid weigh 2.79 kg. What is its specific gravity?
   a. 0.56
   b. 0.86
   c. 1.16
   d. 1.79

3. How much Demerol would be given to a patient if the dose on hand was 50 mg/mL and the patient was to receive 75 mg?
   a. 0.5 mL
   b. 1.0 mL
   c. 1.5 mL
   d. 2.0 mL

4. What is the generic name for the brand-name drug Bactrim DS?
   a. Amoxicillin-clavulanate
   b. Cephalexin
   c. Sulfamethoxazole-trimethoprim
   d. Sulfamethoxazole-trimethoprim DS

5. What is the maximum number of refills allowed for a prescription of oxycodone + APAP if authorized by the prescriber?
   a. None
   b. Five
   c. 12
   d. Unlimited

6. How many grams of 2.5% hydrocortisone cream should be mixed with 240 g of 0.25% hydrocortisone cream to make a 1% hydrocortisone cream?
   a. 120 g
   b. 180 g
   c. 240 g
   d. 360 g

7. What is the maximum number of refills allowed for a Schedule III drug?
   a. None
   b. One
   c. Five
   d. Six

8. Which dosage form is defined as a clear, sweetened, flavored hydroalcoholic, containing water and alcohol, that may be either medicated or not?
   a. Elixir
   b. Emulsion
   c. Enema
   d. Syrup

9. Which interpretation of "ii gtt os bid" is correct?
   a. Instill two drops in right ear twice a day.
   b. Instill two drops in right eye twice a day.
   c. Instill two drops in left ear twice a day.
   d. Instill two drops in left eye twice a day.

10. How many grams of dextrose are in 1 L of D5W?
    a. 50 mcg
    b. 50 mg
    c. 5.0 g
    d. 50 g

11. Which of the following drugs is not a form of estradiol?
    a. Climara
    b. Estrace
    c. Estraderm
    d. Premarin

12. Which of the following would not be used in extemporaneous compounding?
    a. Class A balance
    b. Compounding slab
    c. Graduate cylinder
    d. Laminar flow hood

13. What does a gram measure?
    a. Distance
    b. Vision
    c. Volume
    d. Weight

14. Which dosage form is an aqueous solution with sucrose?
    a. Emulsion
    b. Solution
    c. Suspension
    d. Syrup

15. What does DUE mean?
    a. Directions Under Evaluation
    b. Doctor Under Examination
    c. Drug Used Externally
    d. Drug Utilization Evaluation

16. Approximately how many liters are in 1 qt?
    a. 1 L
    b. 2 L
    c. 3 L
    d. 4 L

17. How many days will a prescription of 60 tablets last if the directions read "i-ii tabs PO q4-6h"?
    a. 5 days
    b. 7 days
    c. 10 days
    d. 15 days

18. Which of the following drugs is a Schedule II drug?
    a. Acetaminophen with codeine
    b. Alprazolam
    c. Cocaine
    d. Flurazepam

19. What does *hypoglycemia* mean?
    a. High blood pressure
    b. High blood sugar
    c. Low blood pressure
    d. Low blood sugar

20. How many days would 40 capsules of a medication last if the directions were "i cap qid ac and hs"?
    a. 4 days
    b. 8 days
    c. 10 days
    d. None of the above

21. How many milliliters of a 10% stock solution of an ingredient are needed to prepare 120 mL of a solution containing 10 mg of the ingredient per milliliter?
    a. 0.12 mL
    b. 1.2 mL
    c. 12 mL
    d. 120 mL

22. In what proportion should 20% zinc oxide be mixed with white petrolatum (diluent) to produce a 3% zinc oxide ointment?
    a. 1 part ZnO and 1 part white petrolatum
    b. 3 parts ZnO and 17 parts white petrolatum
    c. 3 parts ZnO and 14 parts white petrolatum
    d. 17 parts ZnO and 3 parts white petrolatum

23. If 120 mL of a 2% (w/v) are diluted with water to 1 pint, what will be the strength of the dilution?
    a. 0.25%
    b. 0.5%
    c. 1.0%
    d. 8.0%

24. Gentamicin 120 mg in 100 mL D5W is administered over 30 min every 8 hr with a 10-drop kit. What will the rate be?
    a. 2 gtt/min
    b. 4 gtt/min
    c. 16 gtt/min
    d. 33 gtt/min

25. How would one take a medication if the directions said "PO"?
    a. By mouth
    b. By rectum
    c. Left ear
    d. Topically

26. If a child weighs 8 kg and the adult dose is 10 mL, how much medication should the child receive?
    a. 0.5 mL
    b. 1.2 mL
    c. 4.0 mL
    d. 6.7 mL

27. What is a common side effect of ACE inhibitors?
    a. Anaphylaxis
    b. CNS stimulation
    c. Cough
    d. Respiratory depression

28. What is the generic for Lipitor?
    a. Atorvastatin
    b. Fluvastatin
    c. Pravastatin
    d. Simvastatin

29. What type of pharmacy balance is required in all pharmacies?
    a. Class A
    b. Class B
    c. Electronic
    d. Triple-beam

30. In whom is trazodone contraindicated?
    a. Children with enuresis
    b. Elderly women with Alzheimer disease
    c. Elderly men with erectile dysfunction
    d. Young males

31. Amitriptyline is to TCA as venlafaxine is to ___ _____.
    a. Calcium channel blocker
    b. H_2 antagonist
    c. Protease inhibitor
    d. SSRI

32. What term describes the response when two or more drugs combine to provide a response that is greater than the sum of the two individual drugs?
    a. Additive effect
    b. Potentiation
    c. Synergistic effect
    d. None of the above

33. What is the proper dose for a 6-year-old child if the adult dose is 10 mg?
    a. 33 mcg
    b. 3.3 mg
    c. 33 mg
    d. 333 mg

34. What form must be submitted to the DEA to request to destroy controlled substances?
    a. Form 41
    b. Form 49
    c. Form 224
    d. Form 225

35. What is inventory?
    a. Expired merchandise
    b. Merchandise available for sale
    c. Merchandise to be ordered
    d. Overstock merchandise

36. What size syringe should be used to measure 0.6 mL of fluid?
    a. 1 mL
    b. 5 mL
    c. 10 mL
    d. 20 mL

37. A patient receives 5 mL of a 15% solution of a drug. What is the drug dose?
    a. 75 mg
    b. 750 mg
    c. 7.5 g
    d. 75 g

38. In multiples of what number should tablets or capsules be counted at a time using a spatula and a pill tray?
    a. 1
    b. 2
    c. 5
    d. 10

39. How many milligrams are equal to 2 gr?
    a. 1 mg
    b. 13 mg
    c. 130 mg
    d. 1300 mg

40. What temperature is considered room temperature?
    a. 8°C
    b. 8° to 15°C
    c. 15° to 30°C
    d. 30° to 40°C

41. Which of the following drugs will produce an adverse effect if alcohol is consumed during the course of therapy?
    a. Disulfiram
    b. Guaifenesin
    c. Hydrochlorothiazide
    d. Triamcinolone

42. At which part of the liquid does one look when measuring liquids?
    a. A point between the bottom and top of the meniscus
    b. Bottom of the meniscus
    c. Top of the meniscus
    d. None of the above

43. Which dosage form may be either oil-in-water or water-in-oil?
    a. Capsule
    b. Emulsion
    c. Suspension
    d. Suppository

44. What is the generic name for the beta-blocker Tenormin?
    a. Atenolol
    b. Metoprolol
    c. Propranolol
    d. Nadolol

45. What is the direction for airflow in a horizontal laminar airflow hood?
    a. From the back of the hood to the front
    b. From the bottom of the hood to the top
    c. From the front of the hood to the back
    d. From the top of the hood to the bottom

46. How many milliliters of a 1:50 (w/v) stock solution can be prepared from 1 pint of a 5% stock solution?
    a. 96 mL
    b. 192 mL
    c. 720 mL
    d. 1200 mL

47. Which of the following side effects may be attributed to an overdosage of salicylates?
    a. GI upset
    b. Platelet changes
    c. Tinnitus
    d. All the above

48. Which DAW code should be used if the physician authorizes the use of a generic drug but the patient requests the brand-name drug?
    a. 0
    b. 1
    c. 2
    d. 3

49. At what standard time would a patient receive medication if it was 0800 hours military time?
    a. 7 AM
    b. 8 AM
    c. 7 PM
    d. 8 PM

50. Which body system is affected by GERD?
    a. Cardiovascular
    b. Endocrine
    c. Gastrointestinal
    d. Pulmonary

51. Which of the following drugs is not a quinolone?
    a. Ciprofloxacin
    b. Norflex
    c. Norfloxacin
    d. Floxin

52. What is the meaning of the prefix *osteo-*?
    a. Bone
    b. Cell
    c. Lymph
    d. Muscle

53. Which of the following medications could be used as a prophylactic for migraines?
    a. Imitrex
    b. Inderal
    c. Midrin
    d. Stadol

54. Which of the following is not an antiviral agent?
    a. Acyclovir
    b. Clotrimazole
    c. Didanosine
    d. Zidovudine

55. What term refers to the processes involved in the preparation of a sterile product to prevent contamination of the product?
    a. Aseptic technique
    b. Extemporaneous compounding
    c. Geometric dilution
    d. Levigation

56. What is the cost for 24 mg of an active ingredient used in a compound if the bulk bottle of the active ingredient costs $250.00/g?
    a. $1.50
    b. $3.00
    c. $6.00
    d. $9.00

57. A 1000-mL IV bag was hung at 0800 hours and is to run at 100 mL/hr. What time would the next bag be needed?
    a. 1200 hours
    b. 1400 hours
    c. 1600 hours
    d. 1800 hours

58. How many milliliters of water should be added to 100 mL of 10% stock solution of sodium chloride to prepare a 0.9% solution of sodium chloride?
    a. 10.1 mL
    b. 101 mL
    c. 1011 mL
    d. 1111 mL

59. Which of the following professional licenses does not confer the ability to prescribe medications?
    a. DDS
    b. LCSW
    c. MD
    d. PA

60. Which of the following drugs is not available in a transdermal dosage form?
    a. clonidine
    b. estradiol
    c. fentanyl
    d. fexofenadine

61. What is MedWatch?
    a. A device that signals that an another IV bag needs to be hung in an institution
    b. A reporting program available to pharmacies indicating physicians who may be overprescribing narcotics
    c. A reporting program available to health care providers to report adverse events that pose a serious health threat
    d. A service established by the AARP to monitor polypharmacy in the elderly

62. What is the name of the opening of a needle?
    a. Bevel
    b. Hilt
    c. Lumen
    d. Point

63. What is the meaning of the term "non rep"?
    a. Do not repeat
    b. No known allergies
    c. Nothing by mouth
    d. Refill

64. Which form is required to dispense controlled substances?
    a. Form 222
    b. Form 224
    c. Form 225
    d. Form 363

65. Which of the following is not an abbreviation for extended-release forms of medication?
    a. CD
    b. CR
    c. ERF
    d. SR

66. Which DAW code is used when the physician writes "Brand Name Only" on the prescription?
    a. 0
    b. 1
    c. 2
    d. 3

67. What is the generic name for Tenormin?
    a. Atenolol
    b. Carisoprodol
    c. Nadolol
    d. Propranolol

68. Which of the following is not a manner for a new prescription to be presented for filling at a pharmacy?
    a. Called in by the physician
    b. Called in by the patient
    c. Fax
    d. Presented by the patient

69. Which of the following drugs would use "pulse dosing"?
    a. Clotrimazole
    b. Fluconazole
    c. Itraconazole
    d. Ketoconazole

70. What term can be described as "the rules of a facility or institution"?
    a. Policy
    b. Procedure
    c. Protocol
    d. Standard

71. How many days would a prescription of 30 tablets last if the directions were "i tab tid ac"?
    a. 3 days
    b. 6 days
    c. 8 days
    d. 10 days

72. What is the meaning of the abbreviation "BS"?
    a. Blood sugar
    b. Blood in stools
    c. Body surface
    d. Bowel syndrome

73. What is the brand name of enalapril?
    a. Accupril
    b. Monopril
    c. Vasotec
    d. Zestril

74. How would a patient take a medication if the directions read "prn"?
    a. As directed
    b. As needed
    c. By mouth
    d. By rectum

75. Which of the following drugs may be used to counteract the side effects of antipsychotic medications?
    a. Benztropine
    b. Citalopram
    c. Propranolol
    d. Zolpidem

76. What is the generic name for Zyprexa?
    a. Donepezil
    b. Metaxalone
    c. Olanzapine
    d. Risperidone

77. A child weighs 30 kg and is prescribed a 10-mg/kg dose of amoxicillin tid. The pharmacy stocks 50 mg/mL. How much medication would the patient receive each day?
    a. 3 mL
    b. 6 mL
    c. 13 mL
    d. 18 mL

78. To what classification does Tessalon Perles belong?
    a. Antitussive
    b. Antihistamine
    c. Decongestant
    d. Expectorant

79. Which of the following is true about generically equivalent drugs?
    a. Chemically different but are expected to produce the same therapeutic outcome and toxicity
    b. Chemically identical in strength, concentration, dosage form, and route of administration
    c. Contain different active ingredients
    d. Priced exactly the same as brand-name drugs

80. Which of the following is the generic name for Pepcid?
    a. Cimetidine
    b. Famotidine
    c. Nizatidine
    d. Ranitidine

81. How many tablets should be given to a patient with the following prescription?

    Hctz 50 mg 1 month supply
    1 tab PO qod
    ref × 6

    a. 15
    b. 30
    c. 90
    d. 180

82. What is the flow rate of 1000 mL of Ringer's lactate to be infused over 8 hours?
    a. 6.25 mL/hr
    b. 12.5 mL/hr
    c. 62.5 mL/hr
    d. 125 mL/hr

83. What hospital committee is responsible for creating and maintaining the drug formulary?
    a. Infection Control Committee
    b. Nursing and Pharmacy Committee
    c. Pharmacy and Therapeutics Committee
    d. Product Evaluations Committee

84. Interpret the following: "ii caps stat, then i cap q hr, max 5 caps/12 hr"
    a. Take two capsules by mouth immediately, then one capsule at bedtime, maximum of five capsules in 5 hours.
    b. Take two capsules by mouth immediately, then one capsule each hour, maximum of five capsules in 12 hours.
    c. Take 11 capsules by mouth immediately, then one capsule at bedtime, maximum of five capsules within the next 12 hours.
    d. Take 11 capsules by mouth immediately, then one capsule each hour, maximum of five additional capsules in 12 hours.

85. Medications in which schedule have no medical use in the United States and possess an extremely high potential for abuse?
    a. Schedule I
    b. Schedule II
    c. Schedule III
    d. Schedule IV

86. What type of drug is affected by MAC?
    a. Discontinued drugs
    b. Investigational drugs
    c. Nonproprietary drugs
    d. Proprietary drugs

87. What is the generic name for Patanol?
    a. Brimonidine
    b. Ciprofloxacin
    c. Latanoprost
    d. Olopatadine

88. Which of the following is not required on a prescription label?
    a. Directions for usage
    b. Drug name with strength and quantity
    c. Physician's DEA number
    d. Prescription or serial number

89. You have received a medication order for Lasix 40 mg bid for 10 days. You prepare a unit dose of Lasix suspension (10 mg/mL). How much would you dispense for a unit dose?
    a. 4 mL
    b. 8 mL
    c. 10 mL
    d. 18 mL

90. How many pairs of latex gloves should be worn when preparing IV admixtures?
    a. None
    b. One
    c. Two
    d. Three

91. Which of the following is not used to treat depression?
    a. Antipsychotics
    b. MAOIs
    c. SSRIs
    d. TCAs

92. A pharmacy technician is preparing an IV admixture and notices on the medication order the abbreviation "NS." What does NS mean?
    a. Nasal solution
    b. Normal saline
    c. Normal solution
    d. No smoking while the patient is receiving the IV

93. Which of the following topical corticosteroid dosage forms is most potent?
    a. Cream
    b. Gel
    c. Lotion
    d. Ointment

94. Which of the following drugs is not a Schedule II drug?
    a. Codeine
    b. Fentanyl
    c. Lorazepam
    d. Meperidine

95. Which of the following drugs will produce an adverse effect if alcohol is consumed during the course of therapy?
    a. Amoxicillin
    b. Azithromycin
    c. Metronidazole
    d. Nitrofurantoin

96. Which of the following dosage forms bypasses the digestive system?
    a. Capsule
    b. Enteric coated tablet
    c. Oral tablet
    d. Sublingual tablet

97. What may a pharmacy technician do as a result of OBRA 90?
    a. Call a physician and recommend a different drug dosage
    b. Counsel a patient with regard to his or her drug therapy
    c. Offer to counsel a patient, if allowed by state law
    d. Screen patient profiles for drug-disease contraindications

98. A patient weighs 60 lb and has been given a prescription in which he or she is to receive 3 mg/lb each day. How many milligrams will the patient receive each day?
    a. 170 mg
    b. 175 mg
    c. 180 mg
    d. 185 mg

99. Which type of insulin can be added to an IV solution?
    a. Extended insulin zinc
    b. Isophane insulin
    c. NPH insulin
    d. Regular insulin

100. What is another name for a nonproprietary drug?
    a. Brand-name drug
    b. Generic drug
    c. Investigational drug
    d. OTC drug

PRACTICE EXAMINATION III

Select the response that best answers the question.

1. What is the purpose of postmarketing monitoring of new drugs?
    a. Ensure GMP
    b. Monitor the quality of new drugs
    c. Removal of unsafe drugs
    d. Testing for purity and effectiveness of new drugs

2. What does the abbreviation "hs" mean on a prescription?
    a. At bedtime
    b. Hours
    c. House
    d. None of the above

3. What is the maximum number of refills allowed for a Schedule III drug?
   a. None
   b. One
   c. Five
   d. 10

4. Which of the following drugs is not an NSAID?
   a. Colchicine
   b. Celecoxib
   c. Ibuprofen
   d. Oxaprozin

5. Which of the following drugs would be contraindicated with vitamin K therapy?
   a. Glyburide
   b. Heparin
   c. Pentoxifylline
   d. Warfarin

6. What auxiliary label should be included on a container of medication that has the following instruction: "i gtt os bid"?
   a. For external use
   b. For the ear
   c. For the eye
   d. Use rectally

7. Where would a buccal tablet be placed?
   a. Between the cheeks and gum
   b. Orally
   c. Rectally
   d. Under the tongue

8. Which of the following would be found on a hospital medication order but not on a retail prescription?
   a. Dosage schedule
   b. Drug name
   c. Drug strength
   d. Patient name

9. Which of the following is true concerning nitrofurantoin?
   a. It should be taken as a loading dose.
   b. It should be taken at breakfast only.
   c. It should be taken with alcohol.
   d. It should be taken with food.

10. What does the suffix *-ectomy* mean?
    a. Disease
    b. Hardening
    c. Removal
    d. Vomiting

11. Which of the following drugs is not a cephalosporin?
    a. Keflex
    b. Lorabid
    c. Suprax
    d. Vantin

12. A technician is given 120 mL of a 50% (w/v) potassium chloride solution and is told to add 6 oz of sterile water to it. What will be the final w/v percentage concentration of the solution?
    a. 10%
    b. 20%
    c. 33%
    d. 47%

13. How long must a laminar airflow hood be on before being used?
    a. 15 minutes
    b. 30 minutes
    c. 1 hour
    d. 2 hours

14. What disease may result in the formation of a goiter?
    a. Cancer
    b. Hypertension
    c. Hypoglycemia
    d. Hyperthyroidism

15. Why would a pharmacy receive a noncompliance report?
    a. The pharmacy failed to maintain adequate controlled substance records and has been cited by the DEA on an audit.
    b. The pharmacy failed to properly fill out a Form 222.
    c. The pharmacy failed to purchase medications from a specific vendor with whom an agreement had been negotiated by the GPO.
    d. The pharmacy purchased more drugs than it is permitted based on its budget.

16. What is a drug monograph?
    a. A picture of the drug from the manufacturer
    b. A price list for the drug from the manufacturer
    c. Literature on the drug
    d. Literature on the drug manufacturer

17. Which pharmacy reference book contains drug costs?
    a. *Blue Book*
    b. *Orange Book*
    c. *Red Book*
    d. *White Book*

18. How many milliliters are in 1 cubic centimeter?
    a. 1 mL
    b. 2 mL
    c. 5 mL
    d. 10 mL

19. Which of the following drugs must be placed in a child-resistant container?
    a. Inhalation products
    b. Mebendazole tablets
    c. Ranitidine
    d. Sublingual nitroglycerin tablets

20. How much guaifenesin with codeine would you dispense for a 5-day supply if the prescription calls for "Guaifenesin c Codeine 5 cc q4h PO prn"?
    a. 120 mL
    b. 150 mL
    c. 450 mL
    d. 480 mL

21. Which medication should not be prescribed for young males?
    a. Desyrel
    b. Paxil
    c. Prozac
    d. Zoloft

22. How often is a biennial inventory taken in a pharmacy?
    a. Monthly
    b. Twice per year
    c. Yearly
    d. Every 2 years

23. Which of the following drugs could be used prophylactically for dental procedures?
    a. Ampicillin
    b. Amoxicillin
    c. Ibuprofen
    d. Naproxen sodium

24. What size container would you use in dispensing 240 mL of a liquid medication?
    a. 2 oz
    b. 4 oz
    c. 6 oz
    d. 8 oz

25. To prepare 2.5 L of a 1:20 solution from a 30% solution, how much water is added?
    a. 417 mL
    b. 2083 mL
    c. 2500 mL
    d. 15,000 mL

26. The pharmacy technician receives a prescription for Flexeril 10 mg, and the instructions read "i PO tid." What is the total daily dose?
    a. 10 mg
    b. 20 mg
    c. 30 mg
    d. 40 mg

27. Antidepressants in which of the following classifications need to be washed out of the body before a patient switches to another antidepressant?
    a. Lithium
    b. MAOIs
    c. SSRIs
    d. TCAs

28. Which part of the body would be affected by a condition with the word root *arthro*?
    a. Arm
    b. Artery
    c. Joint
    d. Membrane

29. Which of the following is not a disadvantage of an oral dosage form?
    a. Delayed onset of action
    b. Ease of administration
    c. First-pass metabolism
    d. Taste of medication

30. How many grams of fluorouracil will a 154-lb patient receive in 5 successive days at a dosage rate of 12 mg/kg/day?
    a. 0.84 g
    b. 1.848 g
    c. 4.2 g
    d. 9.24 g

31. A 10-year-old child weighs 90 lb. How much medication should the child receive using Young's formula if the adult dose is 30 mg?
    a. 13 mg
    b. 18 mg
    c. 50 mg
    d. 66 mg

32. What are the two methods of pharmacy claims submission to third-party payers?
    a. Electronic and e-mail
    b. Electronic and fax
    c. Electronic and FedEx
    d. Electronic and hard copy

33. Which of the following is not a task a pharmacy technician would perform?
    a. Counting medication
    b. Extemporaneous compounding
    c. Reconstituting medications
    d. Counseling a patient

34. If a patient is to receive 2.4 g of medication per day and the drug is available in 600-mg tablets, how many tablets are needed for a day's dose?
    a. Half a tablet
    b. 1 tablet
    c. 4 tablets
    d. 8 tablets

35. Which of the following drugs should be avoided in the treatment of people with asthma?
    a. Antihistamines
    b. Beta-blockers
    c. NSAIDs
    d. All the above

36. How many 30-mg $KMnO_4$ (potassium permanganate) tablets are needed to prepare the following solution?
    $KMnO_4$ 1 : 5000 600 mL
    a. 2 tablets
    b. 3 tablets
    c. 4 tablets
    d. 6 tablets

37. Which of the following drugs is not available as an OTC product?
    a. Aluminum hydroxide–magnesium hydroxide
    b. Lansoprazole
    c. Omeprazole
    d. Ranitidine

38. What does "NPO" mean on a medication order?
    a. Do not refill
    b. Do not place in mouth
    c. Do not repeat
    d. Nothing by mouth

39. Dissolve 40 g of urea in enough liquid to make a 20% solution. What is the total volume?
    a. 2 mL
    b. 8 mL
    c. 20 mL
    d. 200 mL

40. What is the correct interpretation of "10 mg MS IM q4h prn pain"?
    a. Inhale 10 mg of morphine sulfate every 4 hours as needed for pain.
    b. Insert 10 mL of morphine sulfate intramuscularly every 4 hours as needed for pain.
    c. Inject 10 mg of morphine sulfate intravenously every 4 hours as needed for pain.
    d. Inject 10 mg of morphine sulfate intramuscularly every 4 hours as needed for pain.

41. What should a patient take for a headache if he or she is taking warfarin?
    a. APAP
    b. ASA
    c. Narcotic analgesics
    d. NSAIDs

42. How much water should be added to 1 L of 70% isopropyl alcohol to prepare a 30% solution?
    a. 2.33 mL
    b. 42.86 mL
    c. 1333 mL
    d. 2.33 L

43. What type of alcohol is used to clean a laminar airflow hood?
    a. Ethyl alcohol
    b. Isopropyl alcohol
    c. Methyl alcohol
    d. Rubbing alcohol

44. How many grams of a 10% and 1% ointment should be used to make 45 g of a 2% ointment?
    a. 5 g of the 1%, 40 g of the 2%
    b. 5 g of the 1%, 40 g of the 10%
    c. 5 g of the 10%, 40 g of the 2%
    d. 5 g of the 10%, 40 g of the 1%

45. Which of the following medications is not measured in International Units?
    a. Heparin
    b. Insulin
    c. Vitamin B
    d. Vitamin E

46. Which of the following interpretations of "i cap qid ac and hs" is correct?
    a. Take one caplet by mouth 1 hour before meals and at bedtime.
    b. Take one capsule by mouth 1 hour before meals and at bedtime.
    c. Take one capsule by mouth after meals and before bedtime.
    d. Take one capsule by mouth before meals and at bedtime.

47. Capsules of which of the following sizes contains the smallest quantity?
    a. 0
    b. 1
    c. 2
    d. 4

48. What term refers to a pharmacy receiving a predetermined amount of money for a patient regardless of the number of prescriptions filled or the value of the prescriptions each month?
    a. Capitation
    b. Copayment
    c. Deductible
    d. Fee for service

49. Which of the following would not be found on a CSAR?
    a. Amount of medication administered
    b. Amount of medication wasted
    c. Date and time of the administration of a drug
    d. Expiration date of the drug administered

50. Cephalexin is to cephalosporin as ciprofloxacin is to _____.
    a. Macrolide
    b. Penicillin
    c. Quinolone
    d. Tetracycline

51. What is the meaning of AAC?
    a. Actual acquisition cost
    b. Average acquisition cost
    c. Average assessed cost
    d. Average acquisition cost containment

52. What does PCA stand for?
    a. Patient-calibrated analysis
    b. Patient-controlled analgesia
    c. Partially collapsed artery
    d. Perennial circumvented arteriosclerosis

53. What is the generic name for Zestril?
    a. Enalapril
    b. Fosinopril
    c. Lisinopril
    d. Quinapril

54. How often should a fentanyl patch be changed?
    a. Once per day
    b. Every 3 days
    c. Once per week
    d. Once per month

55. Which of the following drugs, if expired, can result in a fatality?
    a. Amoxicillin
    b. Cephalexin
    c. Clarithromycin
    d. Tetracycline

56. Which term refers to the name of the medication, its strength, and the quantity to be dispensed?
    a. Inscription
    b. Rx
    c. Signa
    d. Subscription

57. Why is it important to follow the procedures of an institution?
    a. Following procedures will result in a promotion.
    b. Following procedures will result in a pay increase.
    c. Procedures are established to prevent errors from occurring in a pharmacy.
    d. The PTCB and State Boards of Pharmacy follow up with pharmacy technicians to ensure that they are following procedures. Failure to follow procedures may result in either a suspension or a revocation of their certification.

58. If a medication has an expiration date of 3/06, when will it expire?
    a. The first day of June 2003
    b. The last day of June 2003
    c. The first day of March 2006
    d. The last day of March 2006

59. How much medication should a 40-lb child receive if the adult dose is 25 mg?
    a. 5.66 mg
    b. 6.66 mg
    c. 7.66 mg
    d. 8.66 mg

60. By what route should Phenergan 25 mg suppository be taken?
    a. PO
    b. PR
    c. SL
    d. TOP

61. How many times a day would a patient take medication if it is prescribed "tid"?
    a. One
    b. Two
    c. Three
    d. Four

62. What should a pharmacy technician do while processing a prescription if he or she receives a contraindication message on the pharmacy terminal screen?
    a. Bypass the screen and continue to process the prescription
    b. Contact the physician and ask that a different drug be prescribed
    c. Inform the patient that you cannot fill the prescription because the physician made an error
    d. Inform the pharmacist of the message

63. Which organization is responsible for drug recalls?
    a. Board of Pharmacy
    b. DEA
    c. FDA
    d. NABP

64. Which of the following is an indication for NSAIDs?
    a. Analgesic
    b. Antiinflammatory
    c. Antipyretic
    d. All the above

65. How many kilograms are in 4.4 lb?
    a. 0.2 kg
    b. 2.0 kg
    c. 20 kg
    d. 200 kg

66. What type of drug recall occurs when a drug is not likely to cause a temporary adverse health consequence?
    a. Class I recall
    b. Class II recall
    c. Class III recall
    d. No recall is required

67. What does the suffix *-osis* mean?
    a. Abnormal condition
    b. Inflammation
    c. Study of
    d. Treatment

68. Where should used needles be placed after use?
    a. In a biohazard container
    b. In a red plastic bag
    c. In a sharps container
    d. With normal trash

69. How many days will the following prescription last?

    Amoxicillin 125 mg/5 mL 75 cc
    i tsp PO tid

    a. 1
    b. 5
    c. 10
    d. 15

70. What do the first 5 digits of an NDC number represent?
    a. Drug item
    b. Drug manufacturer
    c. Drug package
    d. None of the above

71. If 150 mL of a substance weighs 170 g, what is its specific gravity?
    a. 0.88
    b. 1.0
    c. 1.13
    d. 1.25

72. Which of the following is a local anesthetic?
    a. Benzocaine
    b. Butorphanol
    c. Neostigmine
    d. Zolmitriptan

73. Which of the following herbal products would be used as a laxative?
    a. American ginseng
    b. Cascara sagrada
    c. Goldenseal
    d. Melatonin

74. How many grams of a 10% and 2% ointment should be used to make 25 g of a 5% ointment?
    a. 2%: 9.4 g; 10%: 15.6 g
    b. 2%: 10 g; 10%: 15 g
    c. 2%: 12.5 g; 10%: 12.5 g
    d. 2%: 15.6 g; 10%: 9.4 g

75. What is the flow rate of 1 L of NS to be infused over 8 hr?
    a. 8 mL/hr
    b. 12.5 mL/hr
    c. 125 mL/hr
    d. 1000 mL/hr

76. In what schedule is methylphenidate classified?
    a. Schedule I
    b. Schedule II
    c. Schedule III
    d. Schedule IV

77. Which of the following drugs would not be used to treat COPD?
    a. Albuterol
    b. Guaifenesin
    c. Ipratropium bromide
    d. Salmeterol

78. Which of the following drugs is a calcium channel blocker?
    a. Carvedilol
    b. Nadolol
    c. Nifedipine
    d. Valsartan

79. What is the correct dosage for a 25-lb child if the adult dose is 100 mg?
    a. 7.6 mg
    b. 17 mg
    c. 68 mg
    d. 113 mg

80. What are the four elements of medical and pharmaceutical nomenclature?
    a. Prefixes, suffixes, root words, and combining vowels
    b. Prefixes, suffixes, key words, and combining vowels
    c. Prefixes, suffixes, key words, and combining consonants
    d. Prefixes, suffixes, root words, and combining consonants

81. How many 4-oz bottles of an exempt narcotic may be purchased every 48 hr by an individual?
    a. None
    b. 1
    c. 2
    d. None of the above

82. What advice should be given to a patient taking metronidazole?
    a. Avoid alcohol
    b. Take with food
    c. Take all of the medication
    d. All the above

83. What is the maximum number of different items that may be ordered on a Form 222?
    a. 5
    b. 10
    c. 15
    d. 20

84. Which of the following medications should not be given to individuals younger than 18 years?
    a. Cephalexin
    b. Ciprofloxacin
    c. Clarithromycin
    d. Clindamycin

85. Which of the following side effects may result from taking thiazide diuretics?
    a. Hypocalcemia
    b. Hypoglycemia
    c. Hypokalemia
    d. Hypourticaria

86. How many 10-gr tablets are required to make 1000 mL of a 1:1000 solution?
    a. ½ tablet
    b. 1 tablet
    c. 1½ tablets
    d. 2 tablets

87. Which organization ensures a safe environment for employees?
    a. DEA
    b. EPA
    c. FDA
    d. OSHA

88. What condition may result if a child takes aspirin after being exposed to chickenpox?
    a. Glaucoma
    b. Herpes zoster
    c. Reye syndrome
    d. Toxic shock syndrome

89. Which of the following is not a duty performed by a pharmacy technician?
    a. Answering telephones
    b. Accepting a new prescription over the phone from a physician's office
    c. Preparing prescription labels
    d. Pricing prescriptions

90. Which of the following is an example of drug duplication?
    a. Aldactone and Coreg
    b. Calan and Isoptin
    c. Coumadin and Zetia
    d. Dyazide and Vasotec

91. How many days would 40 capsules of a medication last if the directions were "i cap qid"?
    a. 4 days
    b. 6 days
    c. 8 days
    d. 10 days

92. When would you take a medication if the directions stated "ac"?
    a. After a meal
    b. At bedtime
    c. Before a meal
    d. In the morning

93. What does the word root *cardio* mean?
    a. Ears
    b. Eyes
    c. Heart
    d. Skin

94. What is the meaning of the prefix *intra-*?
    a. Below
    b. Between
    c. Equal
    d. Within

95. Which of the following is not a side effect of steroidal medications?
    a. Bruising
    b. Inflammation
    c. Moon face
    d. Weight gain

96. Which dosage form would use the process of inunction to be absorbed into the body?
    a. Capsules
    b. Inhalants
    c. Ointments
    d. Suppositories

97. How many milliliters of water must be added to 250 mL of a 0.9% (w/v) stock solution of sodium chloride to prepare a ½ NS solution?
    a. 125 mL
    b. 250 mL
    c. 375 mL
    d. 500 mL

98. Which of the following is the federal legend that must appear on all prescriptions?
    a. Caution: Federal law prohibits dispensing without a prescription
    b. Caution: Federal law prohibits the transfer of this prescription to anyone other than the intended
    c. Package not child resistant
    d. Warning: May be habit forming

99. Which of the following is not a side effect of decongestants?
    a. Decreased blood pressure
    b. Elevated blood pressure
    c. Increased heart stimulation
    d. Increased CNS stimulation

100. What is D5W?
    a. 5% distilled water
    b. 5% dextrose in water
    c. Discontinue 5% water
    d. Dispense for 5 weeks

PRACTICE EXAMINATION IV

Select the response that best answers the question.

1. You have received a medication order to prepare a 250-mL bag of NS with 1 g of Kefzol. The patient is to receive a 250-mg dose per hour. The infusion is calibrated at 10 gtt/mL. What flow rate is needed to deliver the dose?
    a. 1 gtt/min
    b. 10 gtt/min
    c. 15 gtt/min
    d. 20 gtt/min

2. Which process brings a drug from the administration site into the bloodstream?
   a. Absorption
   b. Distribution
   c. Metabolism
   d. Elimination

3. What is the generic name for Lotensin?
   a. Benazepril
   b. Enalapril
   c. Lisinopril
   d. Prinivil

4. How many inches inside a laminar airflow hood should one prepare a sterile product?
   a. 4 inches
   b. 6 inches
   c. 10 inches
   d. 12 inches

5. How many milliliters are in 1 L?
   a. 1 mL
   b. 100 mL
   c. 1000 mL
   d. 1,000,000 mL

6. Which drug classification of antibiotics should not be taken if the patient is allergic to penicillin?
   a. Aminoglycosides
   b. Cephalosporins
   c. Macrolides
   d. Quinolones

7. What is meant by the half-life of a drug?
   a. The amount of time it takes to dissolve a substance
   b. The amount of time it takes to dispense a package or container of medication
   c. The amount of time necessary to process one half of the number of prescriptions in a given day
   d. The amount of time it takes to eliminate one half of the drug in circulation

8. How many 500-mg doses can be prepared from a 10-g vial of cefazolin?
   a. 15
   b. 20
   c. 25
   d. 50

9. Which of the following drug classifications can be used to treat chronic pain?
   a. H$_2$ blockers
   b. MAOIs
   c. SSRIs
   d. TCAs

10. Which dosage form features a gelatin shell?
    a. Caplet
    b. Capsule
    c. Enema
    d. Suppository

11. Which of the following is considered a solid dosage form?
    a. Cream
    b. Emulsion
    c. Suspension
    d. Tablet

12. Which law is being violated if a drug is dispensed without a valid prescription?
    a. Controlled Substances Act of 1970
    b. Durham-Humphrey Amendment
    c. FDCA 1938
    d. OBRA 90

13. Which of the following is a calcium channel blocker?
    a. Atenolol
    b. Carvedilol
    c. Diltiazem
    d. Lisinopril

14. What does AWP stand for?
    a. Actual warehouse price
    b. Actual wholesale price
    c. Average wholesale price
    d. Average wholesale promotion

15. Which of the following respiratory medications is not a combination product?
    a. Advair
    b. Allegra D
    c. Combivent
    d. Singulair

16. Which of the following might be used to treat arthritis?
    a. Feverfew
    b. Ginger
    c. Ginkgo
    d. Glucosamine

17. When a pharmacy technician is performing geo-metric dilution, when does the technician add the most potent ingredient, which may also have the smallest weight or smallest volume, to the mortar?
    a. Anytime
    b. As the first ingredient
    c. As the last ingredient
    d. Intermittently during the compounding process

18. Which of the following factors does not affect the route of administration?
    a. Disease state
    b. Ease of administration
    c. Rate of action
    d. Shape of the dosage form

19. How many days will the following prescription last?

    Ampicillin 250 mg #40
    i cap PO qid ac and hs

    a. 5 days
    b. 8 days
    c. 10 days
    d. 20 days

20. Which process is the reducing of a substance to small, fine particles?
    a. Blending
    b. Comminution
    c. Sifting
    d. Tumbling

21. Which of the following drugs is safe to take for a headache if the patient has peptic ulcer disease?
    a. Acetaminophen
    b. Acetylsalicylic acid
    c. Ibuprofen
    d. Naproxen sodium

22. Which of the following drugs is the generic name for Micronase?
    a. Glimepiride
    b. Glipizide
    c. Glyburide
    d. Lispro

23. What is the generic name for Fosamax?
    a. Alendronate
    b. Calcitonin-salmon
    c. Etidronate
    d. Raloxifene

24. Which of the therapeutic equivalence codes states that the product meets the necessary bio-equivalence requirements?
    a. AA
    b. AB
    c. B
    d. BC

25. Which of the following is not an example of a dispersion?
    a. Emulsion
    b. Lotion
    c. Ointment
    d. Suppository

26. What is the generic name for Dilantin?
    a. Divalproex
    b. Gabapentin
    c. Phenytoin
    d. Valproic acid

27. Which of the following migraine preparations is a controlled substance?
    a. Butorphanol
    b. Sumatriptan
    c. Tramadol
    d. Zolmitriptan

28. What temperature is equivalent to 98.6°F?
    a. 35°C
    b. 36°C
    c. 37°C
    d. 38°C

29. Which of the following does not increase the level of cholesterol in the body?
    a. Corticosteroids
    b. Loop diuretics
    c. Nitroglycerin
    d. Thiazide diuretics

30. Which of the following drugs is the generic name for Glucotrol?
    a. Glimepiride
    b. Glipizide
    c. Glyburide
    d. Metformin

31. Which of the following drugs is not an SSRI?
    a. Fluoxetine
    b. Paroxetine
    c. Risperidone
    d. Sertraline

32. Which of the following would not be a reason for a prescription to be rejected by an insurance provider?
    a. Compounded drugs with one ingredient being a legend drug
    b. Incorrect NDC number
    c. Invalid ID number
    d. Prescription coverage has expired

33. What is the generic name for Zyprexa?
    a. Nefazodone
    b. Olopatadine
    c. Olanzapine
    d. Trazodone

34. A patient presents a prescription to the pharmacy for Ceclor 125 mg/5 mL with the directions of 1 tsp PO tid × 10 d. How much should be dispensed to the patient?
    a. 75 mL
    b. 100 mL
    c. 150 mL
    d. 200 mL

35. Which insulin has the longest duration of action?
    a. NPH insulin
    b. Lente insulin
    c. Regular insulin
    d. Ultralente insulin

36. What is the sensitivity of a Class A balance?
    a. 1 mg
    b. 6 mg
    c. 10 mg
    d. 20 mg

37. Which of the following is not a brand of verapamil?
    a. Calan
    b. Coreg
    c. Isoptin
    d. Verelan

38. Which dosage form is produced by compression?
    a. Capsule
    b. Lozenge
    c. Suppository
    d. Tablet

39. Which of the following products is not indicated as a smoking-cessation product?
    a. Habitrol
    b. NicoDerm
    c. Wellbutrin
    d. Zyban

40. What is the maximum number of refills for a Schedule IV drug if authorized by the physician?
    a. None
    b. Five
    c. 12
    d. Unlimited

41. What is the generic name for Micronase?
    a. Glimepiride
    b. Glipizide
    c. Glyburide
    d. Pioglitazone

42. Which of the following products is used to induce emesis?
    a. Emetrol
    b. Ipecac
    c. PEG
    d. Simethicone

43. How many grams of boric acid are required to make 4 fl oz of the following boric acid solution?

    Boric acid 50 g
    Purified water qs to make 1000 mL

    a. 0.006 g
    b. 0.06 g
    c. 0.6 g
    d. 6 g

44. What is the purpose of a loading dose of medication?
    a. To control costs
    b. To improve compliance
    c. To obtain a therapeutic level of the medication in the bloodstream as soon as possible
    d. To reduce side effects

45. What is the meaning of "w/v"?
    a. Number of grams per 1 mL
    b. Number of grams per 100 mL
    c. Number of micrograms per 100 mL
    d. Number of milligrams per 100 mL

46. If a patient has a dry, nonproductive cough, what classification of drug should the patient take?
    a. Antihistamine
    b. Antitussive
    c. Decongestant
    d. Expectorant

47. What drug is abbreviated "HCTZ"?
    a. Hycomine
    b. Hycodan
    c. Hydrochlorothiazide
    d. Hydrea

48. What is the percent equivalent of a 1:20 ratio?
    a. 0.05%
    b. 0.5%
    c. 5.0%
    d. 50%

49. What type of label is placed on medications to warn patients or provide additional information?
    a. Auxiliary label
    b. Patient product insert
    c. Patient profile
    d. Prescription label

50. Which of the following products is not used to treat hyperlipidemia?
    a. Aspirin
    b. Fibric acid derivatives
    c. HMG-CoA reductase inhibitors
    d. Metamucil

51. Which of the following is not an input device for a computer?
    a. Bar code technology
    b. Keyboard
    c. Printer
    d. Touchscreen applications

52. Which vitamin deficiency would result in rickets?
    a. Vitamin A
    b. Vitamin B_1
    c. Vitamin C
    d. Vitamin D

53. What is the meaning of CSAR?
    a. Controlled Studies Are Reviewed
    b. Controlled Substance Administration Record
    c. Controlled Substance Audit and Review
    d. Cost, Sales, Allocation, and Resources

54. Which of the following drugs does not need to be packaged in a child-resistant package?
    a. Digoxin
    b. Ibuprofen
    c. Nitroglycerin
    d. Simvastatin

55. Which of the following statements is not true concerning insulin?
    a. Glargine insulin should not be mixed with any other insulins.
    b. Injection sites need to be rotated.
    c. Regular and Lente insulins do not mix.
    d. When insulin is mixed, regular insulin should be drawn up after the first insulin in the syringe.

56. Zidovudine is to AZT as lamivudine is to _____ _____.
    a. a4c
    b. ddI
    c. d4T
    d. 3TC

57. Which of the following drugs should be taken with food?
    a. Amoxicillin
    b. Minocycline
    c. Nitrofurantoin
    d. Tetracycline

58. If 5000 mL of a substance weighs 6565 g, what is the specific gravity of the substance?
    a. 0.76
    b. 0.95
    c. 1.31
    d. 1.5

59. If a patient has a hepatic disorder, which organ is involved?
    a. Heart
    b. Kidney
    c. Liver
    d. Stomach

60. What does "U&C" mean when billing prescriptions?
    a. Unusual customer
    b. Unusual and customary
    c. Usual customer
    d. Usual and customary

61. Who may recommend an OTC product to a patient?
    a. All pharmacy technicians
    b. All PTCB-certified technicians
    c. All technicians who have completed continuing education in OTC products
    d. None of the above

62. The adult dose of a drug is 200 mg. What is the dose for a 5-month-old infant?
    a. 0.267 mg
    b. 0.667 mg
    c. 6.67 mg
    d. 66.7 mg

63. Which of the following drugs is not a selective 5-HT receptor agonist used to treat migraine headaches?
    a. Imitrex
    b. Maxalt
    c. Midrin
    d. Zomig

64. What is the percentage strength of a solution that is made by adding 100 mL of purified water to 600 mL of a 25% solution?
    a. 4.2%
    b. 12.5%
    c. 21.4%
    d. 30.00%

65. Which reference book contains the USP and NF drug standards and dispensing requirements?
    a. *Drug Topics Orange Book*
    b. *Drug Topics Red Book*
    c. *USP DI* Volume I
    d. *USP DI* Volume III

66. Which of the following products can be used as a smoking cessation product and as an antidepressant?
    a. Bupropion
    b. Nicotine
    c. Trazodone
    d. Zolpidem

67. Who makes notations in and signs Medication Administration Records (MARs) in an institution?
    a. Doctors
    b. Nurses
    c. Pharmacists
    d. Pharmacy technicians

68. Which of the following would be a correct DEA number for Dr. A. Shedlock?
    a. AB135426
    b. BS2456879
    c. FS1578926
    d. MS2254235

69. What assumption should a pharmacy technician make if she observes a white, fluffy precipitate in a 250-mL bag of D5W?
    a. The solution has been contaminated.
    b. The solution has been exposed to the cold.
    c. The solution has been exposed to bright light.
    d. The solution should be shaken to disperse the precipitate before dispensing.

70. How many refills may a physician order for a Schedule II drug?
    a. None
    b. One
    c. Five
    d. Unlimited refills in a 1-year time frame

71. For which of the following drugs is it mandatory that a customer receive a PPI?
    a. Amoxicillin
    b. Lithonate
    c. Premarin
    d. Synthroid

72. What do the three sets of numbers in an NDC number reflect?
    a. Drug manufacturer, drug product, and the year an NDA was filed
    b. Drug manufacturer, drug product, and package size
    c. Drug manufacturer, drug name, and drug strength
    d. None of the above

73. Which of the following drugs is not used for asthma?
    a. Albuterol
    b. Ipratropium
    c. INH
    d. Salmeterol

74. Which of the following solutions is the most diluted?
    a. 25%
    b. 20%
    c. 2.5%
    d. 0.25%

75. What is the meaning of "i gtt ou tid ud"?
    a. Instill one drop in each ear three times a day as directed.
    b. Instill one drop in each eye two times a day as directed.
    c. Instill one drop in each eye three times a day as needed.
    d. Instill one drop in each eye three times a day as directed.

76. Levothyroxine is to hypothyroidism as glyburide is to _____.
    a. ACE inhibitor
    b. Beta-blocker
    c. Oral hyperglycemic agent
    d. Oral hypoglycemic agent

77. How many milligrams are in "gr iss"?
    a. 32.5 mg
    b. 65 mg
    c. 97.5 mg
    d. 130 mg

78. Which of the following drugs is not used as a prophylactic product?
    a. Amoxicillin
    b. Imitrex
    c. Norgestimate–ethinyl estradiol
    d. Propranolol

79. How would one administer an "ung"?
    a. Orally
    b. Rectally
    c. Sublingually
    d. Topically

80. What does the term "overhead" refer to in business?
    a. All of the costs associated with a business
    b. Ceilings
    c. Inventory
    d. Payroll

81. How much of a D10W solution contains 100 g of dextrose?
    a. 0.01 L
    b. 0.1 L
    c. 1 L
    d. 2 L

82. In which schedule would you find the combination product oxycodone + acetaminophen?
    a. Schedule II
    b. Schedule III
    c. Schedule IV
    d. Schedule V

83. Which of the following terms is an indication for a potassium chloride supplement?
    a. Hyperkalemia
    b. Hypoglycemia
    c. Hypokalemia
    d. Hyponatremia

84. How many days does a pharmacy have to fill a prescription of Accutane?
    a. 1 day
    b. 7 days
    c. 30 days
    d. 180 days

85. Where would oxycodone with acetaminophen be stored in the pharmacy?
    a. In the refrigerator
    b. In the pharmacy safe
    c. With the "fast movers"
    d. With the pills and tablets

86. You have a solution of heparin 100,000 units/L with an infusion apparatus labeled 60 gtt/mL. What is the flow rate to deliver a dose of 20 units/minute?
    a. 3 gtt/min
    b. 12 gtt/min
    c. 15 gtt/min
    d. 20 gtt/min

87. How many drops per milliliter does a "mini-drip" system provide?
    a. 10 gtt/mL
    b. 15 gtt/mL
    c. 30 gtt/mL
    d. 60 gtt/mL

88. What does an 80/20 report tell a pharmacist or pharmacy technician?
    a. Products that have an 80% gross profit
    b. Products that have a 20% gross profit
    c. Drug products that reflect 80% of the pharmacy's purchasing dollars
    d. Controlled substances that represent 20% of the total number of prescriptions filled

89. Which of the following would not be a correct auxiliary label for a patient taking doxycycline?
    a. Avoid dairy products
    b. Avoid sunlight
    c. Not to be taken by pregnant women or children younger than age 9 years
    d. Take on an empty stomach

90. Which of the following drugs is not a beta-blocker?
    a. Coreg
    b. Inderal
    c. Procardia
    d. Tenormin

91. The cost of 100 tablets of a particular medication is $2.00. What would the retail price be if there were a 30% gross profit?
    a. $0.60
    b. $2.00
    c. $2.30
    d. $2.60

92. What units are used to measure electrolytes?
    a. mEq
    b. mg
    c. mL
    d. units

93. How many grams of 20% zinc oxide ointment would contain 10 g of zinc oxide?
    a. 5 g
    b. 10 g
    c. 20 g
    d. 50 g

94. Where would you prepare hazardous drugs in a pharmacy?
    a. In a biologic safety hood
    b. In a horizontal laminar airflow hood
    c. In a vertical laminar airflow hood
    d. On an ointment slab

95. Deficiency of which vitamin may result in scurvy?
    a. Vitamin A
    b. Vitamin B_1
    c. Vitamin C
    d. Vitamin D

96. What type of drug requires a DEA number?
    a. Controlled substance
    b. Investigational drug
    c. Legend drug
    d. OTC drug

97. Xanax is to anxiety as Lunesta is to _____ ____.
    a. Allergy
    b. Infection
    c. Inflammation
    d. Sleep

98. Rx: Codeine phosphate 30 mg/tsp
    Tussin syrup   30 mL
    Elixophyllin qs 240 mL
    Sig: 5 mL qid pc hs

    If 5 mL of Tussin syrup contains 100 mg of guaifenesin, how many milligrams of the drug would be taken daily?
    a. 2.5 mg
    b. 5 mg
    c. 10 mg
    d. 50 mg

99. What is the route of administration for a prescription with the directions "i supp pr q6h prn"?
    a. Orally
    b. Rectally
    c. Urethrally
    d. Vaginally

100. What type of solution is a total parenteral solution?
    a. Dialysis solution
    b. Hypotonic solution
    c. Hypertonic solution
    d. Isotonic solution

PRACTICE EXAMINATION V

Select the response that best answers the question.

1. What organ would be affected if a patient was experiencing rhinitis?
    a. Bladder
    b. Ear
    c. Eye
    d. Nose

2. What volume does a small-volume parenteral contain?
    a. 100 mL
    b. 250 mL
    c. 500 mL
    d. All the above

3. What process occurs when a drug blocks the activity of metabolic enzymes in the liver?
   a. Additive effects
   b. Inhibition
   c. Potentiation
   d. Synergism

4. The pharmacist asks you to prepare 250 mL of a 25% acetic acid solution. How much acetic acid would you need to make this preparation?
   a. 62.5 mg
   b. 6250 mg
   c. 62.5 g
   d. 6250 g

5. Which of the following dosage forms could a diabetic patient receive?
   a. Elixir
   b. Emulsion
   c. Spirits
   d. Syrups

6. Which organ can be affected by a condition of flutter?
   a. Esophagus
   b. Heart
   c. Intestine
   d. Kidneys

7. Which of the following auxiliary labels would not be appropriate for a prescription of sulfasalazine?
   a. Avoid sunlight
   b. Drink plenty of water
   c. Keep refrigerated
   d. May discolor urine

8. A pharmacy has 300 mL of a 50% solution; 200 mL is added to this solution to decrease the concentration. How many grams of active ingredient would be in the diluted solution?
   a. 7.5 g
   b. 30 g
   c. 150 g
   d. 300 g

9. How much of a 10% and 60% dextrose solution should be mixed to prepare 1 L of a 40% dextrose solution?
   a. 10%: 600 mL; 60%: 400 mL
   b. 10%: 500 mL; 60%: 500 mL
   c. 10%: 400 mL; 60%: 600 mL
   d. 10%: 300 mL; 60%: 700 mL

10. When opening a glass ampule, always use a gauze swab for which of the following reasons?
    a. To protect your finger from cuts
    b. To prevent contamination of the product inside the ampule
    c. To disinfect the ampule
    d. None of the above

11. How many inventory turns would a pharmacy experience if the initial inventory of the accounting period was $225,000, the final inventory of the period was $250,000, and the pharmacy had sales of $2.75 million?
    a. 12.22 turns
    b. 11.58 turns
    c. 11.00 turns
    d. 5.79 turns

12. A solution of haloperidol contains 2 mg/mL of active ingredient. How many grams are in 1 pint of this solution?
    a. 0.0096 g
    b. 0.096 g
    c. 0.96 g
    d. 9.6 g

13. How often should a patient change his or her Catapres TTS patch?
    a. Once per day
    b. Every other day
    c. Weekly
    d. Monthly

14. Which of the following is the generic name for Percocet?
    a. Acetaminophen + codeine
    b. Acetaminophen + hydrocodone
    c. Acetaminophen + oxycodone
    d. Acetaminophen + propoxyphene

15. A 44-lb child is to receive 4 mg of phenytoin per kilogram of body weight daily as a anticonvulsant. How many milliliters of pediatric phenytoin suspension containing 30 mg/5 mL should the child receive?
    a. 13.3 mL
    b. 50 mL
    c. 80 mL
    d. 176 mL

16. Which organization is concerned about employee safety?
    a. HIPAA
    b. TJC
    c. OBRA
    d. OSHA

17. Which dosage form is a clear, sweetened, flavored hydroalcoholic solution containing water and ethanol?
    a. Collodion
    b. Elixir
    c. Suspension
    d. Syrup

18. The abbreviation "ou" is found on a prescription. What does it mean?
    a. Both ears
    b. Both eyes
    c. Both feet
    d. Both hands

19. The product Infants' Mylicon Drops contains 2 g of simethicone in a 30-mL container. How many milligrams of the drug are contained in each teaspoonful dose?
    a. 0.33 mg
    b. 33 mg
    c. 333 mg
    d. 1000 mg

20. What is another term for hyperalimentation?
    a. Aseptic technique
    b. Dietary supplementation
    c. Extemporaneous compounding
    d. TPN

21. Which of the following ophthalmic products should be refrigerated?
    a. Apraclonidine
    b. Brimonidine
    c. Brinzolamide
    d. Latanoprost

22. What is the generic name for Avapro?
    a. Candesartan
    b. Irbesartan
    c. Losartan
    d. Valsartan

23. In how many direction(s) does air flow in a laminar flow hood?
    a. One
    b. Two
    c. Three
    d. Four

24. New OTC drugs are required to go through necessary phases. Which phase occurs when a final review is done on the ingredients of the agent in question and the public is able to give feedback?
    a. Phase I
    b. Phase II
    c. Phase III
    d. Phase IV

25. What is the generic name for Glucophage?
    a. Glimepiride
    b. Glipizide
    c. Glyburide
    d. Metformin

26. What factors should be considered when dealing with elderly patients?
    a. Auditory issues
    b. Chronic conditions
    c. Multiple medications
    d. All the above

27. Which of the following drugs is available as both a tablet and an IV solution?
    a. Accupril
    b. Capoten
    c. Monopril
    d. Vasotec

28. What should one tell a patient with a prescription of griseofulvin suspension?
    a. Be careful of sunlight; it may cause photosensitivity.
    b. Shake well.
    c. Store at room temperature.
    d. All the above.

29. Which of the following products is not available as a transdermal patch?
    a. Catapres
    b. Duragesic
    c. Nitroglycerin
    d. Tegretol

30. What is the nonproprietary name for Deltasone?
    a. Lithium
    b. Methylprednisolone
    c. Prednisolone
    d. Prednisone

31. Which answer best describes the information that should be included in a Schedule V sale log for C-V drugs sold without a prescription?
    a. Dispensing date, printed name, signature and address of buyer, name and quantity of the product sold, and the pharmacist's signature
    b. Dispensing date, signature and phone number of the buyer, product name, and product company with lot number
    c. Dispensing date, signature of the buyer, name and quantity of product sold, price of the product sold, and the lot number of the product sold
    d. Dispensing date, buyer signature, pharmacist signature, product name and amount, and the expiration date of the product

32. What should be done in preparing a prescription for etoposide?
    a. Flush the remaining contents down a sink or toilet
    b. Wear protective clothing if you are allergic to etoposide
    c. Place labels on the container so it has a professional appearance
    d. Prepare it in a biologic safety cabinet

33. Which of the following drugs is not an MAOI?
    a. Bupropion
    b. Phenelzine
    c. Selegiline
    d. Tranylcypromine

34. What would be the infusion rate for a 50-mg/mL magnesium sulfate solution to provide 1.2 g/hr?
    a. 0.4 mL/hr
    b. 2.5 mL/hr
    c. 20 mL/hr
    d. 24 mL/hr

35. Which of the following is not a cardiovascular medication?
    a. Coreg
    b. Diovan
    c. Evista
    d. Plavix

36. What is another term for a Master Formula Sheet?
    a. MAR
    b. MSDS
    c. Pharmacy compounding log
    d. Record log sheet

37. What body organ would be affected by hepatotoxicity?
    a. Intestines
    b. Kidneys
    c. Liver
    d. Thyroid

38. How would a prescriber write a prescription for "Zolpidem 5 mg at bedtime if needed"?
    a. Zolpidem 5 mg q hs prn
    b. Zolpidem 5 mg q hs ad
    c. Zolpidem 5 mg q 9 PM ad lib
    d. Zolpidem 5 mg q hs qs

39. What does ASHP mean?
    a. American Schools of Health Practices
    b. American Society of Health-System Pharmacists
    c. American Society of Hospital Pharmacists
    d. Association of Specialty Health Practitioners

40. What type of hypersensitivity reaction occurs when circulating antibodies of the IgG, IgM, or IgA class react with an antigen associated with a cell membrane?
    a. Type I
    b. Type II
    c. Type III
    d. Type IV

41. What is another term for suggested retail price?
    a. Discounted price
    b. List price
    c. Net price
    d. Sale price

42. A pharmacy must ensure that its pharmacy records are "readily retrievable" for a pharmacy inspector. This means they must be able to be produced within how much time?
    a. 24 hours
    b. 48 hours
    c. 72 hours
    d. 96 hours

43. Which of the following can be used to treat asthma?
    a. Beta-2 agonists
    b. Cromolyn
    c. Corticosteroids
    d. All the above

44. To which organization would an individual report a medication error?
    a. DEA
    b. FDA
    c. MedWatch
    d. State Board of Pharmacy

45. Drugs in which of the following classifications do not interact with phenobarbital?
    a. Beta-blockers
    b. H_2 antagonists
    c. TCAs
    d. Warfarin

46. What is the meaning of "prn"?
    a. As needed
    b. Per rectal needs
    c. Practical registered nurse
    d. Physician requires notice

47. Which dosage form may either be oil-in-water or water-in-oil?
    a. Emulsion
    b. Solution
    c. Suspension
    d. Syrup

48. What factor(s) influence the effect of a drug on an individual?
    a. Age
    b. Disease
    c. Gender
    d. All the above

49. A drug in which schedule of medication may be purchased as an "exempt narcotic"?
    a. Schedule II
    b. Schedule III
    c. Schedule IV
    d. Schedule V

50. Which body system would be affected by an anaphylactic reaction?
    a. Digestive
    b. Endocrine
    c. Respiratory
    d. Musculoskeletal

51. Which of the following medication(s) should not be taken with phenytoin?
    a. Fluoxetine
    b. Oral contraceptives
    c. Theophylline
    d. All the above

52. Where does one contract a nosocomial infection?
    a. At home
    b. In a hospital
    c. At school
    d. At work

53. Which of the following tasks do computers perform?
    a. Communication
    b. Input and output
    c. Processing and storage
    d. All the above

54. What does a red C indicate on a prescription?
    a. Prescription has been canceled by the physician.
    b. Prescription has been copied and transferred to another pharmacy.
    c. Prescription has been processed by the pharmacy and has been picked up by the patient.
    d. Prescription is a controlled substance.

55. Which of the following is the generic name for Capoten?
    a. Captopril
    b. Carvedilol
    c. Clonidine
    d. Clopidogrel

56. What is glaucoma?
    a. A bacterial infection of the eye
    b. A fungal infection of the eye
    c. A viral infection
    d. Increased pressure within the eye

57. Which of the following is not available as an OTC product?
    a. Chlorpheniramine
    b. Diphenhydramine
    c. Fexofenadine
    d. Loratadine

58. Which of the following classifications does not have a drug interaction with oral contraceptives?
    a. Antibiotics
    b. Anticonvulsants
    c. Antifungals
    d. Antihypertensives

59. Which type of diabetes can be controlled through exercise and diet?
    a. Gestational diabetes
    b. Secondary diabetes
    c. Type 1 diabetes
    d. Type 2 diabetes

60. What is another term for a "crash cart"?
    a. Code blue cart
    b. Code orange cart
    c. Code red cart
    d. Code yellow cart

61. Which form is used to document medication being administered to a patient?
    a. MAR
    b. MDR
    c. POS
    d. TAR

62. What document must be completed for every employee hired by a pharmacy?
    a. Application
    b. Background check
    c. I-9
    d. Reference check

63. What is a medication order called when it is presented to a community pharmacy?
    a. Inscription
    b. MAR
    c. Patient profile
    d. Prescription

64. What type of unit-dose system is referred to as *punch cards, bingo cards,* or *blister packs*?
    a. Blended unit-dose system
    b. Modified unit-dose system
    c. Modular cassette
    d. Multiple medication packages

65. What part of the laminar flow hood is responsible for removing contaminants?
    a. The blower
    b. The HEPA filter
    c. The recovery vent
    d. The side walls

66. What medication could be prescribed for a patient with a UTI?
    a. AZT
    b. HCTZ
    c. NTG
    d. SMZ-TMP DS

67. Depakote is to anticonvulsant as Celebrex is to _____.
    a. Antibiotic
    b. Antifungal
    c. Estrogen
    d. NSAID

68. What is the generic name for Prevacid?
    a. Esomeprazole
    b. Lansoprazole
    c. Omeprazole
    d. Pantoprazole

69. What is another name for a troche?
    a. Effervescent tablet
    b. Gelatin capsule
    c. Granule
    d. Lozenge

70. Which law is being violated if a pharmacist prepares a medication under unsanitary conditions?
    a. DSHEA of 1994
    b. FDCA of 1938
    c. OBRA 90
    d. HIPAA

71. Which of the following is not a sulfa drug?
    a. Azulfidine
    b. Azactam
    c. Bactrim
    d. Gantrisin

72. Which reference book is included in *USP DI* Volume III and contains the FDA's approved drug products?
    a. *American Drug Index*
    b. *Blue Book*
    c. *Orange Book*
    d. *Red Book*

73. If 1 g of dextrose provides 3.4 kcal, how many kilocalories will 200 mL of a 25% dextrose solution provide?
    a. 17 kcal
    b. 170 kcal
    c. 340 kcal
    d. 680 kcal

74. Which of the following is not a reason for a third-party claim to be rejected by an insurance carrier?
    a. Drug not covered
    b. Invalid identification number
    c. Generic drug dispensed
    d. Refill too soon

75. What term refers to fragments of a vial closure that contaminate a parenteral solution?
    a. Bevel
    b. Coring
    c. Hub
    d. Lumen

76. What is the brand name for lorazepam?
    a. Ativan
    b. Dalmane
    c. Klonopin
    d. Valium

77. What term describes directions to a pharmacist on a prescription?
    a. DAW indicator
    b. Inscription
    c. Subscription
    d. Signa

78. The larger the needle gauge, the _____ the diameter of the needle.
    a. Larger
    b. Longer
    c. Smaller
    d. Shorter

79. Which of the following terms is a set amount of money that must be paid by the patient before the insurer will cover additional expenses?
    a. Coinsurance
    b. Copayment
    c. Deductible
    d. Maximum allowable cost

80. What is the correct meaning for the signa in the following prescription?

    Timoptic 0.25% 15 mL
    i gtt ou bid

    a. Instill 1 drop in each ear twice per day.
    b. Instill 1 drop in each eye twice per day.
    c. Instill 1 drop in left eye twice per day.
    d. Instill 1 drop in left ear twice per day.

81. Which of the following medications may be used to treat type 2 diabetes?
    a. Estraderm
    b. Isordil
    c. Januvia
    d. Nexium

82. Which of the following medications is available over the counter?
    a. Boniva
    b. Lomotil
    c. Nasacort
    d. Zyrtec

83. Which schedules of controlled substances are monitored through prescription monitoring programs?
    a. Schedule II
    b. Schedule III
    c. Schedule IV
    d. All the above

84. What is the meaning of the pharmacy abbreviation "dtd"?
    a. Daylight time doses
    b. Do not take daily
    c. Give of such doses
    d. Of each

85. Which of the following units of measure for weight is the smallest?
    a. Gram
    b. Kilogram
    c. Microgram
    d. Milligram

86. Which of the following medications is not an antiviral medication?
    a. Symmetrel
    b. Zerit
    c. Zithromax
    d. Zovirax

87. Which of the following routes of administration is administration into a vein?
    a. IA
    b. IM
    c. IV
    d. SL

88. Which of the following medications may not be used to treat osteoporosis?
    a. Actonel
    b. Boniva
    c. Cordarone
    d. Fosamax

89. Which of the following diuretics would not require a prescription for potassium chloride to supplement potassium loss?
    a. Chlorthalidone
    b. Furosemide
    c. Hydrochlorothiazide
    d. Spironolactone

90. What is the meaning of NPI?
    a. National Pharmaceutical Institute
    b. National Pharmacopeia Index
    c. National Provider Identifier
    d. No Provider Identified

91. What is the basic unit of measurement of weight in the metric system?
    a. Gram
    b. Kilogram
    c. Microgram
    d. Milligram

92. What is the unit of measure for insulin?
    a. USP Units
    b. Milliequivalents
    c. Milliliters
    d. Milliosmoles

93. In which drug classification does carbamazepine belong?
    a. Antibiotic
    b. Anticonvulsant agent
    c. Antiparkinsonian agent
    d. Antipsychotic agent

94. To which schedule do anabolic steroids belong?
    a. II
    b. III
    c. IV
    d. V

95. What is the percentage of a 1:25 (w/v) solution?
    a. 0.04%
    b. 0.4%
    c. 4.0%
    d. 40.0%

96. Which of the following medications requires a prescription to treat diarrhea?
    a. Diphenoxylate
    b. Lactulose
    c. Loperamide
    d. Polyethylene glycol

97. Which of the following medications does not require a child-resistant container?
    a. APAP with codeine
    b. Hydrochlorothiazide
    c. Levothyroxine
    d. Nitroglycerin

98. Prescription of which of the following analgesic medications requires a physician to have a DEA number?
    a. Daypro
    b. Motrin
    c. Naprosyn
    d. Vicoprofen

99. Which of the following estrogen medications is not a transdermal dosage form?
    a. Climara
    b. Estraderm
    c. Premarin
    d. Vivelle

100. Prescriptions for drugs in which of the following controlled substance schedules may be faxed to a pharmacy?
    a. Schedule III
    b. Schedule IV
    c. Schedule V
    d. All the above

PRACTICE EXAMINATION VI

Select the response that best answers the question.

1. What part of Medicare reimburses a retail pharmacy for prescription medications?
   a. Part A
   b. Part B
   c. Part C
   d. Part D

2. What type of interaction occurs when a patient takes tetracycline with milk?
   a. Adverse effect
   b. Drug-drug
   c. Drug-food
   d. Synergistic

3. At what standard time would a patient receive a medication if the military time was 1800 hours?
   a. Midnight
   b. 8 AM
   c. 6 PM
   d. 8 PM

4. When does a "code blue" occur?
   a. When a patient is having a heart attack
   b. When a patient stops breathing
   c. A and B
   d. None of the above

5. Which of the following is not used to treat gastrointestinal problems?
   a. Antacids
   b. H_2 receptor agonists
   c. H_2 receptor antagonists
   d. Proton pump inhibitors

6. Which of the following products should not be chewed?
   a. Azatadine
   b. Azelastine
   c. Benzonatate
   d. Fexofenadine

7. What is the generic name for Retrovir?
   a. Didanosine
   b. Lamivudine
   c. Stavudine
   d. Zidovudine

8. How many minutes should a pharmacy be allowed to deliver a "stat" order?
   a. 5 to 15 minutes
   b. 5 to 30 minutes
   c. 30 to 45 minutes
   d. 45 to 60 minutes

9. Which formula for calculating a child's dose is the most accurate?
   a. Body surface area
   b. Clark's rule
   c. Fried's rule
   d. Young's rule

10. Convert 10° Celsius to degrees Fahrenheit.
    a. −12° F
    b. 32° F
    c. 42° F
    d. 50° F

11. An IV order calls for the addition of 45 mEq of $CaCO_3$ (calcium carbonate). You have a 25-mL vial of calcium carbonate 4.4 mEq/mL. How many milliliters of this concentration do you need to add to this IV solution?
    a. 5.6 mL
    b. 8.4 mL
    c. 10.2 mL
    d. 12.8 mL

12. Deficiency of what vitamin may result in beriberi?
    a. Vitamin A
    b. Vitamin B_1
    c. Vitamin C
    d. Vitamin D

13. Who is the person in whose name an insurance policy is held?
    a. Beneficiary
    b. Dependent
    c. Subscriber
    d. Patient

14. Drugs in what classification may yield side effects such as dry mouth, difficult urination, or constipation?
    a. Alpha-blockers
    b. Anticholinergics
    c. Beta-blockers
    d. Cholinergics

15. It is recommended that 25 mg/kg of a drug be given q6h to an infant weighing 13.2 lb. How many milligrams of a drug would be used for each dose?
    a. 75 mg
    b. 150 mg
    c. 330 mg
    d. 600 mg

16. In this formula, how much talc is needed to fill 120 g of the compound?

Nupercainal ointment	4%
Zinc oxide	20%
Talc	2%

    a. 1200 mg
    b. 1500 mg
    c. 2400 mg
    d. 120 g

17. Which of the following is not a method to reduce hypertension?
    a. Increase physical inactivity to regular aerobic physical activity
    b. Increase the amount of sleep an individual receives at night
    c. Reduce high sodium intake to moderate sodium intake
    d. Reduce excess alcohol consumption to moderate alcohol consumption

18. The medications Diovan HCT, Dyazide, Hyzaar, and Zestoretic are combination products used in the treatment of cardiovascular disease. Which medication is found in all of them?
    a. Hydrochlorothiazide
    b. Lisinopril
    c. Triamterene
    d. Valsartan

19. Which of the following is an antidote for an overdose of heparin?
    a. Coumadin
    b. Enoxaparin
    c. Phytonadione
    d. Protamine sulfate

20. What is the percent equivalent of a 1:10 ratio?
    a. 0.01%
    b. 0.1%
    c. 1.0%
    d. 10.0%

21. Which of the following pieces of information is required on a medication order for a patient in a hospital but not for a prescription being filled at a retail pharmacy?
    a. Medical record number
    b. Patient's name
    c. Physician's name
    d. Name and strength of medication

22. What does MDI mean?
    a. Medical diagnosis included
    b. Medical doctor under investigation
    c. Metered-dose inhaler
    d. Multidose inhaler

23. Which term refers to the vehicle that contains a dissolved drug?
    a. Solute
    b. Solution
    c. Solvent
    d. Syrup

24. What term refers to an abnormal heartbeat?
    a. Arrhythmia
    b. Bradycardia
    c. Flutter
    d. Tachycardia

25. How much hydrocortisone is found in a 1-oz tube of hydrocortisone 1% cream?
    a. 0.3 mg
    b. 3.0 mg
    c. 0.3 g
    d. 3.0 g

26. Who licenses pharmacists in each state?
    a. DEA
    b. FDA
    c. Federal government
    d. State board of pharmacy

27. What is fibromyalgia?
    a. Brittle hair and nails
    b. Chronic pain in the muscles
    c. Inflammation of tendon
    d. Lymph node disease

28. What is the minimum weighable quantity for a Class A balance?
    a. 120 mg
    b. 150 mg
    c. 250 mg
    d. 500 mg

29. What type of dosage form is prepared using the "punch method"?
    a. Capsules
    b. Emulsions
    c. Suppositories
    d. Tablets

30. What type of documentation does OSHA require for pharmacies that handle hazardous chemicals?
    a. Manufacturer Safety Documentation Sheets
    b. Manufacturer Sheets for Documentation of Safety
    c. Material Safety Data Sheets
    d. Mixture Safety Documentation Sheets

31. Where should a patient store a prescription of liquid amoxicillin suspension?
    a. In a bathroom vanity
    b. In a kitchen cupboard
    c. In the refrigerator
    d. Does not matter where it is stored

32. A pharmacy wants to mark up a product by 30%. How much would an item with this markup cost if its original cost was $4.50?
    a. $5.85
    b. $6.23
    c. $6.40
    d. $7.10

33. What is the generic name for Depakote?
    a. Divalproex
    b. Gabapentin
    c. Primidone
    d. Valproic acid

34. Which of the following is not found on a Master Formula Sheet used in compounding?
    a. Amount of ingredient needed
    b. Color of ingredient
    c. Manufacturer's lot number and expiration date
    d. Name of individual who weighed or measured ingredient

35. What is the meaning of "ou" on a prescription?
    a. Each ear
    b. Each eye
    c. Left eye
    d. Right ear

36. What piece of equipment reduces the risk of contamination when IV admixtures are prepared?
    a. Foot pedal sinks
    b. Humidifiers
    c. Laminar flow hoods
    d. Ultraviolet lighting

37. What type of formulary is a limited list of drugs?
    a. Closed formulary
    b. Open formulary
    c. Restricted formulary
    d. None of the above

38. What type of copayment is a different dollar amount based on the type of drug being dispensed?
    a. Fixed copayment
    b. Percentage copayment
    c. Variable copayment
    d. None of the above

39. How often is the *Physicians' Desk Reference* published?
    a. Biannually
    b. Biennially
    c. Every 6 months
    d. Yearly

40. What is the meaning of the word root *osteo*?
    a. Artery
    b. Bone
    c. Cell
    d. Muscle

41. A patient has been ordered PB $\frac{1}{4}$ gr; how many 15-mg tablets should the patient receive?
    a. 1
    b. 2
    c. 3
    d. 4

42. A pharmacy technician is preparing heparin 25,000 units in 500 mL of D5W. The appropriate concentration on the label should read _____.
    a. 50 units/mL
    b. 75 units/mL
    c. 100 units/mL
    d. 125 units/mL

43. How many 2-tsp doses can be prepared from 1 L of a solution?
    a. 50
    b. 100
    c. 500
    d. 1000

44. Which method of administration is used to provide medication to an unconscious patient?
    a. Inunction
    b. Inhalation
    c. Parenteral
    d. Peroral

45. What is the purpose of the DEA?
    a. Accepting NDAs from manufacturers
    b. Enforcing the Controlled Substances Act of 1970
    c. Licensing pharmacists
    d. Overseeing the MedWatch program

46. Which liquid form is a dispersion in which one liquid is dispersed in another immiscible liquid?
    a. Emulsion
    b. Lotion
    c. Ointment
    d. Suspension

47. Who may accept new prescriptions phoned in from a physician's office according to federal law?
    a. Pharmacists
    b. Pharmacy aides
    c. Pharmacy clerks
    d. Pharmacy technicians

48. Which term on a prescription is an instruction to the pharmacist?
    a. Inscription
    b. Rx
    c. Signa
    d. Subscription

49. Why are amber vials used to package medications?
    a. To clearly identify oral products from topical products
    b. To prevent an individual from identifying a medication
    c. To prevent moisture from getting inside the container
    d. To protect the medication from ultraviolet light and possible degradation

50. What components would be found in total nutrient admixture?
    a. Amino acids, dextrose, lipids
    b. Amino acids, dextrose, proteins
    c. Amino acids, dextrose, vitamins
    d. Amino acids, dextrose, minerals, vitamins

51. Which law is being violated if an employer discriminates against a potential employee because of medical reasons that would not prevent him or her from properly performing the job?
    a. ADA
    b. Any Willing Provider
    c. OSHA
    d. Prescription Drug Equity Act

52. Which of the following drugs is not a macrolide?
    a. Azithromycin
    b. Clarithromycin
    c. Doxycycline
    d. Erythromycin-sulfisoxazole

53. What does IV mean?
    a. Intravenous
    b. Intravenous piggyback
    c. Intravenous push
    d. Involuntary

54. What is the primary source of medication for community pharmacies?
    a. Chain pharmacy warehouses
    b. GPOs
    c. Manufacturers and wholesalers
    d. Store-to-store vendors

55. Who develops the formulary for a hospital?
    a. Board of directors of the hospital
    b. FDA
    c. GPO
    d. P&T committee

56. Which medication should be dispensed to a pregnant woman with hypertension?
    a. Lisinopril
    b. Methyldopa
    c. Nifedipine
    d. Verapamil

57. What does "qsad" mean on a prescription?
    a. A sufficient quantity
    b. A sufficient quantity for the right ear
    c. A sufficient quantity to make
    d. To make for the right ear

58. Which reference book is the official compendium of pharmaceutical products in the United States?
    a. *Facts and Comparisons*
    b. *Physicians' Desk Reference*
    c. *Remington's Pharmaceutical Sciences*
    d. *USP-NF*

59. What is the purpose of a Group Purchasing Organization?
    a. Negotiates prices for hospital pharmacies
    b. Purchases medications for hospital pharmacies
    c. Purchases medications for community pharmacies
    d. Purchases medications for managed care pharmacies

60. How long must controlled substance records be retained according to federal law?
    a. 6 months
    b. 1 year
    c. 2 years
    d. 7 years

61. Which gland influences water balance, body temperature, appetite, and emotions?
    a. Hypothalamus
    b. Pancreas
    c. Thymus
    d. Thyroid

62. Which of the following drug classifications would use pulse dosing?
    a. Antibiotics
    b. Anticonvulsants
    c. Antidepressants
    d. Antifungal

63. Which pharmacy law clearly defined adulteration and misbranding?
    a. Pure Drug Act of 1906
    b. Food, Drug, and Cosmetic Act of 1938
    c. Durham-Humphrey Amendment
    d. Poison Control Act of 1970

64. Waht type of drug classification ends in "-pril"?
    a. ACE inhibitors
    b. Benzodiazepines
    c. Corticosteroids
    d. H_2 antagonists

65. What advice should not be given to a patient taking penicillin products?
    a. Do not take with juices or colas
    b. May cause drowsiness
    c. Take on an empty stomach
    d. Take with water

66. How much gentian violet is in 100 mL of a 1:10,000 solution?
    a. 0.01 mg
    b. 10 mg
    c. 0.01 g
    d. 10 g

67. A drug is available in the following strengths and dosage forms: 125-mg tablets, 250-mg capsules, 125-mg/5-mL liquid. A child weighs 55 lb; the recommended dose is 10 mg/kg/24 hr, and the drug is to be given in either 6- or 12-hour intervals. Which of the following would not be an appropriate regimen?
    a. One 125-mg tablet q12h
    b. One 250-mg capsule q12h
    c. 1 tsp of 125 mg/5 mL liquid q12h
    d. One half of a 125-mg tablet q6h

68. A dermatologist prescribes 2 oz of the following compound:

    LCD   2%
    Salicylic acid   5%
    Yellow petrolatum   qs ad

    The pharmacy prepares a 500-g bulk container and repackages it in 2-oz containers. How much salicylic acid is needed to compound 500 g?
    a. 0.5 g
    b. 2.5 g
    c. 5 g
    d. 25 g

69. A manufacturer's invoice totals $500.00 with the terms 3% net. How much should be remitted to the manufacturer if it is paid in 30 days?
    a. $15.00
    b. $150.00
    c. $485.00
    d. $500.00

70. A patient is to receive 1 L of D5/0.45 NS with 20 mEq solution over 24 hours. What is the flow rate?
    a. 21 mL/hr
    b. 24 mL/hr
    c. 41 mL/hr
    d. 84 mL/hr

71. What color C should be stamped on controlled-substance prescriptions?
    a. Black
    b. Blue
    c. Green
    d. Red

72. What type of mortar and pestle should be used in mixing liquid compounds?
    a. Glass
    b. Latex
    c. Porcelain
    d. Wedgwood

73. What is the markup rate for a prescription that costs $35.00 and retails for $50.00?
    a. 30%
    b. 43%
    c. 57%
    d. 70%

74. An IV solution is to be infused over a 12-hour period. The total exact volume is 800 mL. What would be the infusion rate?
    a. 0.56 mL/min
    b. 1.11 mL/min
    c. 2.7 mL/min
    d. None of the above

75. You have a 10% solution of dextrose. How many grams of dextrose are in 500 mL of this solution?
    a. 50 mg
    b. 500 mg
    c. 5000 mg
    d. 50 g

76. How many 5-gr tablets are required to make 650 mL of a 1:200 solution?
    a. 5
    b. 10
    c. 15
    d. 20

77. On the state board examination, a label shows that the medication is dispensed in a 4-oz bottle and is a 5% solution. How much medication is present in the bottle?
    a. 6 mg
    b. 24 mg
    c. 6 g
    d. 24 g

78. What is the flow rate to be used to infuse 1000 mL of NS over 4 hours if the set delivers 10 gtt/mL?
    a. 25 gtt/min
    b. 35 gtt/min
    c. 41 gtt/min
    d. 82 gtt/min

79. Two tablespoonfuls of 85% boric acid solution are diluted to 10%. How many 3-oz bottles will the technician be able to fill with the diluted solution?
    a. One
    b. Two
    c. Four
    d. Eight

80. What does Syrup USP contain?
    a. Alcohol in water
    b. Oleaginous fluid in water
    c. PEG in water
    d. Sucrose in water

81. Which of the following statements is false regarding the Isotretinoin Safety and Risk Management Act of 2004?
    a. Females are required to have monthly pregnancy tests.
    b. Patients are required to undergo monthly education regarding the medication.
    c. Prescriptions can be written for a 90-day supply.
    d. Prescriptions cannot be telephoned to the pharmacy from the physician's office.

82. Which of the following is the generic name for Omnicef?
    a. Cefdinir
    b. Cefotaxime
    c. Cefprozil
    d. Ceftriaxone

83. Which of the following medications is an example of a carbacephem?
    a. Azactam
    b. Invanz
    c. Lorabid
    d. Primaxin

84. Which of the following drugs is a ketolide?
    a. Dynabac
    b. Keflex
    c. Ketek
    d. Velosef

85. Which of the following medications is not a protease inhibitor?
    a. Agenase
    b. Crixivan
    c. Invirase
    d. Sustiva

86. What is the route of administration for heparin?
    a. IA
    b. IM
    c. IV
    d. Oral

87. What is the infusion rate in milliliters per hour if a total of 500 mL is infused over 4 hours?
    a. 100 mL/hr
    b. 125 mL/hr
    c. 500 mL/hr
    d. 2000 mL/hr

88. Which classification of drugs has interactions with many foods and OTC products?
    a. MAOIs
    b. MOAs
    c. SSRIs
    d. TCAs

89. Which of the following medications is not a bisphosphonate used to treat osteoporosis?
    a. Actonel
    b. Boniva
    c. Fosamax
    d. Miacalcin

90. Which of the following suffixes designates that a drug is a calcium channel blocker?
    a. -dipine
    b. -mycin
    c. -olone
    d. -pril

91. Which of the following may be a side effect of an antihistamine?
    a. Drowsiness
    b. Rapid heartbeat
    c. Stomach distress
    d. Watery eyes

92. What is an ongoing, systematic process for monitoring, evaluating, and improving the quality of pharmacy services?
    a. Peer review
    b. Pharmacy certification
    c. Process validation
    d. Quality assurance

93. Which of the following is not required on a prescription label?
    a. Name and address of the pharmacy
    b. Name of the prescriber
    c. Serial number of the prescription
    d. Telephone number of the patient

94. What is the maximum number of tablets that can be taken in 1 day with the directions "1–2 tabs PO q4-6h prn pain"?
    a. 4 tablets
    b. 6 tablets
    c. 8 tablets
    d. 12 tablets

95. What does the computer insurance error message "patient not found" or "invalid ID number" indicate?
    a. The customer is not a legitimate patient.
    b. The medication is not covered under the plan.
    c. The patient does not appear to be enrolled in the insurance program.
    d. The patient's condition is not covered under the prescription plan.

96. Which of the following medications should be prepared in a biologic safety cabinet?
    a. Etoposide
    b. IV solution containing insulin
    c. IV solution of gentamycin
    d. Skin cream

97. A mother is waiting for an antibiotic prescription of amoxicillin suspension for her child and asks the pharmacy technician what she should give her child for a fever. What should the pharmacy technician do?
    a. Inform the pharmacist of the parent's question.
    b. Offer to call the physician for a prescription to reduce a child's fever.
    c. Recommend children's aspirin to the mother.
    d. Tell the mother to apply cold compresses to the child's forehead.

98. Which of the following is an indication of Zofran?
    a. Constipation
    b. Diarrhea
    c. Migraine headache
    d. Nausea and vomiting

99. Which of the following provides regulations for compounding sterile preparations?
    a. Pure Food and Drug Act
    b. Food, Drug, and Cosmetic Act
    c. MSDS
    d. USP <797>

100. Which of the following would be appropriate directions for Ambien?
    a. i tab PO q am
    b. i tab PO q hs
    c. i tab sl q hs
    d. i tab PO tid prn anxiety

Pharmacy Technician Certification Examination Test-Taking Skills

PREPARE FOR THE TEST

- Know exactly what you will be tested on. Review test outlines if available.
- Study all key topics that will appear on the examination.
- Spread out your review over a period of weeks. Focused reviews over time are more effective than cramming.
- Outline your text and mark topics that need a more concentrated review.
- Try to predict questions that may be on the test, then test your skills in answering them.

ON THE DAY OF THE TEST

- Get enough sleep the night before the test. Make sure you have gotten adequate sleep the week before the test.
- Arrive early and choose a comfortable working area.
- Dress casually and comfortably. Take extra time planning appropriate clothes.
- Arrive prepared with necessary supplies (pencils, nonprogrammable calculator, admission ticket for the examination, and personal identification).

AS YOU TAKE THE TEST

- Listen, read, and follow the directions carefully.
- Look over the test before answering any questions. Scanning the test will provide you with key information about the scope and difficulty of the test.

- First complete the sections that are easiest for you.
- Answer the questions in order, but postpone questions that challenge you until later in the test. Answer the harder questions later.
- On your second pass through the test, ignore the answered questions and focus only on the questions you did not answer.
- Never leave a question unanswered; there is no penalty for guessing. (Time management is a key to success; it is to your advantage to answer all the items on the test.)
- Change your answers only when you are certain you made a mistake. Your first answer is usually the correct one.

TIPS FOR MULTIPLE-CHOICE QUESTIONS

- Remember that there is only one preferred answer even though more than one answer may appear to be correct.
- Use the process of elimination when you do not know the answer. Eliminate the most obviously wrong answer first, then the second, and then make your best decision between the last two choices.
- If you are still unsure about which is the correct answer, select the longer or more descriptive answer of the remaining answer set.
- If the answer set presents a range of numbers, eliminate the highest and lowest, and then select from the middle range of numbers.

- Slow down when you see negative words in the question. Look for words such as *not, except,* and so on. In this case, you need to identify the false statement instead of the true statement.

- Items that contain "absolutes" such as *always, never, must, all,* and *none* severely limit the meaning of the item. Statements that contain absolutes are usually incorrect.

Pharmacy Technician Certification Examination Information

Certification is the process by which a nongovernmental association or agency grants recognition to an individual who has met certain predetermined qualifications specified by that association or agency. The goal of the certification program of the Pharmacy Technician Certification Board (PTCB) is to enable pharmacy technicians to work more effectively with pharmacists to offer greater patient care and service. The PTCB is responsible for the development and implementation of policies related to national certification for pharmacy technicians.

PROFESSIONAL EXAMINATION SERVICE

The Professional Examination Service (PES), the PTCB's contracted testing company, is a nonprofit testing company founded in 1941. The PES specializes in the development and administration of national certification and licensure examinations. The PES's primary operating principle is to develop examinations of the highest quality and reliability. Examinations are developed using the standards established by the National Commission for Certifying Agencies, the American Psychological Association, and the U.S. Equal Employment Opportunity Commission as guidelines.

CERTIFICATION

There are two parts to being a certified pharmacy technician (CPhT). First, pharmacy technicians must sit for and pass the national Pharmacy Technician Certification Examination (PTCE). After a pharmacy technician has passed the examination, he or she may use the designation "CPhT." Second, to continue to hold certification, a CPhT is required to obtain 20 hours of continuing education for recertification within 2 years of original certification or previous recertification. For more information regarding certification, visit the PTCB Web site (http://www.ptcb.org).

RECERTIFICATION

Renewal of certification is required every 2 years. During the 2-year certification period, a CPhT must earn 20 hours of pharmacy-related continuing education; 1 of the 20 hours must be in pharmacy law. Approximately 60 days before the recertification date, the PTCB will mail a recertification packet to the candidate's mailing address on file. For more information on recertification, visit http://www.ptcb.org and download a copy of *PTCB's Recertification Requirements and Guidelines.*

ELIGIBILITY REQUIREMENTS

You must have received a high school diploma, a General Educational Development (GED) certificate, or the foreign equivalent by the application receipt deadline and must never have been convicted of a felony to sit for the PTCE.

PHARMACY TECHNICIAN CERTIFICATION EXAMINATION CANDIDATE ATTESTATION

1. This examination and the test questions contained herein are the exclusive property of the Pharmacy Technician Certification Board.
2. This examination and the items contained herein are protected by copyright law.
3. No part of this examination may be copied or reproduced in part or whole by any means whatsoever, including memorization.
4. My participation in any irregularity occurring during this examination, such as giving or obtaining unauthorized information or aid, as evidenced by observation or subsequent analysis, may result in termination of my participation, invalidation of the results of my examination, or other appropriate action.
5. Future discussion or disclosure of the contents of the examination orally, in writing, or by any other means is prohibited.
6. My signature below indicates that I have read and understood the statement of confidentiality. Failure to comply can result in termination of my participation, invalidation of the results of my examination, or other appropriate action.
7. I understand that during this examination, I may *not* communicate with other candidates, refer to any materials other than those provided to me, or assist or obtain assistance from any person. Failure to comply with these requirements may result in the invalidation of my examination results as well as other appropriate action.
8. Under penalty of perjury, I declare that the information provided in my examination application and any required accompanying documentation is true and complete. I also declare that I have received a high school diploma (or GED certificate) by the application deadline for this examination and, furthermore, that I have never been convicted of a felony.
9. My signature below and/or on my answer sheet for this examination indicates that I have read and understood the attestation statement. I am aware that failure to comply with the outlined requirements will result in serious consequences,

including the invalidation of my examination results.

REVOCATION POLICY

Basis for revocation: The certification of an individual may be revoked by the PTCB for any of the following reasons:

- Documented material deficiency in the current knowledge base necessary to achieve pharmacy technician certification
- Documented gross negligence or intentional misconduct in the performance of services as a pharmacy technician
- Conviction of a felony or a crime involving moral turpitude (including but not limited to the illegal sale, distribution, or use of controlled substances and other prescription drugs)
- Irregularity in taking, cheating on, or failing to abide by the rules regarding confidentiality of the PTCE (including postexamination conduct)
- Failure to cooperate with the PTCB during the investigation of another CPhT
- Making false or misleading statements in connection with certification or recertification

For additional information on the procedure for Revocation of Certification, contact the PTCB at 202-429-7576, http://www.ptcb.org, or 2215 Constitution Avenue, NW, Washington, DC 20037.

AMERICANS WITH DISABILITIES ACT

Arrangements for persons with disabilities will be made on request in conformance with the Americans with Disabilities Act (ADA). Physicians or other professionals submitting documentation in support of your request for accommodation may be contacted by the PTCB for clarification of any information provided in regard to your testing needs. If you have a documented disability (including a visual, orthopedic, or hearing impairment; health impairment; learning disability; emotional disability; or multiple disabilities) and need modification to the usual testing conditions, you may request special testing accommodations (e.g., magnifying lens) to take the national PTCE. You will still be required to take the examination on regularly scheduled national test dates.

On the application, fill in the appropriate space in Box 18 that identifies the accommodation you are requesting, including extra time if needed. If you are requesting an accommodation other than those listed on the application, fill in the space for "Other" and provide a specific description of your needs. Appropriate documentation must be enclosed with your application and must sufficiently explain your disability and the need for the accommodation(s). You may include a letter from an appropriate professional (e.g., physician, psychologist, occupational therapist, educational specialist) or evidence of prior diagnosis or accommodation (e.g., special education services). Previous school records may also be submitted to document your disability. Any professional providing documentation should know of your disability, have diagnosed or evaluated you, or have provided the accommodation for you.

The documentation letter you obtain from that professional must be on official stationery and include the following information:

1. Identification of the specific disability or diagnosis
2. The approximate date when the disability was first diagnosed or identified
3. A brief history of the disability
4. Identification of the tests or protocols used to confirm the diagnosis
5. A brief description of the disability
6. A description of past accommodations made for the disability
7. An explanation of the need for the testing accommodation(s)
8. Signature and title of the professional

If you have been diagnosed as having an emotional disability, your letter from the appropriate professional should include identification of the DSM-IV classification of the diagnosis.

Your request for special accommodations will be reviewed, and the PES will notify you of the status and disposition of your request at least 5 weeks before the examination date. If you have specific questions regarding the provisions of a testing accommodation, please contact the PES at 475 Riverside Drive, New York, NY 10115 or at 877-782-2888 for details.

If you do not notify the PES of needed accommodations at the time of application, the accommodations will not be available at the time of the examination.

The PTCB acknowledges the provisions of the ADA and will offer the examination in a center and manner that is accessible to persons with disabilities or will offer alternative arrangements for candidates with disabilities.

AFFIRMATIVE ACTION

The PTCB does not discriminate against any individual because of race, gender, age, religion, disability, veteran status, or national origin. The PTCB and PES endorse the principles of equal opportunity. Eligibility criteria for examination and certification under the national pharmacy technician certification program are applied equally to all applicants regardless of race, religion, sex, national origin, veteran status, age, or disability.

PASSING SCORE

A panel of content experts establishes a passing score for the national PTCE using appropriate standard-setting procedures, under the guidance of the PES. The passing score for the PTCE is criterion referenced rather than normative; that is, it is based on a standard of performance that experts in the profession have determined to be acceptable for certification. It is not based on a "curve," as are some academic tests.

Candidates must obtain a scaled score of at least 650 to pass the PTCE. The passing score was established by a panel of content experts who used the modified-Angoff method. According to this method, each question is individually evaluated and rated by the panelists. Panelists estimate the percentage of qualified candidates who will answer each item correctly. The overall passing score is computed by averaging the panelists' ratings. The PTCB Certification Council recommends the passing score to the Board of Governors.

To ensure the security and integrity of the PTCE, multiple forms of the examination with different questions are used in different years. The passing score is not set as a specific raw score or number of questions answered correctly because some of these examination forms may be slightly easier or more difficult than other forms. Because of the variations in difficulty, the PTCE is equated. After the test forms have been equated, the raw scores are converted to scaled scores, which are equivalent for all administrations of the PTCE. Thus a given scaled score reflects the same level of ability regardless of the form of the PTCE that was taken. The range of total scaled scores for the PTCE is 300 to 900.

Equating is a statistical process by which scores on different forms of the PTCE are calibrated onto a common scale. Equating ensures that candidates of comparable proficiency will be likely to obtain approximately the same-scaled scores regardless of fluctuations in the overall difficulty level from one examination administration to another.

After each examination administration, individual test items are evaluated for their performance. Items identified as being ambiguous may be scored with multiple correct answers with no penalty to the candidates.

Many quality-control procedures are used during the scoring process to ensure the accuracy of score reports. Answer sheets are electronically scored and the data stored on computer files from which score reports are generated. A preliminary item analysis is conducted and reviewed by the PTCB Certification Council to ensure that the examination items perform as expected and are psychometrically sound. In addition, comments from candidates on examination questions are considered at this time. This review allows adjustments to scoring if there are flawed test items. All the answer sheets are scored after the production of a final scoring key. Score reports are then printed and mailed.

Each candidate will receive a score report that will provide feedback from the three main function areas of the examination content outline. This is done to give the candidate an idea of how well he or she performed in each area and to identify areas of weakness. The passing score, however, is based on the candidate's performance on all questions. There is no passing score for each of the functions.

RECOGNITION OF CERTIFICATION

After you have met all eligibility requirements and have passed the national PTCE, you may use the designation "CPhT" after your name. CPhTs have demonstrated their knowledge and skills related to the work of pharmacy technicians. A certificate and wallet card will be sent to newly certified pharmacy technicians approximately 60 days after their certification examination. Certification is valid for 2 years. CPhT designation lapel pins and uniform patches may also be purchased.

A listing of CPhTs will be maintained by the PTCB and may be reported in its publications.

CONFIDENTIALITY OF SCORES

The application to take the national PTCE constitutes written authorization for the test developer to release that candidate's scores to the PTCB and to the candidate only. Access to candidate scores is limited to staff members at the PTCB and PES who are involved in the production and mailing of these reports. Group performance data will be used by the PES, the PTCB, or others designated by the PTCB for purposes of research and development and reporting to the profession. Individual test scores are provided to the candidate only.

RECERTIFICATION

CPhTs are required to complete 20 hours of pharmacy-related continuing education (1 hour must be in pharmacy law) during each 2-year certification period. For more information regarding the recertification process, download a copy *PTCB's Recertification Requirements and Guidelines.*

PERSONAL INFORMATION UPDATE

Each examination candidate must notify the PES in writing of any changes in name or address. Changes in name must be accompanied by appropriate documentation (e.g., notarized copy of marriage certificate, divorce decree). The PES cannot notify you of examination admission or test results if your information is not current.

PREPARING FOR THE EXAMINATION

The national PTCE applies to all practice settings. In preparing for the national PTCE, familiarity with the material contained in any basic pharmacy technician training manuals or books may be helpful. Your supervising pharmacist may also be helpful in designing a study plan. The PTCB does not endorse, recommend, or sponsor any review course, manuals, or books for the PTCB examination.

The PTCB encourages pharmacy technicians to visit the "Exam Information" portion of the PTCB Web site (http://www.ptcb.org). Candidates are able to access a full-length practice test, a list of texts used to assist in writing questions for the examination, and a "Useful Numbers" section that provides the contact numbers for publishers of examination study materials.

FREQUENTLY ASKED QUESTIONS REGARDING COMPUTER-BASED EXAMINATIONS

WHY DID PTCB CHANGE FROM PENCIL-AND-PAPER EXAMINATIONS TO COMPUTER-BASED TESTING?

The implementation of computer-based testing (CBT) strengthens PTCB's commitment to serving the pharmacy technician profession through a valid and reliable computer-based examination process. CBT provides numerous benefits to candidates, educators, and other PTCB stakeholders, including availability of examination results within a few weeks of testing; increased flexibility, that is, more choices of when and where to take the examination; scheduling flexibility, allowing candidates to reschedule up to 24 hours before the examination; and professional, state-of-the-art, distraction-free testing centers.

DO ALL CANDIDATES TAKE THE SAME EXAMINATION, OR DOES EACH CANDIDATE TAKE A DIFFERENT EXAMINATION?

Each candidate will be presented with a unique set of test items, but all candidates will be tested on the same subject matter based on PTCB test specifications.

DOES IT TAKE MORE TIME TO COMPLETE THE COMPUTERIZED EXAMINATION COMPARED WITH THE PAPER-AND-PENCIL VERSION?

No. PTCB's examination in CBT format will take less time to complete than the paper-and-pencil version. There is no test booklet or answer sheet to manage, and there are no "bubbles" to fill in with a pencil.

WHEN ARE THE COMPUTERIZED EXAMINATION RESULTS AVAILABLE?

When candidates complete their examination, they will receive a printout that indicates the date their examination results will be available. Individual examination results will be available based on the date that each candidate tests. They will be available on a rolling basis and can be seen online and will be mailed to the candidate within a few weeks of the test date.

WHAT IS PTCB'S POLICY FOR RETAKING THE EXAMINATION AFTER AN UNSUCCESSFUL ATTEMPT?

Candidates who fail the examination will not be allowed to retake the examination during the same testing window. These candidates will be required to apply to take the PTCE in a future testing window or at least 90 days after their initial attempt.

DO I HAVE TO BE AN EXPERIENCED COMPUTER USER AND BE ABLE TO TYPE TO TAKE THE COMPUTER-BASED EXAMINATION?

No. The computerized testing system has been designed so that those with minimal computer experience and typing skills can use it. A tutorial will be available to each candidate at the testing center before he or she takes the examination. Candidates can download the CBT tutorial that is available on test day at http://www.pearsonvue.com/ptcb.

WHEN WILL EXAMINATIONS BE ADMINISTERED?

The examination will be offered during four testing periods called "testing windows" throughout the year, giving candidates a choice of times and locations. Please check the application PDF to obtain your own copy of this year's scheduled examination windows.

WHERE WILL THE COMPUTERIZED EXAMINATIONS BE ADMINISTERED?

PTCB will offer the examination through Pearson VUE's extensive network of more than 200 test center locations in all 50 of the states and Puerto Rico. You may search for a Pearson Professional Center (PPC) near you at http://ptcb.org/AM/Template/cfm.

CAN EXAMINATIONS BE SCHEDULED ONLINE?

Yes, and candidates are encouraged to apply and schedule their examinations online. Once a candidate has completed the application and received an Authorization to Test (ATT) letter, the candidate may then schedule an examination appointment online at the Pearson VUE Web site (http://www.pearsonvue.com/ptcb) or by calling 866-902-0593.

WHAT IS THE COST TO TAKE THE COMPUTER-BASED PTCE?

The fee to apply to take the PTCE is $129.00.

ONCE AN EXAMINATION APPOINTMENT IS SCHEDULED, CAN IT BE CHANGED OR EVEN CANCELED?

Yes. Candidates can cancel or reschedule their examination appointment up to 24 hours before their scheduled appointment at no charge. To cancel or reschedule an examination appointment, call Pearson VUE at 866-902-0593 or go to http://www.pearsonvue.com/ptcb.

You must cancel your appointment at least 1 business day (24 hours) in advance to qualify for a refund. For example, if your appointment is at 11 AM on a Monday, you must cancel by 11 AM the previous Friday. If you wish to cancel your application completely, you must also withdraw your application by contacting the PES at http://www.proexam.org/ptcb or by calling 877-782-2888.

OTHER PHARMACY TECHNICIAN CERTIFICATION ORGANIZATIONS

INSTITUTE FOR THE CERTIFICATION OF PHARMACY TECHNICIANS MISSION STATEMENT

The mission of the Institute for the Certification of Pharmacy Technicians (ICPT) is to recognize pharmacy technicians who are proficient in the knowledge and skills needed to assist pharmacists to safely, accurately, and efficiently prepare and dispense prescriptions and to promote high standards of practice for pharmacy technicians. In support of this mission, ICPT does the following:

- Promotes high standards of practice for pharmacy technicians
- Promotes safe and effective patient care by encouraging the use of highly qualified pharmacy technicians in all pharmacy practice settings
- Develops and conducts examinations that evaluate the knowledge and skills associated with the performance of tasks required for professional practice as a pharmacy technician
- Provides a means for recognizing pharmacy technicians who continue to demonstrate their qualifications by complying with ICPT continuing education requirements and adhering to high professional standards

ExCPT NATIONALLY RECOGNIZED ASSOCIATIONS

The Exam for the Certification of Pharmacy Technicians (ExCPT) is recognized by the National Community Pharmacists Association, the National Organization for Competency Assurance, and the National Association of Chain Drug Stores as a psychometrically sound pharmacy technician certification examination.

ExCPT RECERTIFICATION INFORMATION

Pharmacy technician certification must be renewed every 2 years. During the 2-year period before recertification, CPhTs must participate in at least 20 hours of continuing education, including at least 1 hour of pharmacy law. To recertify, technicians must complete the ICPT Recertification Application form and send it to ICPT along with full payment by the postmark deadline.

FREQUENTLY ASKED QUESTIONS

EXAMINATION

When are you offering your next test?
Tests can usually be taken within 2 to 3 business days after registration. LaserGrade provides affordable and efficient computer-based testing through its network of testing centers located throughout North America. LaserGrade's comprehensive testing programs include delivery of tests for federal and state agencies as well as corporate clients and national certification organizations. Once you call LaserGrade,

you will schedule a specific time and place for your test. Visit http://www.Lasergrade.com for a location near you, and call 800-211-2754 to register for the ExCPT.

I just took my examination. When will I get my certificate?
Certificates are mailed within 4 weeks. However, a candidate receives the results immediately on completion of the examination on a printout. The printout can be used at your pharmacy until the certificate comes in the mail.

Do I need to do anything else to be registered as a certified technician in my state?
Requirements for technician education, registration, licensing, and certification vary by state. You may check the state-by-state requirements posted on http://www.nationaltechexam.org for more information, or contact the state board of pharmacy for your state. A list of state boards of pharmacy is found in Appendix K and also on the Web site at http://www.nationaltechexam.org.

Is the ExCPT examination accepted in my state?
Requirements for technician education, registration, licensing, and certification vary by state. You may check the state-by-state requirements for more information or contact the state board of pharmacy for your state.

Do you have a practice test online that I can practice with before I take the examination?
A self-assessment test can be found on the ICPT Web site, located under the Virginia Exam. ICPT offers two practice tests that can be taken online. One practice test tests all knowledge areas. Another practice test focuses just on math questions. Each test, offered for $25 each, is a timed test of 50 questions. Candidates have 90 minutes to complete the test. One purpose of these tests is to allow the technician to practice with questions of the type typically seen on a certification examination but taken under similar timed conditions. You can access these practice tests at http://nationaltechexam.coursehost.com.

I would like to practice my math. Do you have some sample math questions I can take before the examination?
ICPT offers a practice test that is all math. This practice test offers 50 math and calculation questions that are similar to those that might be seen on a national

certification examination. This test can be accessed at http://nationaltechexam.coursehost.com.

How do I register for the test?

Call 800-211-2754 to register for the ExCPT at a nearby location. Available sites can also be located by visiting http://www.Lasergrade.com and clicking on "Locate a Test Center." Next, type in your zip code and click on "Find Testing Center." Then call 800-211-2754 to register for the ExCPT.

Where can I take the ExCPT examination?

Available sites can be located by visiting http://www.Lasergrade.com and clicking on "Locate a Test Center." Next, type in your zip code and click on "Find Testing Center." Then call 800-211-2754 to register for the ExCPT.

What are the testing conditions like?

All testing centers must follow strict requirements, which can be found on the http://www.Lasergrade.com Web site.

Do I get to use my calculator and scratch paper or will these be provided?

A calculator on the computer, two pieces of paper, and a pencil will be provided.

When do I get my test results?

Immediately on completion of the examination.

How much does the examination cost?

$95, which can be paid with a credit card at the time of registration.

How many times can I take the examination if I do not pass the first time?

You must wait a month before taking the examination a subsequent time. You may take it as many times as needed. A fee is required for each examination session.

How long am I certified for?

Certification is for a 2-year period, after which you must recertify to keep your certification current. Recertification information is available as part of the Candidate's Guide at http://www.nationaltechexam.org/excptinfo.shtml.

How much time do I get to take the examination?

The examination must be completed within 2 hours.

RECERTIFICATION

I am licensed through October and I think I need to recertify. What do I need to do?

You must complete a recertification form and send the appropriate renewal fee. To recertify you can download an application form or complete the online application process. Please note that recertifications are subject to random audit and review. Please keep your documentation of continuing education and recertification in order. Information on recertification is located at http://www.nationaltechexam.org/excptinfo.shtml#Recertification.

Can I recertify online?

Yes, you can recertify online, and you will receive a discount.

I think my certification has lapsed. Do I need to take the test again?

Pharmacy technician certification must be renewed every 2 years. If you have not recertified within the 90-day grace period after the expiration date on your certificate, you are no longer certified. You may, however, be eligible to have your recertification status reinstated if you do so within 18 months of the expiration date. Reinstated certification will expire on the same date that it would have expired had you recertified on time; there is no extension of the expiration date. To reinstate your certification status, you must complete at least 20 hours of continuing education, including at least 1 hour of pharmacy law. All continuing education requirements are the same as for recertification. To recertify, technicians must complete the ICPT Reinstatement Form (available at http://www.nationaltechexam.org) and send it to ICPT along with full payment by the postmark deadline. The fee for reinstatement is $80. Applications not completed correctly will be returned and will require an additional $10 reapplication fee. Reinstatement is not available in the following circumstances:

- Certification has been expired for more than 18 months.
- Certification has been revoked.
- The pharmacy technician has been convicted of or pled guilty to a felony.

If recertification lapsed more than 18 months ago, you must retake the ExCPT.

Appendix C

Pharmaceutical Conversions

METRIC PREFIXES

Nano: 1/1,000,000,000 of the unit of measure
Micro: 1/1,000,000 of the unit of measure
Milli: 1/1000 of the unit of measure
Kilo: 1000 × the unit of measure

Another way to understand this relationship is shown below:

Nano- (smallest)	Micro-	Milli-	Unit	Kilo- (largest)

To move from a smaller unit to a larger unit, divide in multiples of 1000. To move from a larger unit to a smaller unit, multiply in multiples of 1000.

METRIC UNITS OF MEASURE

WEIGHT

gram (g or gm), basic unit

VOLUME

liter (L)

HOUSEHOLD UNITS OF MEASURE

VOLUME

5 mL = 1 teaspoon (tsp)
3 tsp = 1 tablespoon (tbsp)
2 tbsp = 1 fluid ounce (fl oz)
8 fl oz = 1 cup

2 cups = 1 pint (pt)
2 pt = 1 quart (qt)
4 qt = 1 gallon (gal)

mL (smallest)		tsp	tbsp	oz	cup	pint	quart	gallon (largest)

WEIGHT

1 pound (lb) = 16 oz

APOTHECARY

VOLUME

1 fluid dram (fl dr) = 1 tsp
3 fl dr = 1 tbsp

WEIGHT

28.35 grams (g) = 1 ounce (oz)
16 oz = 1 lb
2.2 lb = 1 kilogram (kg)

MILITARY TIME

STANDARD TIME	MILITARY TIME
1:00 AM	0100
2:00 AM	0200
3:00 AM	0300
4:00 AM	0400
5:00 AM	0500

STANDARD TIME	MILITARY TIME	STANDARD TIME	MILITARY TIME
6:00 AM	0600	4:00 PM	1600
7:00 AM	0700	5:00 PM	1700
8:00 AM	0800	6:00 PM	1800
9:00 AM	0900	7:00 PM	1900
10:00 AM	1000	8:00 PM	2000
11:00 AM	1100	9:00 PM	2100
Noon	1200	10:00 PM	2200
1:00 PM	1300	11:00 PM	2300
2:00 PM	1400	Midnight	2400
3:00 PM	1500		

Appendix D

Pharmaceutical Abbreviations

Abbreviation	Meaning
aa	of each
ad	up to, so as to make
cc	cubic centimeter (mL)
dtd	dispense such doses or give of such doses
Eq	equivalent
g	gram
gal	gallon
gr	grain
gtt	drop(s)
h	hour
hr	hour
kg	kilogram
L	liter
lb	pound
mcg	microgram
mEq	milliequivalent
mg	milligram
mg/kg	milligram of drug per kilogram of body weight
mL	milliliter (cc)
mOsm	milliosmole
#	number
qs	a sufficient quantity
qs ad	a sufficient quantity to make up to
pt	pint
qt	quart
ss	one-half
tbsp	tablespoonful

Abbreviation	Meaning
tsp	teaspoonful
U*	unit

Dosage Form	Meaning
amp	ampule
cap	capsule
ECT	enteric-coated tablet
elix	elixir
fl	fluid
fl oz	fluid ounce
inj	injection
IV	intravenous
IVP	intravenous push
IVPB	intravenous piggyback
MDI	metered-dose inhaler
oint	ointment
sol	solution
supp	suppository
susp	suspension
syr	syrup
tab	tablet
TDS	transdermal delivery system
TPN	total parenteral nutrition
ung	ointment

*The pharmacy abbreviation appears on the "Do Not Use List" of the Joint Commission (TJC) and Institute for Safe Medication Practices (ISMP). Despite the recommendation of both TJC and ISMP, pharmacy technicians may continue to see prescriptions or medication orders with these abbreviations.

Solution	Meaning	Time of Administration	Meaning
D5LR	5% dextrose in lactated Ringer's solution	a	before
		ac	before meals
D5NS	5% dextrose in normal saline solution	ad lib	at pleasure, freely
		AM	morning, before noon
D5W	5% dextrose in water	ATC	around the clock
D10W	10% dextrose in water	bid	twice per day
		h, hr	hour
D20W	20% dextrose in water	hs	at bedtime
		noct	at night
DW	distilled water	p	after
NS	normal saline (0.9% sodium chloride)	pc	after meals
		PM	evening, afternoon
		postop	postoperative
½ NS	half-strength normal saline (0.45%)	pp	after meals
		prn	as needed
o/w	oil-in-water	q	each, every
RL	Ringer's lactate solution	qd	every day
		q4h	every 4 hr
R/L	Ringer's lactate solution	q6h	every 6 hr
		q8h	every 8 hr
SWFI	sterile water for injection	qh	every hour
		qid	four times per day
w/o	water-in-oil	qod	every other day
		tid	three times per day
		wk	week

Site of Administration	Meaning	Medication†	Meaning
abd	abdomen	ABC	abacavir
ad*	right ear	APAP	acetaminophen (Tylenol)
as*	left ear	ASA	aspirin
au*	each ear	ATV	atazanavir
buc	in the cheek	AZT	zidovudine (Retrovir)
IA	intraarterial	BCP	birth control pill
ID	intradermal	CBV	zidovudine and lamivudine
IM	intramuscular		
IT	intrathecal	ddC	zalcitabine
IV	intravenous	ddI	didanosine (Videx)
NPO	nothing by mouth	d4T	stavudine (Zerit)
od*	right eye	DES	diethylstilbestrol
os*	left eye	DLV	delavirdine
ou*	each eye	EES	erythromycin ethylsuccinate
per	by or through		
PO	by mouth	EFV	efavirenz
PR	by rectum	5FU	fluorouracil (Efudex)
PV	by vagina	FPV	fosamprenavir
R	rectum	FTC	emtricitabine
SC, SQ, subq*	subcutaneous (under the skin)	HC	hydrocortisone
SL	sublingual (under the skin)	HCTZ	hydrochlorothiazide (Diuril)
top	topical		
vag	vaginal		

*Appears on the "Do Not Use List" of TJC and the ISMP.

†TJC and ISMP discourage the use of medication abbreviations; however, the pharmacy technician may continue to see abbreviations for medications on prescription or medication orders.

Medication†	Meaning	Body Condition	Meaning
HRT	hormone replacement therapy	DJD	degenerative joint disease
IDV	indinavir	DM	diabetes mellitus
INH	isoniazid	DT	delirium tremens
LPV/r	lopinavir with ritonavir	GERD	gastroesophageal reflux disease
MOM	Milk of Magnesia	GI	gastrointestinal
MS	morphine sulfate	GT	gastrostomy tube
MTX	methotrexate	GU	genitourinary
MVI	multiple vitamins	HA	headache
NFV	nelfinavir	HBP	high blood pressure
NTG	nitroglycerin	HIV	human immunodeficiency virus
NVP	nevirapine		
PCN	penicillin		
PTU	propylthiouracil	HR	heart rate
RTV	ritonavir	HT, HTN	hypertension
SMZ/TMP	sulfamethoxazole and trimethoprim (Bactrim or Septra)	JRA	juvenile rheumatoid arthritis
		NKA	no known allergies
SQV-HGC	saquinavir	NKDA	no known drug allergies
SQV-SGC	saquinavir		
3TC	lamivudine (Epivir)	N&V, N/V	nausea and vomiting
T-20	enfuvirtide	OA	osteoarthritis
TDF	tenofovir DF	OCD	obsessive-compulsive disorder
TRZ	zidovudine, lamivudine, and abacavir	P	pulse
		PTT	prothrombin time
		PVC	premature ventricular contraction
TVD	emtricitabine		
ZnO	zinc oxide	RA	rheumatoid arthritis
		RBC	red blood cell
Body Condition	**Meaning**	SCT	sickle-cell trait
AIDS	acquired immunodeficiency syndrome	SOB	shortness of breath
		Sx	symptom
		TED	thromboembolic disease
BM	bowel movement		
BP	blood pressure	Tx	treatment
BPH	benign prostatic hypertrophy	UA	uric acid, urinalysis
		URI	upper respiratory infection
BS	blood sugar		
CA	cancer	UTI	urinary tract infection
CAD	coronary artery disease	VS	vital sign
		WBC	white blood cell
CHF	congestive heart failure		
		Miscellaneous Pharmacy Abbreviation	**Meaning**
COPD	chronic obstructive pulmonary disease	C	Celsius
CP	chest pain	c	with
CVA	cerebrovascular accident	DAW	dispense as written
		D/C*	discontinue or discharge

†TJC and ISMP discourage the use of medication abbreviations; however, the pharmacy technician may continue to see abbreviations for medications on prescription or medication orders.

*Abbreviation appears on the "Do Not Use" list of TJC and the ISMP.

Miscellaneous Pharmacy Abbreviation	Meaning	Miscellaneous Pharmacy Abbreviation	Meaning
dil	dilute, dissolve	RN	registered nurse
disp	dispense	Rx	take
div	divide	s	without
F	Fahrenheit	sig	write on label
KVO	keep vein open	T	temperature
m ft	mix and make	ut dict	as directed
non rep	do not repeat	ud	as directed
NR	no refill		

Institute for Safe Medication Practices List of Error-Prone Abbreviations, Symbols, and Dose Designations

Abbreviation	Meaning	Possible Error	Solution
µg	Microgram	Mistaken as "mg"	Use mcg
AD, AS, AU	Right ear, left ear, each ear	Mistaken as OD, OS, OU (right eye, left eye, each eye)	Use right ear, left ear, or each ear
OD, OS, OU	Right eye, left eye, each eye	Mistaken as AD, AS, AU (right ear, left ear, each ear)	Use right eye, left eye, or each eye
BT	Bedtime	Mistaken as BID (twice daily)	Use bedtime
cc	Cubic centimeter	Mistaken as "u" (units)	Use mL
D/C	Discharge or discontinue	Premature discontinuation of medications if D/C (intended to mean discharge) has been misinterpreted as "discontinued" when followed by a list of discharge medications	Use discharge and discontinue
IJ	Injection	Mistaken as IV or intrajugular	Use injection
IN	Intranasal	Mistaken as IM or IV	Use intranasal
HS	Half-strength	Mistaken as bedtime	Use half-strength
hs	At bedtime, hour of sleep	Mistaken as half-strength	Use bedtime

Abbreviation	Meaning	Possible Error	Solution
IU	International Unit	Mistaken as IV (intravenous) or 10 (ten)	Use units
o.d. or OD	Once daily	Mistaken as "right eye" (OD, oculus dexter), leading to oral liquid medications administered in the eye	Use daily
OJ	Orange juice	Mistaken as OD or OS (right or left eye); drugs meant to be diluted in orange juice may be given in the eye	Use orange juice
Per os	By mouth; orally	The "os" can be mistaken as "left eye" (OS, oculus sinister)	Use PO, by mouth, or orally
q.d. or QD	Every day	Mistaken as "qid," especially if the period after the "q" or the tail of the "q" is misunderstood as an "i"	Use daily
qhs	Nightly at bedtime	Mistaken as "qhr" (every hour)	Use nightly
qn	Nightly at bedtime	Mistaken as "qh" (every hour)	Use nightly or at bedtime
q.o.d. or QOD	Every other day	Mistaken as "qd" (daily) or "qid" (four times daily) if the "o" is poorly written	Use every other day
q1d	Daily	Mistaken as q.i.d. (four times daily)	Use daily
q6PM	Every evening at 6 PM	Mistaken as every 6 hours	Use 6 PM nightly or 6 PM daily
SC, SQ, sub q	Subcutaneous	SC mistaken as SL (sublingual); SQ mistaken as "5 every"; the "q" in "sub q" has been mistaken as "every" (e.g., a heparin dose ordered "sub q 2 hours before surgery" misunderstood as every 2 hours before surgery)	Use subcut or subcutaneously
ss	Sliding scale	Mistaken as "55"	Spell out sliding scale; use one-half or ½
SSRI	Sliding scale regular insulin	Mistaken as selective-serotonin reuptake inhibitor	Spell out sliding scale (insulin)
SSI	Sliding scale insulin	Mistaken as strong solution of iodine	Spell out sliding scale (insulin)
i/d	Once daily	Mistaken as "tid"	Use 1 daily
TIW or tiw	Three times a week	Mistaken as "3 times a day" or "twice in a week"	Use 3 times weekly

Abbreviation	Meaning	Possible Error	Solution
U or u	Unit	Mistaken as the number 0 or 4, causing a tenfold overdose or greater (e.g., 4U seen as "40" or 4u seen as "44"); mistaken as "cc" so dose given in volume instead of units (e.g., 4u seen as 4 cc)	Use unit
Trailing zero after decimal point (e. g., 1.0 mg)	1 mg	Mistaken as 10 mg if the decimal point is not seen	Do not use trailing zeros for doses expressed in whole numbers
Naked decimal point (e.g., .5 mg)	0.5 mg	Mistaken as 5 mg if the decimal point is not seen	Use zero before a decimal point when the dose is less than a whole unit
Drug name and dose run together; especially problematic for drug names that end in "l" (e.g., Inderal40 mg or Tegretol300 mg)	Inderal 40 mg Tegretol 300 mg	Mistaken as Inderal 140 mg Mistaken as Tegretol 1300 mg	Place adequate space between the drug name, dose, and unit of measure
Numeric dose and unit of measure together (e.g., 10mg, 100mL)	10 mg 100 mL	The "m" is sometimes mistaken as a zero or two zeros, risking a tenfold to 100-fold overdose	Place adequate space between the dose and the unit of measure
Abbreviations such as mg or mL with a period following the abbreviation	mg mL	The period is unnecessary and could be mistaken as the number 1 if written poorly	Use mg, mL, and so on without a terminal period
Large doses without properly placed commas (e.g. 100000 units or 1000000 units)	100,000 units 1,000,000 units	100000 has been mistaken as 10,000 or 1,000,000; 1000000 has been mistaken as 100,000	Use commas for dosing units at or above 1000, or use words such as 100 "thousand" or 1 "million" to improve readability
ara-A	vidarabine	Mistaken as cytarabine (ARA-C)	Use complete drug name
AZT	zidovudine (Retrovir)	Mistaken as azathioprine or aztreonam	Use complete drug name
CPZ	Compazine (prochlorperazine)	Mistaken as chlorpromazine	Use complete drug name
DPT	Demerol-Phenergan-Thorazine	Mistaken as diphtheria-pertussis-tetanus (vaccine)	Use complete drug name
DTO	diluted tincture of opium, or deodorized tincture of opium (Paregoric)	Mistaken as tincture of opium	Use complete drug name

Abbreviation	Meaning	Possible Error	Solution
HCl	hydrochloric acid or hydrochloride	Mistaken as potassium chloride (the "H" is misinterpreted as "K")	Use complete drug name unless expressed as a salt of a drug
HCT	hydrocortisone	Mistaken as hydrochlorothiazide	Use complete drug name
HCTZ	hydrochlorothiazide	Mistaken as hydrocortisone	Use complete drug name
MgSO$_4$	magnesium sulfate	Mistaken as morphine sulfate	Use complete drug name
MS, MSO$_4$	morphine sulfate	Mistaken as magnesium sulfate	Use complete drug name
MTX	methotrexate	Mistaken as mitoxantrone	Use complete drug name
PCA	procainamide	Mistaken as patient-controlled analgesia	Use complete drug name
PTU	propylthiouracil	Mistaken as mercaptopurine	Use complete drug name
T3	Tylenol with Codeine No. 3	Mistaken as liothyronine	Use complete drug name
TAC	triamcinolone	Mistaken as tetracaine, adrenalin, cocaine	Use complete drug name
TNK	TNKase	Mistaken as TPA	Use complete drug name
ZnSo$_4$	zinc sulfate	Mistaken as morphine sulfate	Use complete drug name
Stemmed Drug Names			
Nitro drip	nitroglycerin infusion	Mistaken as sodium nitroprusside infusion	Use complete drug name
Norflox	norfloxacin	Mistaken as Norflex	Use complete drug name
IV Vanc	intravenous vancomycin	Mistaken as Invanz	Use complete drug name

Drug Nomenclature: Stems Used by the U.S. Adopted Names Council

Stem Example	Definition	Stem Example	Definition
-ac	antiinflammatory	-azoline	antihistamine or local vasoconstrictor
-actide	synthetic corticotropin		
-adol or -adol-	analgesic	-azosin	antihypertensive
-adox	quinolone antibacterial	-bactam	beta-lactamase inhibitor
-aj-	antiarrhythmic	-bamate	tranquilizer
-aldrate	antacid aluminum salt	-barb or -barb-	barbituric acid derivative
-alol	combined alpha- and beta-blocker	-bendazole	antihelmintic
		bol- or -bol-	anabolic steroid
-amivir	neuraminidase inhibitor	-butazone	antiinflammatory
-andr-	androgen	-caine	local anesthetic
-anserin	serotonin 5-HT receptor antagonist	calci- or -calci-	vitamin D analog
		-camsule	camphor sulfonic acid derivative
-antel	antihelmintic		
-arabine	antineoplastic	-carbef	carbacephem antibiotic
-aril, -aril-	antiviral	cef-	cephalosporin
-arit	antirheumatic	-cept	receptor
-arol	anticoagulant	-cic	hepatoprotective
-arot-	arotinoid	-cidin	natural antibiotic
arte-	antimalarial	-cillin	penicillin
-ase	enzyme	-citabrine	nucleoside antiviral or antineoplastic
-ast	antiasthmatic		
-astine	antihistamine	-clidine	muscarinic agonist
-atadine	tricyclic antiasthmatic	-clone	hypnotic tranquilizer
-azenil	benzodiazepine receptor agonist or antagonist	-cog	blood coagulation factor
		-conazole	systemic antifungal
-azepam	antianxiety	-cort-	cortisone derivative
-azepide	cholecystokinin	-crinat	diuretic
-azocine	narcotic antagonist	-crine	acridine derivative

Stem Example	Definition	Stem Example	Definition
-cromil	antiallergic	-giline	monoamine oxidase inhibitor
-curium	neuromuscular blocking agent	-gillin	antibiotic
-cycline	tetracycline antibiotic	gli-	oral hypoglycemic agent
-dan	positive isotropic agent	-glitazone	antidiabetic
-dapsone	antimicrobacterial	-gramostim	granulocyte macrophage colony-stimulating factor
-dar	multidrug inhibitor		
-dil, dil-, or -dil-	vasodilator	-grastim	granulocyte colony-stimulating factor
-dipine	phenylpyridine		
-dismase	superoxide dismutase activity	-grel- or -grel	platelet antiaggregant
-ditan	antimigraine 5-HT receptor agonist	guan-	antihypertensive
		-icam	antiinflammatory
-dopa	dopamine receptor agonist	-ifen	antiestrogens
		-ilide	class III antiarrhythmic
-dralazine	antihypertensive	-imex	immunostimulant
-dronate	calcium metabolism receptor	-imib	Acyl-CoA:cholesterol acetyltransferase inhibitor
-ectin	antiparasitic		
-entan	endothelin receptor antagonist	-imode	immunomodulator
		-imus	immunosuppressive
-erg-	ergot alkaloid derivative	io-	iodide-containing contrast medium
-eridine	analgesic		
-ermin	growth factor	-irudinem	anticoagulant
estr- or -estr-	estrogen	-isomide	antiarrhythmic
-etanide	diuretic	-iurn	quaternary ammonium derivative
-ezolid	oxazolidinone antibacterial		
		-kacin	antibiotic
-fenamate	fenamic acid ester or salt	-kalant	potassium channel agonist
-fenin	diagnostic aid	-kef- or -keph-	encephalin agonist
-fenine	analgesic	-kin	interleukin-type substance
-fentanil	narcotic analgesic		
-fiban	fibrinogen receptor antagonist	-kinra	interleukin receptor antagonist
-fibrate	clofibrate-type compound	-kiren	renin inhibitor
-filcon	hydrophilic contact lens material	-lazad	lipid peroxidation inhibitor
-fingol	sphingosine	-leukin	interleukin-2–type compound
-flapon	5-lipoxygenase activating protein inhibitor	-lubant	leukotriene antagonist
-flurane	general inhalation anesthetic	-lukast	leukotriene receptor antagonist
-focon	hydrophobic contact lens material	-lutamide	antiandrogen
		-mab	monoclonal antibody
-formin	oral hypoglycemic agent	-mantadine or -mantine-	adamantine derivative
-fradil	calcium channel blocker		
-fungin	antifungal antibiotic	-mastat	antineoplastic
-fylline or -phylline	theophylline derivative	-meline	cholinergic agonist
-gab-	gamma-aminobutyric acid (GABA) mimetic	-mer	polymer
		-mesine	sigma receptor ligand
-gado-	gadolinium derivative	-mestane	antineoplastic
-ganan	antibacterial	-metacin	antiinflammatory
-gest	progestin	-micin	aminoglycoside antibiotic

Stem Example	Definition	Stem Example	Definition
-monam	monobactam antibiotic	-porfin	benzoporphyrin
-mostim	monocyte macrophage colony-stimulating factor	-pramine	imipramine-type antidepressant
-motine	antiviral	-prazole	antiulcer
-moxin	monoamine oxidase inhibitor	pred-, -pred-, or -pred	prednisone derivative
		-pressin	vasoconstrictor
-mustine	antineoplastic	-priode	antipsychotic
-mycin	macrolide antibiotic	-pril	antihypertensive
-nab or -nab-	cannabinol derivative	-prilat	antihypertensive
nal-	narcotic agonist or antagonist	-prim	antibacterial
		-profen	antiinflammatory
		-prost or -prost-	prostaglandin derivative
-navir	human immunodeficiency virus protease inhibitor	-queside	cholesterol sequestrant
		-ractam	nootrope substance
		-relin	prehormone
		-relix	hormone release–inhibiting agent
-nidap	nonsteroidal antiinflammatory	-renone	aldosterone antagonist
-nidazole	antiprotozoal	-restat- or -restat	aldose reductase inhibitor
nifur-	5-nitrofuran derivative		
-nixin	antiinflammatory	-retin	retinol derivative
-olol	beta-blocker	-ribine	ribofuranil
-olone	steroid	rifa-	antibiotic
-onoid	topical steroid	-rinone	cardiotonic
-orex	anorexiant	-rozole	aromatase inhibitor
-orphan	morphinan derivative	-rubicin	antineoplastic antibiotic
-oxacin	quinolone antibiotic	-sal, -sal-, or sal-	salicylic acid derivative
-oxan	alpha-adrenoreceptor antagonist	-sartan	angiotensin II receptor antagonist
-oxanide	antiparasitic	-semide	diuretic
-oxef	antibiotic	-serpine	derivatives of Rauwolfia alkaloid
-oxetine	antidepressant		
-pafant	platelet-activating factor antagonist	-setron	serotonin (5-HT3) antagonist
-pamide	diuretic	-sidomine	antianginal
-pamil	coronary vasodilator	som-	growth hormone derivative
-pamine	dopaminergic		
-parcil	antithrombotic	som-, -bove	bovine somatotropin derivative
-parcin	glycopeptide antibiotic		
-parin	heparin derivative	som-, por-	porcine somatotropin derivative
-paroid	heparinoid-type substance		
		-spirone	anxiolytic
-penem	antibiotic	-sporin	immunosuppressant
perfl(u)-	perfluorochemical	-stat or -stat-	enzyme inhibitor
-peridol	antipsychotic	-ster-	steroid (androgen, anabolic)
-pirox	antimycotic pyridine derivative		
		-steride	testosterone reductase inhibitor
-plact	platelet factor 4 analog		
		-stigmine	anticholinesterase
-planin	antibacterial	-stinmel	N-methyl D-aspartate receptor antagonist
-platin	antineoplastic		
-plon	nonbenzodiazepine anxiolytic	sulfa-	sulfonamide antibacterial
		-sulfan	antineoplastic alkylating agent
-poetin	erythropoietin		

Stem Example	Definition	Stem Example	Definition
-tant	tachykinin receptor antagonist	-troline	antipsychotic
		trop- or -trop-	atropine derivative
-tecan	antineoplastic	-udine	antineoplastic
-tepa	antineoplastic	-uplase	urokinase-type plasminogen activator
-teplase	tissue-type plasminogen activator	-uracil	uracil derivative used as thyroid antagonist or as antineoplastic
-terol	bronchodilator		
-tesinol	thymidylate synthetase inhibitor	-uridine	uridine derivative used as antiviral agent or as antineoplastic
-thiazide	diuretic		
-tiapine	antipsychotic	-vastatin	antihyperlipidemic
-tiazem	calcium channel blocker	-verine	spasmolytic
-tibant	antiasthmatic	vin- or -vin-	vinca alkaloid
-tide	peptide	-vir-, -vir, or vir-	antiviral
-tidine	H$_2$-receptor antagonist	-virsen	antisense
-tocin	oxytocin derivative	-vudine	antineoplastic or antiviral
-toin	antiepileptic		
-trexate	folic acid analog	-xanox	antiallergic respiratory tract drug
-trexed	antineoplastic		
-tricin	antibiotic	-zolamide	carbonic anhydrase inhibitor
-triptan	antidepressant		
-triptyline	antidepressant	-zolast	benzoxazole antiasthmatic
-troban	antithrombotic		
-trodast	thromboxane A receptor antagonist		

Top 200 Prescription Drugs and Their Classifications

Brand Name	Generic Name	Indication (Drug Classification)
Abilify	aripiprazole	Psychosis
Accupril	quinapril	Hypertension (angiotensin-converting enzyme [ACE] inhibitor)
AcipHex	rabeprazole	Gastrointestinal reflux disease (GERD) (proton pump inhibitor)
Actonel	risedronate	Paget's disease, osteoporosis
Actos	pioglitazone	Diabetes
Adderall	amphetamine mixed salts	Narcolepsy, attention deficit disorder
Advair Diskus	salmeterol and fluticasone	Asthma (bronchodilator, corticosteroid)
Aldactone	spironolactone	Diuretic (potassium sparing)
Allegra	fexofenadine	Antihistamine
Alphagan P	brimonidine tartrate	Glaucoma
Altace	ramipril	Hypertension (ACE inhibitor)
Amaryl	glimepiride	Diabetes type 2 (sulfonylurea)
Ambien	zolpidem	Insomnia
Amoxil	amoxicillin	Infection (penicillin)
Anaspaz, Cystospaz	hyoscyamine sulfate	Peptic ulcer, spasms
Antivert	meclizine	Motion sickness, vertigo
Apri, Aviane	ethinyl estradiol and desogestrel	Oral contraceptive
Aricept	donepezil	Alzheimer's disease, dementia
Armour Thyroid	thyroid tablets	Hormone replacement
Arthrotec	diclofenac and misoprostol	Arthritis
Astelin	azelastine	Allergies
Atacand	candesartan cilexetil	Hypertension (angiotensin II antagonist)
Atarax	hydroxyzine HCl	Itching
Ativan	lorazepam	Anxiety, sedation

Brand Name	Generic Name	Indication (Drug Classification)
Augmentin	amoxicillin and clavulanate	Bacterial infection (penicillin combination)
Avalide	irbesartan and hydrochlorothiazide	Hypertension (angiotensin II antagonist, thiazide diuretic)
Avandia	rosiglitazone	Diabetes
Avapro	irbesartan	Hypertension (angiotensin II antagonist)
Avelox	moxifloxacin	Bacterial infection (quinolone)
Azmacort, Nasacort	triamcinolone	Respiratory allergies
Bactrim (DS), Septra (DS)	trimethoprim and sulfamethizole	Bacterial infection (sulfa)
Bactroban	mupirocin	Infection
Benicar HCT	olmesartan medoxomil and hydrochlorothiazide	Hypertension (angiotensin II antagonist thiazide diuretic)
Bentyl	dicyclomine hydrochloride	Irritable bowel syndrome
Biaxin XL	clarithromycin	Bacterial infection (macrolide)
BuSpar	buspirone	Depression
Calan	verapamil	Hypertension (calcium channel blocker)
Capex	fluocinolone acetonide	Psoriasis
Capoten	captopril	Hypertension (ACE inhibitor)
Cardura	doxazosin	Hypertension (beta-blocker)
Cartia XT	diltiazem	Angina (calcium channel blocker)
Catapres	clonidine	Hypertension (alpha-blocker)
Cefzil	cefprozil	Bacterial infection (cephalosporin)
Celebrex	celecoxib	Inflammation (cyclooxygenase [COX]-2 inhibitor)
Celexa	citalopram	Depression (selective serotonin reuptake inhibitor [SSRI])
Cialis	tadalafil	Erectile dysfunction
Clarinex	desloratadine	Respiratory allergies
Cleocin	clindamycin	Bacterial infection
Cogentin	benztropine	Parkinson's disease
Colchicine	colchicine	Gout
Combivent	ipratropium and albuterol	Asthma (bronchodilator, anticholinergic)
Concerta	methylphenidate	Attention deficit disorder, narcolepsy
Cordarone	amiodarone	Cerebrovascular accident
Coreg	carvedilol	Hypertension (beta-blocker)
Cosopt	dorzolamide and timolol	Glaucoma
Coumadin	warfarin	Blood clot prophylaxis
Cozaar	losartan	Hypertension (angiotensin II antagonist)
Crestor	rosuvastatin	Cholesterol (HMG-CoA reductase inhibitor)
Cymbalta	duloxetine	Depression (SSRI)
Cytotec	misoprostol	Gastric ulcers
Darvocet N	propoxyphene and acetaminophen	Analgesic
Deltasone	prednisone	Inflammation
Depakote	divalproex sodium	Convulsions
Desyrel	trazodone	Depression
Detrol LA	tolterodine	Incontinence

Brand Name	Generic Name	Indication (Drug Classification)
Diflucan	fluconazole	Fungal infection
Dilantin	phenytoin	Convulsions
Diovan	valsartan	Hypertension (angiotensin II antagonist)
Ditropan XL	oxybutynin	Reflex neurogenic bladder
Duragesic	fentanyl citrate	Narcotic analgesic
Dyazide	triamterene and hydrochlorothiazide	Hypertension (combination diuretic)
Dynacin	minocycline	Bacterial infection (tetracycline)
Effexor XR	venlafaxine	Depression (SSRI)
Elavil	amitriptyline	Depression (tricyclic antidepressant [TCA])
Elidel	pimecrolimus	Atopic dermatitis
Estrace	estradiol and ethinyl estradiol	Hormone replacement
Evista	raloxifene	Osteoporosis
Femiron	ferrous fumarate	Iron deficiency
Fioricet	butalbital, acetaminophen, and caffeine	Nonnarcotic analgesic
Flagyl	metronidazole	Anaerobic infection
Flexeril	cyclobenzaprine	Muscle spasms
Flomax	tamsulosin	Benign prostatic hypertrophy
Flonase	fluticasone	Allergic rhinitis
Floxin	ofloxacin	Bacterial infection (quinolone)
Folvite	folic acid	Folate deficiency
Fosamax	alendronate	Osteoporosis
Glucophage	metformin	Diabetes type 2
Glucotrol	glipizide	Diabetes type 2 (sulfonylurea)
Glucovance	glyburide and metformin	Diabetes type 2
GoLYTELY	polyethylene glycolectrolyte	Constipation, bowel cleansing
Hytrin	terazosin	Hypertension (alpha-blocker)
Hyzaar	losartan and hydrochlorothiazide	Hypertension (angiotensin II antagonist, thiazide diuretic)
Imitrex	sumatriptan	Migraine headache
Inderal	propranolol	Cardiovascular disorders (beta-blocker)
Insulin	insulin	Diabetes type 1
Isordil	isosorbide	Angina (nitrate)
Keflex	cephalexin	Bacterial infection (cephalosporin)
Klonopin	clonazepam	Convulsions
Klor-Con	potassium chloride	Potassium replacement
Lamictal	lamotrigine	Epilepsy
Lanoxin	digoxin	Arrhythmia, myocardial infarction (cardiac glycoside)
Lantus	insulin glargine	Diabetes type 1
Lasix	furosemide	Edema (loop diuretic)
Lescol	fluvastatin	Cholesterol (HMG-CoA reductase inhibitor)
Levaquin	levofloxacin	Bacterial infection (quinolone)
Lexapro	escitalopram	Depression (SSRI)
Lioresal	baclofen	Muscle spasms
Lipitor	atorvastatin	Cholesterol (HMG-CoA reductase inhibitor)

Brand Name	Generic Name	Indication (Drug Classification)
Lopid	gemfibrozil	Cholesterol (fibric acid)
Lopressor	metoprolol	Hypertension (beta-blocker)
Lotrel	amlodipine and benazepril	Hypertension (ACE inhibitor, calcium channel blocker combination)
Lotensin	benazepril	Hypertension (ACE inhibitor)
Lunesta	eszopiclone	Insomnia
Macrobid, Macrodantin	nitrofurantoin	Bacterial infection
Mevacor	lovastatin	Cholesterol (HMG-CoA reductase inhibitor)
Micronase	glyburide	Diabetes type 2 (sulfonylurea)
Monopril	fosinopril	Hypertension (ACE inhibitor)
Motrin	ibuprofen	Inflammation (nonsteroidal antiinflammatory drug [NSAID])
Naprosyn	naproxen	Inflammation (NSAID)
Nasonex	mometasone furoate	Nasal inflammation
Neurontin	gabapentin	Convulsions
Nexium	esomeprazole	GERD (proton pump inhibitor)
Niaspan	niacin	Cholesterol
Norvasc	amlodipine	Hypertension (calcium channel blocker)
Omnicef	cefdinir	Bacterial infection (cephalosporin)
Ortho Tri-Cyclen	ethinyl estradiol and norgestimate	Oral contraceptive
Ortho-Evra	ethinyl estradiol and norelgestromin	Oral contraceptive
Oxycontin	oxycodone	Narcotic analgesic
Patanol	olopatadine	Ophthalmic allergies
Paxil	paroxetine	Depression (SSRI)
Penicillin VK	penicillin	Bacterial infection (penicillin)
Pepcid	famotidine	GERD (proton pump inhibitor)
Percocet	oxycodone and acetaminophen	Narcotic analgesic
Phenergan	promethazine	Antiemetic
Plavix	clopidogrel	Atherosclerosis
Pravachol	pravastatin	Cholesterol (HMG-CoA reductase inhibitor)
Premarin	conjugated estrogens	Hormone replacement
Prempro	conjugated estrogens and medroxyprogesterone	Hormone replacement
Prevacid	lansoprazole	GERD (proton pump inhibitor)
Prilosec	omeprazole	GERD (proton pump inhibitor)
Protonix	pantoprazole	GERD (proton pump inhibitor)
Proventil	albuterol	Asthma (bronchodilator)
Prozac	fluoxetine	Depression (SSRI)
Pulmicort	budesonide	Asthma (corticosteroid)
Quinamm	quinine sulfate	Arrhythmias, malaria
Reglan	metoclopramide	Antiemetic
Remeron	mirtazapine	Depression
Restoril	temazepam	Insomnia
Rhinocort	budesonide	Respiratory allergies
Risperdal	risperidone	Psychosis
Seroquel	quetiapine fumarate	Psychotic, bipolar disorders
Sinemet	carbidopa and levodopa	Parkinson's disease

Brand Name	Generic Name	Indication (Drug Classification)
Sinequan	doxepin	Anxiety, depression (TCA)
Singulair	montelukast	Asthma (leukotriene receptor antagonist)
Skelaxin	metaxalone	Skeletal muscle relaxant
Solu-Medrol	methylprednisolone	Inflammation (steroid)
Soma	carisoprodol	Skeletal muscle relaxant
Strattera	atomoxetine	Attention deficit–hyperactivity disorder
Synthroid	levothyroxine sodium	Hormone replacement
Tegretol	carbamazepine	Seizures
Temovate	clobetasol	Psoriasis
Tenoretic	atenolol and chlorthalidone	Hypertension (beta-blocker, diuretic)
Tenormin	atenolol	Hypertension (beta-blocker)
Tessalon Perles	benzonatate	Cough suppressant
Topamax	topiramate	Seizures
Tricor	fenofibrate	Cholesterol
Tylenol with Codeine	acetaminophen and codeine	Analgesic
Ultracet	tramadol and acetaminophen	Analgesic
Ultram	tramadol	Analgesic
Valium	diazepam	Anxiety (benzodiazepine)
Valtrex	valacyclovir	Viral infection
Vasotec	enalapril	Hypertension (ACE inhibitor)
Viagra	sildenafil	Erectile dysfunction
Vibramycin	doxycycline	Bacterial infection (tetracycline)
Vicodin	hydrocodone and acetaminophen	Analgesic
Viracept	nelfinavir	Human immunodeficiency virus, acquired immunodeficiency syndrome
Vistaril	hydroxyzine pamoate	Anxiety
Wellbutrin SR	bupropion	Depression
Xalatan	latanoprost	Glaucoma (prostaglandin agonist)
Xanax	alprazolam	Anxiety (benzodiazepine)
Zantac	ranitidine	Ulcer (H_2 blocker)
Zestoretic	lisinopril and hydrochlorothiazide	Hypertension (ACE inhibitor, diuretic)
Zinacef	cefuroxime	Bacterial infection (cephalosporin)
Zithromax	azithromycin	Bacterial infection (macrolide)
Zocor	simvastatin	Cholesterol (HMG-CoA reductase inhibitor)
Zoloft	sertraline	Depression (SSRI)
Zovirax	acyclovir	Viral infection
Zyloprim	allopurinol	Gout
Zyprexa	olanzapine	Psychosis
Zyrtec	cetirizine	Allergies

Vitamins

Vitamin	Name	Use
A	Retinol	Retinal function and bone growth
B_1	Thiamine	Carbohydrate metabolism
B_2	Riboflavin	Tissue respiration
B_3	Niacin	Lipid metabolism
B_6	Pyridoxine	Amino acid metabolism
B_9	Folic acid	Red blood cell formation
B_{12}	Cyanocobalamin	Red blood cell formation
C	Ascorbic acid	Collagen formation, tissue repair
D_2	Ergocalciferol	Absorption and use of calcium and phosphate
D_3	Cholecalciferol	Absorption and use of calcium and phosphate
E		Antioxidant
K_1	Phytonadione	Blood clotting
K_3	Menadione	Blood clotting

Common Over-the-Counter Products

Brand Name	Generic Name	Classification
Actifed	pseudoephedrine and triprolidine	Decongestant
Advil	ibuprofen	Analgesic, antipyretic
Afrin	oxymetazoline	Decongestant
Aleve	naproxen sodium	Analgesic
Anbesol	benzocaine and phenol	Topical anesthetic
Aspercreme	trolamine salicylate	Topical analgesic
Bayer Aspirin	aspirin	Analgesic, antipyretic, antiinflammatory
Benadryl	diphenhydramine	Antihistamine
Benylin	diphenhydramine	Antitussive
Betadine	povidone iodine	Topical antiseptic
Bonine	meclizine	Antiemetic
Bufferin	aspirin	Analgesic, antipyretic, antiinflammatory
Caladryl	pramoxine, camphor, and calamine	Protectant
Carmex	menthol, camphor, alum, and salicylic acid	Protectant
Cepastat	phenol	Anesthetic
Chlor-Trimeton	chlorpheniramine	Antihistamine
Chloraseptic	benzocaine and menthol	Topical anesthetic
Citrucel	methylcellulose	Laxative
Claritin	loratadine	Antihistamine
Colace	docusate sodium	Stool softener
Compound W	salicylic acid	Keratolytic
Cortaid	hydrocortisone	Allergic reactions
Delsym	dextromethorphan	Antitussive
Dimetapp	brompheniramine	Antihistamine
Donnagel	attapulgite	Antidiarrheal
Doxidan	docusate calcium	Stool softener
Dramamine	dimenhydrinate	Antiemetic
Dulcolax	bisacodyl	Laxative
DuoFilm	salicylic acid	Keratolytic

Brand Name	Generic Name	Classification
Ecotrin	aspirin	Analgesic, antipyretic, antiinflammatory
Emetrol	phosphorated carbohydrates	Antiemetic
Excedrin	acetaminophen, aspirin, and caffeine	Analgesic
Femstat-3	butoconazole	Antifungal
Fibercon	polycarbophil	Laxative
Gas-X	simethicone	Antiflatulent
Gaviscon	aluminum hydroxide and magnesium trisilicate	Antacid
Gly-Oxide	carbamide peroxide	Topical anesthetic
Gyne-Lotrimin	clotrimazole	Antifungal
Imodium AD	loperamide	Antidiarrheal
Ivy Dry	tannic acid, benzocaine, menthol, and camphor	Astringent
Kaopectate	attapulgite	Antidiarrheal
Lactinex	*Lactobacillus*	Lactose intolerance
Listerine	thymol, eucalyptol, methyl salicylate, and menthol	Oral antiseptic
Lotrimin AF	clotrimazole	Antifungal
Maalox	aluminum hydroxide and magnesium hydroxide	Antacid
Metamucil	psyllium hydrophilic mucilloid	Laxative
Micatin	miconazole	Antifungal
Mineral Ice	menthol	Topical muscle relaxant
Monistat	miconazole	Antifungal
Motrin IB	ibuprofen	Analgesic
Motrin	ibuprofen	Analgesic, antipyretic
Mylanta	aluminum hydroxide and magnesium hydroxide	Antacid
Mylanta Gas	simethicone	Antiflatulent
Mylicon Drops	simethicone	Antiflatulent
Myoflex	trolamine salicylate	Topical analgesic
Naphcon A	pheniramine and naphazoline	Decongestant
NasalCrom	cromolyn sodium	Antihistamine
Neo-Synephrine	phenylephrine	Decongestant
Neosporin	polymyxin B sulfate, neomycin, and bacitracin	Topical antibiotic
Nicoderm	nicotine transdermal	Smoking cessation
Nicorette	nicotine polacrilex	Smoking cessation
Nicotrol	nicotine transdermal	Smoking cessation
Nix	permethrin	*Pediculus* infestation
NoDoz	caffeine	Central nervous system stimulant
Ocean	normal saline	Nasal moisturizer
Orabase-B	benzocaine	Oral anesthetic
Orajel	benzocaine	Oral anesthetic
Orudis KT	ketoprofen	Analgesic
Oxy 5, Oxy 10	benzoyl peroxide	Acne agent
Pepcid AC	famotidine	Antiulcer
Pepto-Bismol	bismuth subsalicylate	Gastrointestinal distress
Percogesic	phenyltoloxamine citrate and acetaminophen	Analgesic
Peri-Colace	docusate sodium and casanthranol	Stool softener and laxative
Peroxyl	hydrogen peroxide	Topical antiseptic

Brand Name	Generic Name	Classification
Phazyme	simethicone	Antiflatulent
Phillips Milk of Magnesia	magnesium hydroxide	Laxative
Primatene Mist	epinephrine	Bronchodilator
RID	pyrethrin	*Pediculus* infestation
Riopan	hydroxy magnesium and simethicone	Antacid
Robitussin	guaifenesin	Expectorant
Rogaine	minoxidil	Hair replacement
Senokot	senna concentrate	Laxative
Sominex	diphenhydramine	Sleep
Sucrets	hexylresorcinol and dyclonine	Oral anesthetic
Sudafed	pseudoephedrine	Decongestant
Tagamet	cimetidine	Antiulcer
Tavist-D	clemastine fumarate and pseudoephedrine	Antihistamine, decongestant
Tears Naturale	hydroxypropyl methylcellulose	Lubricant
Tinactin	tolnaftate	Antifungal
Tums	calcium carbonate	Antacid
Tylenol	acetaminophen	Analgesic, antiinflammatory
Zantac 75	ranitidine	Antiulcer
Zilactin	tannic acid	Cold sores
Zostrix	capsaicin	Topical muscle relaxant

Laboratory Values

The normal ranges are for reference only.

Serum Plasma

Albumin	3.2-5 g/dL
Bicarbonate	19-25 mEq/L
Blood urea nitrogen/creatinine ratio	10:1-20:1
Calcium	8.6-10.3 mg/dL
Chloride	98-108 mg/L
Creatinine	0.5-1.4 mg/dL
Creatinine clearance	75-125 mL/min
Glucose	80-120 mg/dL
Hemoglobin	4%-8%
Magnesium	1.6-2.5 mg/dL
Potassium	3.5-5.2 mEq/L
Sodium	134-149 mEq/L
Blood urea nitrogen	7-20 mg/dL
Cholesterol	
Total	<200 mg/dL
Low-density lipoprotein	65-170 mg/dL
High-density lipoprotein	40-60 mg/dL
Triglycerides	45-150 mg/dL

Liver Enzymes

Gamma-glutamyl transferase	
Male	11-63 IU/L
Female	8-35 IU/L
Serum glutamic-oxaloacetic transaminase or aspartate transaminase	<35 IU/L (20-48)
Serum glutamic pyruvic transaminase or alanine transaminase	<35 IU/L (10-35)

Complete Blood Cell Count

Hemoglobin	
Male	13.5-16.5
Female	12.0-15.0
Hematocrit	
Male	41-50
Female	36-44

State Boards of Pharmacy*

Alabama State Board of Pharmacy
Jerry Moore, Executive Director
1 Perimeter Park South, Suite 425 South,
  Birmingham, AL 35243
(205) 967-0130
http://www.albop.com

Alaska Board of Pharmacy
Deborah Stovern, Licensing Examiner
PO Box 110806, Juneau, AK 99811-0806
(907) 465-2589
http://www.dced.state.ak.us/occ/ppha.htm
(through the Division of Occupational Licensing)

Arizona State Board of Pharmacy
Llyn A. Lloyd, Executive Director
4425 W. Olive Avenue, Suite 140, Glendale, AZ
  85302
(623) 463-2727
http://www.pharmacy.state.az.us
E-mail: info@azsbp.com

Arkansas State Board of Pharmacy
Charles S. Campbell, Executive Director
101 E. Capitol, Suite 218, Little Rock, AR 72201
(501) 682-0190
http://www.state.ar.us/asbp
Email: sheila.castin@mail.state.ar.us

California State Board of Pharmacy
Patricia F. Harris, Executive Officer
400 R Street, Suite 4070, Sacramento, CA 95814
(916) 445-5014
http://www.pharmacy.ca.gov

Colorado State Board of Pharmacy
Susan L. Warren, Program Administrator
1560 Broadway, Suite 1310, Denver, CO 80202
(303) 894-7750
http://www.dora.state.co.us/pharmacy
Email: kent.mount@dora.state.co.us

Connecticut Commission of Pharmacy
Michelle Sylvestre, Board Administrator
State Office Building, 165 Capitol Avenue,
  Room 147, Hartford, CT 06106
(860) 713-6070
Fax: (860) 713-7242
http://www.ctdrugcontrol.com/rxcommision.htm
E-mail: michelle.sylvestre@po.state.ct.us

Delaware State Board of Pharmacy
David W. Dryden, Executive Secretary
P.O. Box 637, Dover, DE 19901
(302) 739-4798
http://www.dpr.delaware.gov/boards/pharmacy/
  index.shtml

District of Columbia Board of Pharmacy
Graphelia Ramseur, Health Licensing Specialist
825 N. Capitol Street, N.E., Room 2224, Washington,
  DC 20002
(202) 442-9200
Fax: (202) 442-9431
http://hpla.doh.dc.gov/hpla/cwp/view,A,1195,Q,4
  88414,hplaNav,%7C30661%7C,.asp

Florida Board of Pharmacy
John D. Taylor, Executive Director
4052 Bald Cypress Way, Bin #C04,
    Tallahassee, FL 32399-3254
(850) 245-4292
http://www.doh.state.fl.us/mqa/pharmacy/ph_
    home.html

Georgia State Board of Pharmacy
Anita O. Martin, Executive Director
237 Coliseum Drive, Macon, GA 31217-3858
(478) 207-1686
http://www.sos.state.ga.us/ebd-pharmacy

Guam Board of Examiners for Pharmacy
Teresita Villagomez, Acting Administrator
P.O. Box 2816, Hagatna, GU 96932
(671) 475-0251
http://www.dphss.guam.gov/about/licensing.
    htm

Hawaii State Board of Pharmacy
Lee Ann Teshima, Executive Officer
P.O. Box 3469, Honolulu, HI 96801
(808) 586-2694
http://www.state.hi.us/doca.pvl

Idaho Board of Pharmacy
Richard "Mick" Markuson, Executive Director
P.O. Box 83720, Boise, ID 83720-0067
(208) 334-2356
http://www.state.id.us/bop

Illinois Department of Professional Regulation
Kim Scott, Pharmacy Coordinator
320 W. Washington Street, Third Floor,
    Springfield, IL 62786
(217) 785-8159
http://www.dpr.state.il.us
(through Department of Professional
    Regulation)

Indiana Board of Pharmacy
Mark Bina, Director
402 W. Washington Street, Room 041,
    Indianapolis, IN 46204-2739
(317) 234-2067
http://www.in.gov/hpb/boards/isbp/

Iowa Board of Pharmacy Examiners
Lloyd K. Jessen, Executive Secretary/Director
400 S.W. Eighth Street, Suite E,
    Des Moines, IA 50309-4688
(515) 281-5944
http://www.state.ia.us/ibpe

Kansas State Board of Pharmacy
Susan Linn, Executive Director
Landon State Office Building, 900 Jackson, Room
    513, Topeka, KS 66612
(785) 296-4056
http://www.ink.org/public/pharmacy

Kentucky Board of Pharmacy
Michael A. Moné, Executive Director
23 Millcreek Park, Frankfort, KY 40601-9230
http://www.state.ky.us.boards/pharmacy

Louisiana Board of Pharmacy
Malcolm J. Broussard, Executive Director
5615 Corporate Boulevard, Suite 8E,
    Baton Rouge, LA 70808-2537
(225) 925-6496
http://www.labp.com

Maine Board of Pharmacy
Geraldine "Jeri" Betts, Board Administrator
35 State House Station, Augusta, ME 04333
(207) 624-8603
Direct line: (207) 624-8625
Fax: (207) 624-8637
http://www.maineprofessionalreg.org

Maryland Board of Pharmacy
LaVerne George Nasea, Executive Director
4201 Patterson Avenue, Baltimore, MD 21215-2299
(410) 764-4755
http://www.dhmh.state.md.us/pharmacyboard/
Email: md_pharmacy_board@yahoo.com

Massachusetts Board of Registration in Pharmacy
Charles R. Young, Executive Director
239 Causeway Street, Boston, MA 02113
(617) 727-9953
http://www.state.ma.us/reg/boards/ph
E-mail: charles.r.young@state.ma.us

Michigan Board of Pharmacy
Cathy Seyka, Licensing Manager
611 W. Ottawa, First Floor, P.O. Box 30670,
    Lansing, MI 48909-8170
(517) 373-9102
http://www.cis.state.mi.us

Minnesota Board of Pharmacy
David E. Holmstrom, Executive Director
2829 University Avenue S.E., Suite 530,
    Minneapolis, MN 55414-3251
(612) 617-2201
http://www.phcybrd.state.mn.us
E-mail: pharmacy.board@state.mn.us

Mississippi State Board of Pharmacy
William L. "Buck" Stevens, Executive Director
P.O. Box 24507, Jackson, MS 39225-4507
(601) 354-6750
http://www.mbp.state.ms.us

Missouri Board of Pharmacy
Kevin E. Kinkade, Executive Director
P.O. Box 625, Jefferson City, MO 65102
(573) 751-0091
http://www.ecodev.state.mo.us/pr/pharmacy
E-mail: kkinkade@mail.state.mo.us

Montana Board of Pharmacy
Rebecca Deschamps, RPh, Executive Director
P.O. Box 200513, 111 N. Jackson,
    Helena, MT 59620-0513
(406) 841-2356
Fax: (406) 841-2343
http://discoveringmontana.com/dli/bsd/license/
    bsd_boards/pha_board/board_page.html

Nebraska Board of Examiners in Pharmacy
Becky Wisell, Executive Secretary
P.O. Box 94986, Lincoln, NE 68509
(402) 71-2115
http://www.hhs.state.ne.us

Nevada State Board of Pharmacy
Keith W. Macdonald, Executive Secretary
555 Double Eagle Court, Suite 1100,
    Reno, NV 89511-8991
(775) 850-1440
http://www.state.nv.us/pharmacy

New Hampshire Board of Pharmacy
Paul G. Boisseau, Executive Secretary
57 Regional Drive, Concord, NH 03301-8518
(603) 271-2350
http://www.state.nh.us/pharmacy
Email: nhpharmacy@nhsa.state.nh.us

New Jersey State Board of Pharmacy
Deborah (Debbie) Whipple, Executive Director
P.O. Box 45013, Newark, NJ 07101
(973) 504-6450
http://www.state.nj.us/lps/ca/brief/pharm.htm

New Mexico Board of Pharmacy
Jerry Montoya, Chief Inspector/Director
1650 University Boulevard N.E., Suite 400B,
    Albuquerque, NM 87102
(505) 841-9102
http://www.state.nm.us/pharmacy
E-mail: nmbop@nm-us.campuscwix.net

New York Board of Pharmacy
Lawrence H. Mokhiber, Executive Secretary
89 Washington Avenue, 2nd Floor West,
    Albany, NY 12234-1000
(518) 474-3817 ext. 130
Fax: (518) 473-6995
http://www.nysed.gov/prof/pharm.htm
E-mail: pharmbd@mail.nysed.gov

North Carolina Board of Pharmacy
David R. Work, Executive Director
P.O. Box 459, Carrboro, NC 27510-0459
(919) 942-4454
http://www.ncbop.org

North Dakota State Board of Pharmacy
Howard C. Anderson, Jr., Executive Director
P.O. Box 1354, Bismarck, ND 58502-1354
(701) 328-9535
http://www.nodakpharmacy.com/

Ohio State Board of Pharmacy
William T. Winsley, Executive Director
77 S. High Street, Room 1702,
    Columbus, OH 43215-6126
(614) 466-4143
http://www.state.oh.us/pharmacy
E-mail: exec@bop.state.oh.us

Oklahoma State Board of Pharmacy
Bryan H. Potter, Executive Director
4545 Lincoln Boulevard, Suite 112,
    Oklahoma City, OK 73105-3488
(405) 521-3815
http://www.pharmacy.state.ok.us
E-mail: pharmacy@oklaosf.state.ok.us

Oregon State Board of Pharmacy
Gary A. Schnabel, Executive Director
800 N.E. Oregon Street, #9, State Office Building,
    Room 425, Portland, OR 97232
(503) 731-4032
http://www.pharmacy.state.or.us
E-mail: pharmacy.board@state.or.us

Pennsylvania State Board of Pharmacy
Melanie Zimmerman, Executive Secretary
124 Pine Street, P.O. Box 2649,
    Harrisburg, PA 17105-2649
(717) 783-7156
http://www.dos.state.pa.us/bpoa/phabd/
    mainpage.htm

Puerto Rico Board of Pharmacy
Beverly Davila Morales, Executive Director
800 Avenida Robert T. Todd, Office #201, Stop 18,
    Santurce, PR 00908
(787) 725-8161

Rhode Island Board of Pharmacy
Richard A. Yacino, Chief
3 Capitol Hill, Room 205, Providence, RI 02908
(401) 222-2837
http://www.health.ri.gov/hsr/professions/
    pharmacy.php

South Carolina Board of Pharmacy
Cheryl A. Ruff, Administrator
P.O. Box 11927, Columbia, SC 29211-1927
(803) 896-4700
http://www.llr.state.sc.us

South Dakota State Board of Pharmacy
Dennis M. Jones, Executive Secretary
4305 S. Louise Avenue, Suite 104,
    Sioux Falls, SD 57106
(605) 362-2737
Fax: (605) 362-2738
http://www.state.sd.us/dcr/pharmacy

Tennessee Board of Pharmacy
Kendall M. Lynch, Director
Second Floor, Davy Crockett Tower, 500 James
    Robertson Pkwy, Nashville, TN 37243
(615) 741-2718
http://www.state.tn.us/commerce/boards/pharmacy/

Texas State Board of Pharmacy
Gay Dodson, Executive Director/Secretary
333 Guadalupe, Tower 3, Suite 600, Box 21, Austin,
    TX 78701-3942
(512) 305-8000
http://www.tsbp.state.tx.us
E-mail: kay.wilson@tsbp.state.tx.us

Utah Board of Pharmacy
Diana L. Baker, Bureau Director
160 E. 300 South, P.O. Box 146741, Salt Lake City,
    UT 84114-6741
(801) 530-6767
http://www.commerce.state.ut.us/dopl/dopl1.htm
(through Division of Occupational and Professional
    Licensing)

Vermont Board of Pharmacy
Carla Preston, Staff Secretary
26 Terrace Street, Drawer 09,
    Montpelier, VT 05609-1106
(802) 828-2875
http://www.vtprofessionals.org/pharmacists
E-mail: cpreston@sec.state.vt.us

Virgin Islands Board of Pharmacy
Lydia T. Scott, Commissioner of Health
Roy L. Schneider Hospital, 48 Sugar Estate,
    St. Thomas, VI 00802
(340) 774-0117

Virginia Board of Pharmacy
Elizabeth Scott Russell, Executive Director
6606 W. Broad Street, Suite 400,
    Richmond, VA 23230-1717
(804) 662-9911
http://www.dhp.state.va.us/levelone/pharm.
    htm
E-mail: pharmbd@dhp.state.va.us

Washington State Board of Pharmacy
Donald H. Williams, Executive Director
P.O. Box 47863, Olympia, WA 98504-7863
(360) 236-4825
http://www.doh.wa.gov/pharmacy
E-mail: Don.Williams@doh.wa.gov

West Virginia Board of Pharmacy
William T. Douglass, Jr., Executive Director
232 Capitol Street, Charleston, WV 25301
(304) 558-0558
http://www.wvbop.com/

Wisconsin Pharmacy Examining Board
Patrick D. Braatz, Director
1400 E. Washington, P.O. Box 8935,
    Madison, WI 53708
(608) 266-2812
http://www.state.wi.us/agencies/drl
E-mail: dorl@mail.state.wi.us

Wyoming State Board of Pharmacy
James T. Carder, Executive Director
1720 S. Poplar Street, Suite 4, Casper, WY 82601
(307) 234-0294
http://pharmacyboard.state.wy.us
E-mail: pharmbd@trib.com

Technician Professional Membership Organizations

American Association of Colleges of Pharmacy (http://www.aacp.org)
American Association of Pharmacy Technicians (http://www.pharmacytechnician.com)
American Pharmacists Association (http://www.pharmacist.com)
American Society of Health-System Pharmacists (http://www.ashp.org)
Canadian Association of Pharmacy Technicians (http://www.capt.ca)
National Pharmacy Technician Association (http://www.pharmacytechnician.org)

Answers

1. b—An intravenous injection will result in the quickest onset of action.
2. d—The patient is to receive 20 mL per day. A 10-day supply would be 200 mL.
3. c—One dose is equal to two capsules, and the patient would be receiving three doses a day for 10 days (2 capsules/dose × 3 doses/day × 10 days = 60 capsules).
4. c—Convert the ratio to a fraction, then convert the fraction to a decimal and multiply by 100.
5. d—Nitrostat is available in a sublingual dosage form.
6. b—One grain is equal to 65 mg; therefore 30 grains is equal to 1950 mg. To convert milligrams to grams, divide by 1000.
7. b—Lorazepam is a Schedule IV controlled substance; the maximum number of refills permitted is five.
8. c—*Drug Topics Orange Book* provides therapeutic equivalences of medications.
9. b—Paroxetine is the generic name for Paxil.
10. b—Etodolac is the generic name for Lodine.
11. a—0.25% means there is 0.25 g in every 100 g. One pound is equal to 454 g. 0.25 g/100 g = X g/454; X = 1.135, which would be rounded to 1.14 g.
12. a—The term "ut dict" is a Latin abbreviation meaning "as directed."
13. d—The term "dipsia" means thirst.
14. b—The American College of Pharmacy Education (ACPE) accredits pharmacy education programs.
15. d—A total of 112 tablets are needed to fill this prescription.
16. a—Augmentin is a combination product consisting of amoxicillin and clavulanate.
17. c—The *Physicians' Desk Reference* (PDR) is not a required reference book for a pharmacy; however, many pharmacies have a copy.
18. c—A patient should be tapered off prednisone because of its possible side effects.
19. b—Robitussin A-C would be considered an "exempt" narcotic.
20. d—120 g (approximately 4 oz) is the maximum weighable amount on a Class A (III) balance.
21. b—Tylenol with codeine (acetaminophen with codeine) is a Schedule III medication.
22. d—Acyclovir (Zovirax) is an antiviral agent.
23. c—5% (w/v) means 5 g are dissolved in 100 mL. The problem can be solved using a proportion: 5 g/100 mL = X g/1000 mL, where X = 50.
24. c—Estrace is not a combination drug. Bactrim DS is sulfamethoxazole-trimethoprim; Dyazide is triamterene-hydrochlorothiazide; and Prempro is conjugated estrogens plus medroxyprogesterone.
25. c—10 g (solute)/400 g (solvent) × 100% = 2.5%.
26. b—A filter needle prevents glass from entering the final solution when an ampule is drawn from it. Depth filters trap particles as a solution moves through channels; filter straws are used for pulling medication from ampules; and a final filter is used before a solution enters the patient's body.
27. c—Singulair (montelukast) is a leukotriene inhibitor.

28. c—Use the following formula: Final volume (600 mL) × % expressed as a decimal (1:200 or 1/200) = Amount of active ingredient (X grams).

29. b—Rotating medications is an inventory management tool and is done to minimize obsolescence of a medication.

30. d—A "STAT" order means that the medication is needed immediately.

31. d—The Medicaid Tamper-Resistant Prescriptions Act of 2008 requires that all Medicaid prescriptions that are handwritten by the prescriber appear on a tamper-resistant prescription pad.

32. d—A midlevel practitioner such as a physician's assistant or nurse practitioner would have a DEA number beginning with an "M."

33. d—Remeron (mirtazapine) is not a combination product. Estratest (esterified estrogens and methyl testosterone), Hyzaar (losartan and hydrochlorothiazide), and Lotrel (amlodipine and benazepril) are combination products.

34. b—Class A balances have a sensitivity of 6 mg.

35. d—Insulin syringes are available as 30 units/mL, 50 units/mL, and 100 units/mL.

36. b—D5W and 0.9% NS are the two most common intravenous vehicles.

37. c—The Controlled Substances Act requires that all prescribers and dispensers of controlled substances have a DEA number. The requirement of having the physician's DEA number on a prescription shows the pharmacist that the physician has the authority to prescribe controlled substances.

38. a—According to the Controlled Substances Act of 1970, meperidine (Demerol) is a Schedule II drug.

39. c—NACDS stands for the National Association of Chain Drug Stores.

40. b—Discrimination occurs when a decision is made based on an individual's age, gender, race, or sexual orientation.

41. b—Adding the totals of all of the different ingredients gives 2270 mg. Divide 2270 mg/tablet by 1000 mg/g to determine the number of grams.

42. c—Serevent (salmeterol). Proventil or Ventolin is albuterol, Vanceril or Vancenase is beclomethasone, and Azmacort is triamcinolone.

43. b—Specific gravity is a ratio between the weight of a substance and the weight of an equal volume of water. One milliliter of water weighs 1 g; 4 fl oz = 120 mL. Therefore 0.84 = weight of substance/120 g.

44. c—Nifedipine (Procardia or Adalat) is a calcium channel blocker.

45. c—The problem can be solved by using the following formula: Final volume × % (expressed as a decimal) = Amount of active ingredient (g). The final volume is 30 mL, and 1:200 can be expressed as 1/200 or 0.005. The answer is 0.15 g. Multiplying 0.15 g × 1000 mg/g will yield 150 mg.

46. d—Zyloprim is the brand name for allopurinol. Other brand names and generic names are Anturane (sulfinpyrazone), Colchicine (colchicine), and Col-Probenecid (probenecid-colchicine).

47. b—Cubucin is not indicated as a smoking cessation aid.

48. a—Amantadine (Symmetrel) is used in the prevention of influenza and the treatment of Parkinson's disease.

49. b—Doxepin is found in the topical product Zonalon.

50. d—According to the Controlled Substances Act, a physician has up to 7 days to provide a pharmacy a handwritten prescription for a Schedule II medication if it was called in to the pharmacy. The quantity prescribed should be enough to last only until the patient can see the physician.

51. b—Clark's rule is used to calculate a child's dose based on weight using the following formula: Child's dose = Weight (lb)/150 × Adult dose (54/150 × 650 = 234 mg). Because the problem is asking for the dose in milliliters, a proportion should be used: 160 mg/5 mL = 234 mg/X mL, where X = 7.31 mL.

52. a—Generic and brand names are as follows: Celexa (citalopram), Nardil (phenelzine), Eldepryl (selegiline), and Parnate (tranylcypromine).

53. d—HIPAA does not discuss consequences for violations of the law.

54. c—MERF stands for Medication Error Reporting Form, which informs manufacturers of errors caused by commercial packaging and labeling. USP-ISMP stands for the United States Pharmacopeia–Institute for Safe Medication Practices. MedWatch is the FDA Medical Products Reporting Program.

55. b—This is a dilution problem that can be solved by using the formula (IS)(IV) = (FS)(FV), where IS is 80%, FS is 1:5000, or 0.2%, and FV is 500 mL. Substituting these values into the equation results in 1.25 mL of the 80% solution to be used.

56. d—Solve using a proportion: 2 mEq/mL = 40 mEq/X mL, where X = 20 mL.

57. d—Use the following formula: (IS)(IV) = (FS)(FV), or (100%)(X mL) = (2%)(1000 mL). One will need 20 mL of the 100% solution. The

amount of diluent needed can be calculated by subtracting the initial volume from the final volume: 1000 mL − 20 mL = 980 mL of diluent.

58. a—Solve using a proportion: 0.5 mcg/2 mL = 0.125 mcg/X mL, where X = 0.5 mL.

59. c—Normal saline is a 0.9% (w/v) solution; %w/v is the number of grams/100 mL × 100.

60. a—Januvia has been approved for the treatment of type 2 diabetes.

61. d—Medicare Part D pays for prescriptions for Medicare patients enrolled in the plan.

62. a—Quinapril (Accupril) is an ACE inhibitor.

63. b—Sales of pseudoephedrine must be recorded in a book that is retained in the pharmacy for a minimum of 2 years.

64. c—Nitrostat is an example of a sublingual medication used in the treatment of angina.

65. c—Losartan is an angiotensin II receptor antagonist.

66. b—Because of the acidic nature of fruit juices and colas, penicillin is inactivated by both of them.

67. c—An individual experiencing nausea and vomiting may have difficulty taking an oral solution and keeping it down. Nausea and vomiting would not affect a person using a suppository. Unfortunately, not many products are available as a suppository.

68. d—Theophylline is a xanthine derivative.

69. a—Diovan (valsartan) is an angiotensin II receptor antagonist. Isoptin (verapamil), Plendil (felodipine), and Tiazac (diltiazem) are calcium channel blockers.

70. c—Rhinitis medicamentosa is a rebound effect caused by nasal decongestants.

71. c—1 kg = 2.2 lb; therefore 154 lb = 70 kg. Set up a proportion: 12 mg/1 kg = X mg/70 kg. Multiply the number of milligrams × 5 days and the answer will be 4.2 g.

72. d—Oral syringes are used to administer small volumes of oral solutions.

73. b—Concerta (methylphenidate) is used in the treatment of ADHD and ADD. Proton pump inhibitors are used to treat ulcers and gastroesophageal reflux disease.

74. d—Solve using the alligation method, where 95% is the highest concentration, 30% is the lowest concentration, and you are making a 50% solution. Calculate the number of parts of each solution needed for this compound. Next, calculate the volume by using proportions.

75. c—Convert the weight in pounds to kg (187 lb/2.2 lb/kg = 85 kg). Multiply the daily dose by the weight of the individual (50 mg/kg/day × 85 kg = 4250 mg/day). Multiply the daily amount by the length of therapy (4250 mg × 10 days = 42,500 mg). Calculate the number of capsules by dividing the total weight by the weight per capsule (42,500 mg/250 mg per capsule = 170 capsules).

76. b—A diagnostic agent is used in making a diagnosis of a condition.

77. c—Glycosuria, polydipsia, and polyuria are characteristic signs of diabetes.

78. c—Lisinopril is an ACE inhibitor and is not indicated in the treatment of angina. Isosorbide dinitrate, isosorbide mononitrate, and nitroglycerin are nitrates used to treat angina.

79. b—Pharmacy technicians perform technical duties. This is an example of a judgmental activity performed by pharmacists.

80. b—With any insurance plan, a formulary will be set up stating which drugs will be covered or excluded under the plan. "NDC Not Covered" means that the product is not recognized by the insurance plan.

81. b—Generic and brand names are Intron (interferon alfa-2b), interferon alfa-2a (Roferon), interferon beta-1a (Avonex), and interferon beta-1b (Betaseron).

82. d—All the information should be collected to ensure the patient profile is accurate and to reduce the possibility of drug interactions and contraindications associated with medications.

83. c—Drugs and classifications are as follows: misoprostol (Cytotec is a prostaglandin E analog), alginic acid (Gaviscon—coating agent), mesalamine (Rowasa and Asacol are antiinflammatory agents), and sucralfate (Carafate—coating agent).

84. c—Solve using the following equation: Final volume × Percentage (expressed as a decimal) = Amount of active ingredient. (10 mL × 0.004 = 0.04 g). Convert grams to milligrams by multiplying by 1000: (0.04 g × 1000 mg/g = 40 mg).

85. c—Using the formula (IS)(IV) = (FS)(FV), where the initial strength (IS) is 17%, the final strength (FS) is 1:750, or 0.13%, and the final volume (FV) is 1 gal, or 128 fl oz. Solving for the initial volume (IV) will result in 1 fl oz being required to make this dilution.

86. a—Folic acid is also known as vitamin B_9 and is necessary for the creation of new cells.

87. c—Estrace is an estrogen hormone.

88. a—Chocolate or regular milk and orange juice may be mixed with Sandimmune at room temperature. Carbonated beverages should not be mixed with Sandimmune.

89. d—Nasonex is a topical corticosteroid used to treat respiratory allergies.

90. b—Convert 143 lb to kg: 143 lb × 1 kg/2.2 lb. Multiply patient weight in kilograms by dosage by the number of minutes in 1 hr: 65 kg × 5 mcg/kg/min × 60 min/hr = 19,500 mcg. Convert mcg to mg: 19,500 mcg × 1 mg/1000 mcg = 19.5 mg.

91. b—A rapid onset is beneficial because a therapeutic level and response occur more quickly in the body.

92. a—Multiply the total weight of the compound by the percentage of each ingredient expressed as a decimal (HC: 60 g × 0.01 = 0.6 g; precipitated sulfur: 560 g × 0.2 = 12 g).

93. b—Ultralente has a duration of 18 to 20 hr; NPH, 10 to 16 hr; regular, 5 to 6 hr; and Humalog, 1 hr.

94. a—Adderall (amphetamine-dextroamphetamine), Norpramin (desipramine), and Ritalin (methylphenidate) are used to treat ADHD. Even though amitriptyline is a tricyclic antidepressant, as is desipramine, amitriptyline is not used for ADHD.

95. d—Beta-blockers should not be used because they will reduce the action of the heart and cause a pooling of blood in the lower chambers.

96. c—1 tsp = 5 mL; therefore Total quantity (120 mL)/Dose quantity (5 mL/tsp) = 24 tsp. Solve using the following proportion: 15 mg/1 tsp = X mg/24 tsp, where X = 360 mg. To calculate the number of tablets, divide the total weight of codeine: 360 mg/weight per tablet (30 mg per tablet) = 12 tablets.

97. d—The therapeutic window shows the optimum range of therapeutic effects, whereas underdosing produces very few effects and overdosing can lead to severe side effects or even toxicity.

98. b—Net profit = Selling price – Acquisition price – Expenses: $55.00 – $3.75 – $45.00 = $6.25.

99. b—Injectable diazepam is the drug of choice for status epilepticus. If results are not obtained, phenytoin may be used.

100. c—Set up a proportion: 1 g/1,000,000 mcg = 0.12 g/X g, where X = 120,000 mcg. Divide the total weight by the weight per capsule: 120,000 mcg/150 mcg per capsule = 800 capsules.

CHAPTER 1 REVIEW ANSWERS

ANSWERS TO REVIEW QUESTIONS

1. d—The Joint Commission (TJC) is a nonprofit organization whose standards are set to ensure high-quality services in hospitals and long-term care facilities. The Drug Enforcement Agency (DEA) was formed as a result of the Controlled Substances Act of 1970 and is part of the Department of Justice. The DEA is responsible for enforcing the Controlled Substances Act. The Environmental Protection Agency (EPA) is responsible for maintaining the environment and is concerned with pharmacy handling, storage, and destruction of substances such as hazardous waste and controlled substances. The Food and Drug Administration (FDA) is responsible for ensuring that all medications, whether legend or over-the-counter (OTC), are pure, safe, and effective for use in the United States.

2. b—Medicare is a federal health care coverage program for those 65 years of age and older, certain disabled persons, and persons with end-stage renal disease as mandated by Title XVIII of the Social Security Act of 1965. Parts A and B of Medicare cover both hospital care and outpatient services.

3. c—A deductible is a set amount that must be paid by the patient for each benefit period before the insurer will cover additional expenses. Per diem is a predetermined amount of money that is paid to an individual or institution for a daily service. Patient assistance programs are special programs offered by pharmaceutical manufacturers for patients with specific needs who may be unable to afford their medication. A fixed copayment is one in which the patient pays a fixed or set dollar amount for each prescription.

4. b—Documentation that provides detailed information about the hazards of a particular substance. Information found on a Material Safety Data Sheet includes composition of the substance, hazards identified, first-aid measures, and toxicology. This document must be provided by the drug manufacturer.

5. d—Used syringes and needles should be placed in the red plastic sharps container to prevent an individual from being injured by a used needle.

6. c—Jewelry should not be worn while preparing IV admixtures because it may puncture the latex gloves.

7. c—Reconstitution involves mixing a liquid and solid to form a suspension or solution. Geometric dilution is a technique for mixing two powders of unequal quantity. Levigation is the mixing of particles with a base vehicle, in which they are insoluble, to produce a smooth dispersion of the drug by rubbing with a spatula on a tile. Trituration is the process of reducing the particle size and mixing one powder with another.

8. c—Absorption bases are characterized as being greasy, occlusive, difficult to spread, nonwashable, and anhydrous.

9. a—An automatic stop order can be found in both hospitals and long-term nursing facilities. The order will stop for a particular classification after a predetermined period unless otherwise specified by the physician. A STAT order needs to be filled as soon as possible—in a hospital, usually within 5 to 15 minutes; an ASAP order is not as urgent as a STAT order but takes priority over an incoming order; a prn order can be filled whenever needed by the patient.

10. b—*Drug Topics Red Book* provides information regarding drug costs; *Orange Book* provides information about therapeutic equivalence; *National Formulary* sets standards for pharmaceutical ingredients; and the *United States Pharmacopoeia* is an official compendium of monographs setting official national standards for drug substances and dosage forms.

11. c—A hermetic container is impervious to air under normal handling, shipment, storage, and distribution. A child-resistant container is a container that cannot be opened by 80% of children younger than 5 years but can be opened by 90% of adults. An easy-open container is one that has been requested by an individual or a physician. A light-resistant container protects the contents from light through the use of an opaque covering.

12. d—Room temperature is between 15° and 30°C (59° and 86°F); cold is not greater than 8°C (46°F); cool is between 8° and 15°C (46° and 59°F); and excessively hot is above 40°C (greater than 104°F).

13. c—A lot number identifies a particular batch or run of a specific medication. A drug schedule is assigned by the Drug Enforcement Agency (DEA) based on a potential for abuse of the product. A UPC is a universal product code assigned to over-the-counter (OTC) drugs and is similar to a NDC number. An NDC number identifies the drug manufacturer, the drug product, and the packaging of the product.

14. c—The lot number of the medication dispensed is not required on a prescription label. The following information is required: name of pharmacy, address of pharmacy, telephone number of pharmacy, prescriber's name, date prescription was filled, patient's name, name and strength of medication, quantity of medication, directions for use, refill information, and auxiliary labeling.

15. b—A Patient Package Insert is not required to be given to patients receiving prescriptions of ACE inhibitors.

16. b—Emulsions can be prepared by one of three methods: the continental (dry gum method), the wet gum method, or the beaker method.

17. b—Seventy-percent isopropyl alcohol should be used in cleaning the bench of either a vertical or horizontal laminar airflow hood.

18. c—Total parenteral solutions are composed of 50% dextrose, 20% fat, and 10% amino acids. Peripheral parenteral nutrition solutions are composed of 25% dextrose, 10% amino acids, and 10% fat.

19. b—Geometric dilution is the mixing of two ingredients of unequal quantities. During geometric dilution, one begins with the ingredient in the smaller quantity and adds an equal quantity of the next substance in a mortar. Blending is the act of combining two ingredients; levigation is the process of reducing the particle size during the preparation of an ointment; and spatulation is the process of combining substances with a spatula.

20. d—A thickening agent is used in the preparation of a suspension to increase its viscosity; emulsifiers are stabilizers in emulsions; a flocculating agent is an electrolyte used in the preparation of an emulsion; and a mucilage is a wet, slimy liquid formed in the wet gum method of preparing an emulsion.

21. a—Aquaphor is an example of an absorbent base; hydrophilic ointment is an example of an oil-water base; Eucerin is an example of a water-oil base; and PEG is an example of a water-miscible base.

22. a—A fixed copayment is a predetermined amount of money to be paid on each prescription; a percentage copayment is a predetermined percentage of the negotiated price of a prescription; a variable copayment is used when a prescription is not covered under the formulary or may be considered a "lifestyle drug," such as Retin-A, Renova, or Viagra.

23. b—The cost of a hazardous substance is not found on an MSDS form; accidental release measures, exposure controls and personal protection, and handling and storage are found on the MSDS form.

24. a—Absorption bases are anhydrous; water-oil emulsion bases, oil-water bases, and water-miscible bases are hydrous.

25. a—The drug manufacturer is responsible for providing the MSDS form to the purchaser.

26. b—Federal law allows a pharmacy to transfer a prescription for Schedule III to V medications to another pharmacy only once. The patient must

have the remaining refills processed at the pharmacy to which the prescription was transferred.

27. b—A therapeutic code of A means that the medication is therapeutically equivalent to other pharmaceutically equivalent product. B ratings mean the Food and Drug Administration (FDA) does not consider the drug at this time to be therapeutically equivalent to other pharmaceutically equivalent products. AB ratings indicate that the product meets bioequivalence requirements. AA ratings indicate that the product does not present bioequivalence problems in conventional forms.

28. a—Angina occurs when an imbalance in oxygen supply and demand occurs; hypertension occurs when the systolic pressure is greater than 140 mm Hg and diastolic pressure is greater than 90 mm Hg; myocardial infarction occurs when the heart is deprived of oxygen; and a stroke occurs when the brain is deprived of oxygen.

29. c—Potentiation occurs when one drug prolongs the effect of another drug; addition is the combined effect of two drugs; antagonism occurs when a medication works against another medication; and synergism occurs when the combined effect of two drugs is greater than the sum of both drugs' effects.

30. d—Secondary diabetes is caused by another medication; gestational diabetes occurs during pregnancy; type 1 diabetes occurs when the body is unable to produce insulin; and type 2 diabetes occurs later in life and can be controlled by diet, exercise, and oral hypoglycemics.

31. a—A patient experiencing bipolar disease has periods of both depression and mania; an individual with epilepsy will have abnormal electrical discharges occurring in the cerebral cortex; individuals with mania will have extreme excitement, hyperactivity, and possible increased psychomotor activity; people with schizophrenia exhibit extreme psychotic behavior.

32. b—*Drug Facts and Comparisons* has monthly updates issued; *Drug Topics Red Book* and the *Physicians' Desk Reference* (PDR) are updated yearly.

33. c—A physician's Drug Enforcement Agency (DEA) number begins with two letters and is followed by seven numbers. The first letter is an A, B, F, or M. The second letter is the first letter of the physician's last name. If the sum of the first, third, and fifth numbers is added to twice the sum of the second, fourth, and sixth numbers, the total should be a number whose last digit is the same as the last digit of the DEA number.

34. b—Amoxicillin Pediatric Drops is an oral suspension and can be administered to the patient using an oral syringe; low-dose and U-100 syringes are used to inject insulin; and tuberculin syringes are used to inject various parenteral substances into the body.

35. d—A sphygmomanometer is used to measure the vital capacity of an individual; nebulizers are used to generate very fine particles of liquid in a gas and are used in providing inhalation therapy; peak flow meters are used to measure and manage asthma in an individual; pneumograms are two-channel recordings of heart rate and respiration in the monitoring of apnea.

36. a—The CADD Prizm PCS Pump is an example of a patient-controlled analgesia (PCA) device; the CADD-Plus Pump is used to infuse antibiotics; CADD-TPN is used to infuse total parenteral nutrition; and an elastometric balloon system is an infusion device where the medication is inside a pressurized balloon reservoir and is infused by deflating the balloon.

37. a—Glucometers are used by diabetics to measure glucose in the blood; echocardiograms and electrocardiograms are used in cardiac patients; and in a syringe infusion system, medication is contained in a special syringe and is infused by a special infusion pump.

38. c—A single-dose container is a single-unit container for parenteral administration only; a tight container protects the contents from contamination by liquids, other solids, or vapors during normal shipping, handling, storage, and distribution; a single-unit container holds a specific quantity of drug for one dose; and a unit-dose container contains articles for administration other than the parenteral dose, coming directly from the container.

39. b—Emulsions can be prepared by either the dry gum method, the wet gum method, or the beaker method.

40. c—Syrups can be made by the heat method; suppositories can be made by either the compression or fusion mold method.

41. b—Suppositories can made either by the compression or fusion mold method.

42. b—White petrolatum is an oleaginous base.

43. d—Used needles and syringes should be placed in a sharps container; used gloves, gowns, and masks may be placed in a biohazard bag.

44. a—AAC is an abbreviation for actual acquisition cost, which is the price the pharmacy actually paid for a medication after receiving discounts and rebates; AWP stands for the average wholesale price; capitation is a type of reimbursement program; and MAC stands for maximum allowable cost, which is used in billing generic medications.

45. d—A standing order is one in which the patient receives a medication at a specific time each day

while in the hospital; an ASAP order is an urgent order, but not as urgent as a STAT order, which must be filled within 15 minutes of receipt.

46. c—A warm temperature is 30° to 40°C; a cool temperature is 8° to 15°C; room temperature is 15° to 30°C; and excessive heat occurs above 40°C.

47. c—Pyxis Medstation is an automated dispensing device kept on the nursing unit; Baker cells are used in an outpatient pharmacy; Omni Link Rx is a physician's order entry system; and Safety Pak is an automated barcode medication packaging system.

48. c—A medication number (prescription or serial number) is not required on a medication label.

49. b—Expiration date and lot number of a medication are not found on a patient package insert.

50. a—A centralized pharmacy is one where all functions occur in the main area. Medications are transferred to the floors at predetermined times. Decentralized and satellite pharmacies are synonymous and are located near the nursing unit. A floor stock system places all responsibility on the nursing staff.

ANSWERS TO ABBREVIATIONS QUESTIONS

1. a. ac = before meals
   b. amp = ampoule
   c. bid = twice a day
   d. cap = capsule
   e. emuls = emulsion
   f. hs = at bedtime or at hour of sleep
   g. npo = nothing by mouth
   h. oint = ointment
   i. pc = after meals
   j. po = by mouth
   k. pr = per rectum
   l. q4h = every 4 hr
   m. q6h = every 6 hr
   n. q8h = every 8 hr
   o. qd = every or each day
   p. qid = four times per day
   q. qod = every other day
   r. stat = immediately
   s. supp = suppository
   t. syr = syrup
   u. tab = tablet
   v. tid = three times per day

2. a. tsp = teaspoon
   b. tbsp = tablespoon
   c. qt = quart
   d. pt = pint
   e. oz = ounce
   f. NS = normal saline (0.9%)
   g. mL = milliliter

h. mg = milligram
i. mEq = milliequivalent
j. mcg = microgram
k. lb = pound
l. kg = kilogram
m. gr = grain
n. g = gram
o. gal = gallon
p. fl oz = fluid ounce
q. DW = distilled water
r. D5W = 5% dextrose in water
s. D5LR = 5% dextrose in lactated Ringer's solution
t. D20W = 20% dextrose in water
u. D10W = 10% dextrose in water
v. cc = cubic centimeter
w. 1/2 NS = 1/2 normal saline (0.45%)

3. a. APhA = American Pharmaceutical Association
   b. ASAP = as soon as possible
   c. AWP = average wholesale price
   d. CMS = Centers for Medicare and Medicaid Services
   e. DAW = dispense as written
   f. DEA = Drug Enforcement Agency
   g. EPA = Environmental Protection Agency
   h. FDA = Food and Drug Administration
   i. GERD = gastroesophageal reflux disease
   j. GPO = Group Purchasing Organization
   k. HIPAA = Health Insurance Portability and Accountability Act
   l. TJC = The Joint Commission
   m. MI = myocardial infarction
   n. NABP = National Association of Boards of Pharmacy
   o. NF = National Formulary
   p. OSHA = Occupational Safety and Health Administration
   q. OTC = over the counter
   r. P&T Committee = Pharmacy and Therapeutics Committee
   s. PI = protease inhibitor
   t. U & C = usual and customary
   u. USP = United States Pharmacopeia

4. 3TC = lamivudine
   APAP = acetaminophen
   ASA = aspirin
   AZT = azidothymidine
   ddi = didanosine
   D4T = stavudine
   $FeSO_4$ = ferrous sulfate
   HCTZ = hydrochlorothiazide
   INH = isoniazid
   KCl = potassium chloride

MOM = Milk of Magnesia
NTG = nitroglycerin
Pb = phenobarbital
PCN = penicillin
SMZ-TMP = sulfamethoxazole-trimethoprim
TCN = tetracycline

ANSWERS TO PRACTICE LAW QUESTIONS

1. b—The first five numbers identify the drug manufacturer, the middle four numbers identify the drug product, and the last two numbers identify the packaging.
2. b—The Food, Drug, and Cosmetic Act of 1938 defined adulteration and misbranding. Misbranding involves labeling.
3. b—The Occupational Safety and Health Act of 1970 required that work sites be safe for the employees.
4. d—The Poison Prevention Act of 1970 required that all prescriptions be prepared in child-resistant containers except in five different situations. The patient requesting an easy-open container is one of the situations.
5. b—This is an example of adulteration.
6. c—The Durham-Humphrey Act of 1950 allowed a prescription for a noncontrolled substance to be telephoned from a physician's office.
7. d—Nitroglycerin is one of the medications that does not need to be in a child-resistant container according to the Poison Control Act.
8. c—The Durham-Humphrey Act clearly defined legend and OTC medications.
9. c—The Durham-Humphrey Act stated that all legend medications must bear the following: "Federal law prohibits the dispensing of this medication without a prescription."
10. c—The Controlled Substances Act allows a DEA Form 222 to be valid for 60 days after it is signed by the pharmacist in charge or an individual with the power of attorney.
11. c—The Occupational Safety and Health Act of 1970 was written to protect the worker from hazards in the workplace. Material Safety Data Sheets are required to inform an individual of the hazards of handling a particular product and the appropriate treatment if one comes in contact with the substance.
12. b—The Controlled Substances Act allows for the partial filling of a Schedule II medication prescription, with the remaining medication to be provided to the patient within 72 hours or the quantity becomes void.
13. d—The Controlled Substances Act allows for the partial filling of a Schedule III to V medication on the request of the patient. The remaining balance of medication can be dispensed only if the physician has indicated a refill on the prescription. The total number of units of medication or refills cannot exceed what is indicated on the prescription.
14. a—The first letter of a physician's DEA number will be A, B, F, or M. The second letter is the first letter of the physician's last name at the time he or she applied for the DEA number. DEA numbers are required as a result of the Controlled Substances Act.
15. c—The Controlled Substances Act requires that a pharmacy use DEA Form 222 to purchase Schedule II medications. The DEA Form 222 issued to a pharmacy is specific to that pharmacy for the use of ordering or transferring Schedule II medications.
16. c—DEA Form 222 can be used to transfer Schedule II medications, such as Percocet, to another pharmacy.
17. b—On discovery of a theft of controlled substances, the local law enforcement agency needs to be notified and DEA Form 106 needs to be submitted.
18. c—HIPAA is concerned with insurance reform, patient confidentiality, and security of computer systems.
19. b—Centers for Medicare and Medicaid Services (CMS) oversees the operation and reimbursement of these two federal programs.
20. d—The Food, Drug, and Cosmetic Act (FDCA 1938) created the FDA, and one of its duties is to review Investigational New Drug Applications.
21. d—The Harrison Narcotic Act required a prescription for opium-containing products.
22. b—Comprehensive Drug Abuse Prevention and Control Act.
23. c—The Omnibus Reconciliation Act of 1990 (OBRA 90) required drug utilization on all prescriptions and medication orders and an offer to counsel patients on their prescriptions. Failure to perform these tasks may result in monetary penalties and the loss of Medicaid funds.
24. a—The Durham-Humphrey Act allowed prescriptions to be called to the pharmacy from a physician's office.
25. c—Tax-free saving accounts were created under the Medicare Drug Improvement and Modernization Act of 2003.
26. c—The Omnibus Reconciliation Act of 1987 was concerned with care in long-term care facilities; one of the items it addresses is the use of unnecessary medications.

27. d—The Poison Control Act of 1970 allows certain medications to be dispensed without a child-resistant container.
28. d—The Medicare Drug Improvement and Modernization Act of 2003 lowered the reimbursement rate for durable medical equipment.
29. d—The Prescription Drug Marketing Act prohibits the reimportation of medication into the United States. This law is being re-examined.
30. d—The state boards of pharmacy (BOP) oversee the practice of pharmacy in their respective states.

ANSWERS TO PHARMACOLOGY REVIEW QUESTIONS

1. a. Premarin = conjugated estrogens
   b. Lipitor = atorvastatin
   c. Norvasc = amlodipine
   d. Lanoxin = digoxin
   e. Zithromax = azithromycin
   f. Zocor = simvastatin
   g. Zestril = lisinopril
   h. Tenormin = atenolol
   i. Xanax = alprazolam
   j. Cardizem = diltiazem
   k. Glucotrol = glipizide
   l. Allegra = fexofenadine
   m. Procardia = nifedipine
   n. Dilantin = phenytoin
   o. Wellbutrin = bupropion
   p. Relafen = nabumetone
   q. Risperdal = risperidone
   r. Serevent = salmeterol
   s. Zantac = ranitidine
   t. Plavix = clopidogrel
   u. Azmacort = triamcinolone
   v. Amaryl = glimepiride
   w. Phenergan = promethazine
   x. Nolvadex = tamoxifen
   y. Lasix = furosemide
   z. Vasotec = enalapril

2. a. cephalexin = Keflex
   b. fluoxetine = Prozac
   c. paroxetine = Paxil
   d. mupirocin = Bactroban
   e. acetaminophen + codeine = Tylenol with Codeine
   f. propoxyphene N/APAP = Darvocet N
   g. triamterene/HCTZ = Dyazide or Maxzide
   h. alendronate = Fosamax
   i. losartan = Cozaar
   j. fluconazole = Diflucan
   k. amitriptyline = Elavil
   l. rosiglitazone = Avandia
   m. esomeprazole = Nexium
   n. olanzapine = Zyprexa
   o. montelukast = Singulair
   p. nefazodone = Serzone
   q. tolterodine = Detrol
   r. oxycodone = OxyContin
   s. acyclovir = Zovirax
   t. propranolol = Inderal
   u. doxycycline = Vibramycin
   v. nortriptyline = Pamelor
   w. etodolac = Daypro
   x. clindamycin = Cleocin
   y. metronidazole = Flagyl
   z. naproxen = Naprosyn

3. a. Vicodin:
      Do Not Drink Alcoholic Beverages
      May Cause Drowsiness
      Caution: Federal law prohibits the transfer of this drug to any person other than the patient for whom it was prescribed.
   b. Glucophage:
      Do Not Drink Alcoholic Beverages
      Take with Food or Milk
   c. Coumadin:
      Do Not Take with Aspirin
      Take Exactly as Directed by Physician
      Do Not Drink Alcoholic Beverages
   d. Cipro:
      Do Not Take with Antacids
      Avoid Sunlight
   e. Tetracycline:
      Avoid Sunlight
      Do not take Dairy Products and Antacids 1 Hour before Meals or 2 Hours after Meals
   f. Deltasone:
      Take with Food or Milk
      Take Exactly as Directed by Physician
   g. Biaxin:
      Shake Well
      Store at Room Temperature and Discard after 14 Days
   h. Ambien:
      Do Not Drink Alcoholic Beverages
      May Cause Drowsiness
      Caution: Federal law prohibits the transfer of this drug to any person other than the patient for whom it was prescribed.
   i. Motrin:
      Take with Food or Milk
      Do Not Drink Alcoholic Beverages
      May Cause Drowsiness
   j. Depakote:
      Take with Food or Milk
      May Cause Drowsiness

k. Xalatan:
    Refrigerate
    For Ophthalmic Use Only
l. Antivert:
    Do Not Drink Alcoholic Beverages
    May Cause Drowsiness
m. TobraDex:
    For Ophthalmic Use Only
n. Proventil:
    Shake Well
o. Bactrim Suspension:
    Shake Well
    Avoid Sunlight
    Store at Room Temperature
p. Augmentin:
    Take with Food or Milk
q. Benzamycin:
    Keep refrigerated
    Discard after 3 months
r. Minocin:
    Avoid Sunlight
    Do Not Take Dairy Products and Antacids
    1 Hour before Meals or 2 Hours after
    Meals
s. Amoxicillin suspension:
    Shake Well
    Refrigerate and Discard after 14 Days
t. Lotrisone cream:
    For External Use Only
u. Feldene:
    Take with Food or Milk
    Do Not Drink Alcoholic Beverages
v. Ritalin:
    Caution: Federal law prohibits the transfer of
    this drug to any person other than the patient
    for whom it was prescribed.
w. Vicoprofen:
    Take with Food or Milk
    May Cause Drowsiness
    Caution: Federal law prohibits the transfer of
    this drug to any person other than the patient
    for whom it was prescribed.
x. Hydrochlorothiazide:
    Take with Orange Juice or Banana
y. Ultram:
    May Cause Drowsiness
    Do Not Drink Alcoholic Beverages
z. Humulin N:
    Keep Refrigerated
    Shake Well

4. a. Premarin: hormone replacement
   b. Synthroid: hypothyroidism
   c. Lipitor: hyperlipidemia
   d. Prilosec: stomach ulcers
   e. Vicodin: analgesic

   f. Proventil: asthma
   g. Norvasc: hypertension
   h. Amoxil: antibiotic
   i. Prozac: depression
   j. Zoloft: depression
   k. Glucophage: diabetes
   l. Lanoxin: arrhythmias
   m. Prempro: hormone replacement
   n. Paxil: depression
   o. Zithromax: macrolide antibiotic
   p. Zestril: hypertension
   q. Zocor: hyperlipidemia
   r. Prevacid: stomach ulcers
   s. Augmentin: antibiotic
   t. Celebrex: analgesic
   u. Coumadin: anticoagulant
   v. Vasotec: hypertension
   w. Lasix: diuretic
   x. Cipro: antibiotic
   y. Keflex: antibiotic
   z. Deltasone: inflammation

5. a. pravastatin: hyperlipidemia
   b. clarithromycin: antibiotic
   c. norgestimate–ethinyl estradiol: birth control
   d. acetaminophen-codeine: analgesic
   e. atenolol: hypertension
   f. cetirizine: respiratory allergies
   g. zolpidem: hypnotic
   h. alprazolam: anxiety
   i. tramadol: analgesic
   j. quinapril: hypertension
   k. diltiazem: hypertension
   l. glipizide: diabetes
   m. fexofenadine: respiratory allergies
   n. triamterene-HCTZ: diuretic
   o. doxazosin: hypertension
   p. alendronate: osteoporosis
   q. benazepril: hypertension
   r. nifedipine: hypertension
   s. sildenafil citrate: erectile dysfunction
   t. ibuprofen: analgesic
   u. valproate: epilepsy
   v. phenytoin: epilepsy
   w. bupropion: depression; smoking cessation
   x. gabapentin: epilepsy
   y. losartan: hypertension
   z. fluconazole: fungus

6. a. sulfasalazine: sulfa drug
   b. erythromycin stearate: macrolide
   c. doxycycline: tetracycline
   d. ranitidine: H_2 blocker
   e. ampicillin: penicillin
   f. acyclovir: antiviral
   g. lamivudine: NRTI

h. promethazine: antiemetic
i. azelastine: antihistamine
j. codeine: narcotic analgesic
k. carbamazepine: antiepileptic
l. albuterol: bronchodilator
m. beclomethasone: corticosteroid
n. diphenoxylate + atropine: antidiarrheal
o. simethicone: antiflatulent
p. doxazosin: alpha-blocker
q. quinidine: membrane-stabilizing agent
r. amlodipine: calcium channel blocker
s. verapamil: calcium channel blocker
t. captopril: ACE inhibitor
u. hydrochlorothiazide: thiazide diuretic
v. lovastatin: HMG-CoA reductase inhibitor
w. sumatriptan: selective 5-HT receptor agonist
x. estradiol: estrogen replacement
y. fluconazole: antifungal
z. terbinafine: antifungal

7. a. fluoxetine: SSRI
   b. omeprazole: proton pump inhibitor
   c. cephalexin: cephalosporin antibiotic
   d. pravastatin: HMG-CoA reductase inhibitor
   e. celecoxib: COX-2 inhibitor
   f. sertraline: SSRI
   g. atenolol: beta-blocker
   h. furosemide: loop diuretic
   i. metformin: biguanide
   j. digoxin: cardiac glycoside
   k. sulfamethizole-trimethoprim: sulfa antibiotic
   l. ibuprofen: NSAID
   m. rosiglitazone: glitazone
   n. salmeterol: bronchodilator
   o. cefprozil: cephalosporin
   p. quinapril: ACE inhibitor
   q. amitriptyline: TCA
   r. lisinopril: ACE inhibitor
   s. imipramine: TCA
   t. fluvastatin: HMG-CoA reductase inhibitor
   u. ciprofloxacin: quinolone antibiotic
   v. indomethacin: NSAID
   w. hydroxyzine HCl: antihistamine
   x. carbamazepine: antiepileptic
   y. diltiazem: calcium channel blocker
   z. triamcinolone: corticosteroid

8. To what drug classification does each drug belong?
   a. esomeprazole: proton pump inhibitor
   b. prednisone: corticosteroid
   c. acetaminophen + codeine: analgesic
   d. zolpidem: hypnotic
   e. alprazolam: antianxiety agent
   f. fexofenadine: antihistamine
   g. doxazosin: alpha-blocker

   h. citalopram: SSRI
   i. naproxen: NSAID
   j. oxycodone: narcotic
   k. carvedilol: beta-blocker
   l. etodolac: NSAID
   m. piroxicam: NSAID
   n. acetaminophen + hydrocodone: analgesic
   o. levofloxacin: quinolone antibiotic
   p. enalapril: ACE inhibitor
   q. lansoprazole: proton pump inhibitor
   r. acetaminophen + oxycodone: analgesic
   s. tramadol: analgesic
   t. clotrimazole: antifungal
   u. nelfinavir: protease inhibitor
   v. butalbital/codeine/APAP: analgesic
   w. ketoconazole: antifungal
   x. clonidine: CNS agent
   y. nadolol: beta-blocker
   z. doxycycline: tetracycline antibiotic

9. a. Aloe vera: wound and burn healing
   b. Cascara sagrada: laxative
   c. St. John's wort: depression
   d. Melatonin: insomnia
   e. Gingko: memory improvement
   f. Glucosamine: osteoarthritis
   g. Cranberry: urinary tract infection
   h. Chondroitin: osteoarthritis
   i. Goldenseal: antimicrobial
   j. Echinacea: antiviral

ANSWERS TO PRACTICE MATH QUESTIONS

Conversions
1. 1 kg = 2.2 lb
2. 5.5 kg = 5500 g
3. 2500 mg = 2.5 g
4. 350 mcg = 0.350 mg
5. 75 mL = 75 cc
6. 120 mL = 24 tsp
7. 6 tsp = 2 tbsp
8. 7.5 fl oz = 45 tsp
9. 1.5 cups = 12 fl oz
10. 2 gal = 8 qt
11. 6.5 qt = 13 pt
12. 7.5 gr = 487.5 mg
13. 2 g = 30.7 gr
14. 1 L = 200 tsp
15. 650 mg = 10 gr
16. 125 mg = 0.125 g
17. 2.4 g = 2,400,000 mcg
18. 12 tsp = 4 tbsp
19. 2.5 qt = 80 fl oz

20. 75 mg = 0.075 g
21. 2 gal = 7680 mL
22. 8 cups = 0.5 gal
23. 1 lb = 454 g
24. 6 fl oz = 12 tbsp
25. 2 fl oz = 12 tsp

Calculations

Note: There may be more than one way to do many of these problems.

1. **Answer = 50,000 tablets.** Convert 30 g to mcg by multiplying by 1,000,000. Divide 30,000,000 mcg by 600 mcg/tablet.
2. **Answer = 200 mcg.** Convert mg to mcg by multiplying 0.2 mg by 1000 mcg/mg.
3. **Answer = 25 mg.** Multiply 5 mg by 3 days. Multiply 2½ mg by 4 days. Add the sum of these two products.
4. **Answer = 50 mcg.** Convert 0.05 mg to micrograms. Multiply 0.05 mg by 1000 mcg.
5. **Answer = 1.33 mL.** This is a proportion problem that uses both Arabic and Roman numerals (V = 5 and VIISS = 7.5). Set the proportion up as 7.5 gr/2 mL = 5 gr/X mL.
6. **Answer = 6.25 g.** Multiply 250 mcg/tablet by 25,000 tablets. Divide the product 1,000,000 mcg/g.
7. **Answer = 0.4 mg.** 1 grain is equal 65 mg. Solve by using the following proportion: 65 mg/1 gr = X mg/1/150 gr.
8. **Answer = 3.0 g of antipyrine.** Use the following formula: Final weight × % (expressed as a decimal) = Amount of active ingredient, where 60 g is the final weight and 5% is equal to 0.05.
9. **Answer = 7 mL.** This problem can be solved by using the following proportion: 50 mg/5 mL = 70 mg/X mL.
10. **Answer = 5000 mcg.** Solve using a proportion: 20 mg/2 mL = X mg/0.5 mL, where X = 5 mg. Convert 5 mg to micrograms by multiplying by 1000 mcg/mg.
11. **Answer = 187.5 to 375 mg.** Convert pounds to kilograms (165 lb × 1 kg/2.2 lb). Multiply the weight in kilograms by 2.5 mg to obtain the lower dose and multiply the weight in kilograms to obtain the upper dose.
12. **Answer = 49 capsules.** Convert pounds to kilograms (154 lb × 1 kg/2.2 lb). Multiply the weight in kilograms by 25 mg/kg to obtain the dose per day. Multiply the daily dose by 7 days. Divide the total dose by 250 mg per capsule to obtain the number of capsules needed.
13. **Answer = 9.54 mL.** Convert pounds to kilograms (140 lb × 1 kg/2.2 lb). Multiple the weight in kilograms by 15 mg/kg to obtain the daily dosage required. To calculate volume desired, solve using a proportion: 100 mg/mL = daily dosage/X mL.
14. **Answer = 0.6 mL.** This can be solved using a proportion: 250 mg/10 mL = 15 mg/X mL. Cross-multiplying and dividing will provide you with the answer.
15. **Answer = 12.5 mg.** Convert weight in pounds to kilograms (55 lb × 1 kg/2.2 lb). Multiply weight in kilograms by 500 mcg/kg to obtain the correct dose in micrograms. Convert micrograms to milligrams by multiplying micrograms by 1 mg/1000 mcg.
16. **Answer = 0.05 mL.** The problem can be solved by using two proportions. First, convert 330 mcg to milligrams (1000 mcg/1 mg = 330 mcg/X mg, where X = 0.330 mg). Next, calculate the number of milliliters by using the following formula: 6.6 mg/mL = 0.330 mg/X mL.
17. **Answer = 0.58 mL.** This can be solved using a proportion: 2.5 mg/2 mL = 0.725 mg/X mL.
18. **Answer = 1.2 mL.** This can be solved using a proportion: 80 mg/mL = 100 mg/X mL.
19. **Answer = 10 g.** Convert 20 mg to grams by using the following proportion: 1000 mg/1 g = 20 mg/X g, where X = 0.02 g. Next, determine the number of mL in 0.5 L by using a proportion: 1 L/1000 mL = 0.5 L/X mL, where X = 500 mL. Next, use a proportion to solve for the number of grams: 0.02 g/1 mL = X g/500 mL, where X = 10 g.
20. **Answer = 32 doses.** One tablespoon is equal to 15 mL, and 1 pint is equal to 480 mL. Solve using a proportion: 15 mL/1 dose = 480 mL/X doses, where X = 32 doses.
21. **Answer = 56 tablets.** Solve using the following proportion: 75 mg dose/1 tablet = 300 mg dose/X tablets, which is 4 tablets. The abbreviation "bid" means twice per day. Solve for the number of tablets: 4 tablets/dose × 2 doses/day × 7 days = 56 tablets.
22. **Answer = 4%.** Convert the ratio to a proportion (1:25 is equal to 1/25). Next, multiply 1/25 by 100 to obtain the answer of 4%.
23. **Answer = 0.5%.** Convert the ratio to a proportion (1:200 is equal to 1/200). Next, multiply 1/200 by 100 to obtain the answer of 0.5%.
24. **Answer = 77° F.** Solve by using the formula 9C = 5F − 160, where you replace the C with 25: (9)(25) = (5)(F) − 160, and perform the necessary operations.
25. **Answer = 18.33° C.** Solve by using the formula 9C = 5F − 160, where you replace the F with 65: (9)(C) = (5)(65) − 160, and perform the necessary operations.
26. **Answer = 104° F.** Solve by using the formula 9C = 5F − 160, where you replace the C with 40:

$(9)(40) = (5)(F) - 160$ and perform the necessary operations.

27. **Answer = 7°C.** Solve by using the formula $9C = 5F - 160$, where you replace the F with 45: $(9)(C) = (5)(F) - 160$ and perform the necessary operations.

28. **Answer = 0.48 mL.** This can be solved as a proportion using international units: 500,000 units/1.2 mL = 200,000 units/X mL.

29. **Answer = 1.0 mL.** This is a proportion problem. 50 units/2 mL = 25 units/X mL, where X = 1.0 mL.

30. **Answer = 3.5 mL.** This is a proportion problem. 50,000 units/1 mL = 175,000 units/X mL, where X = 3.5 mL.

31. **Answer = 3 packets.** This is a proportion problem using mEq: 20 mEq/1 packet = 60 mEq/X packets, where X = 3 packets.

32. **Answer = 7.5 mL.** Solve this problem using the following proportion: 40 mEq/tbsp = 20 mEq/X mL, where X = 7.5 mL.

33. **Answer = 800 doses.** Convert 0.120 g to mcg (1,000,000 mcg/1 g = X mcg/0.120 g, where X = 120,000 mcg). Calculate the number of doses using a proportion: 150 mcg/1 dose = 120,000 mcg/X doses, where X = 800 doses.

34. **Answer = 200 mL.** The patient is to take 250 mg four times per day for 10 days. 250 mg is contained in a 1-tsp (5-mL) dose: (5 mL/dose)(4 doses/day)(10 days) = 200 mL.

35. **Answer = 7.5 mL.** Convert 25 lb to kilograms using the following proportion: 2.2 lb/1 kg = 25 lb/X kg, where X = 11.36 kg. Multiply patient's weight (kg) by the dose (4 mg/kg) or (4 mg/kg)(11.36 kg) = 45.45 mg. Calculate the number of milliliters needed: 30 mg/5 mL = 45.45 mg/X mL, where X = 7.5 mL.

36. **Answer = 108 mg/kg.** Convert the weight of the child in pounds to kilograms by dividing 33 lb by 2.2 lb/kg, which equals 15 kg. Calculate the amount of aspirin the child consumed by multiplying 20 tablets by 81 mg/tablet, which equals 1620 mg. Solve using a proportion: 1620 mg/15 kg = X mg/1 kg, which equals 108 mg/kg.

37. **Answer = 166.67 mg/kg.** Calculate the weight in kilograms by dividing 44 lb by 2.2 lb/kg, which equals 20 kg. Calculate the number of milligrams per day by multiplying 25 mg/kg/day by 20 kg, which equals 500 mg. The patient is to receive three equal doses. Divide the total amount of medication by three doses (500 mg/3 doses = 166.67 mg/dose).

38. **Answer = 25 mg.** Solve using Young's rule. Young's rule = {Age (in years)/[Age (in years) + 12]} × Adult dose. In this problem the child is 4 years old and the adult dose is 100 mg. Substituting into the equation will result in the following: [4/(4 + 12)] × 100 mg = 25 mg.

39. **Answer = 50 mg.** Solve by using Young's rule. 36 months/12 months/year = 3 years. [(3)/(3 + 12)] × 250 mg = 50 mg.

40. **Answer = 17 mg.** Solve using Young's rule: [2.5/(2.5 + 12)] × 100 mg = 17 mg.

41. **Answer = 15 mg.** Solve using Clark's rule. Clark's rule = [Weight (lb)/150] × Adult dose = Amount of dose (45/150) × 50 mg = 15 mg.

42. **Answer = 5 mL.** Solve using Clark's rule: (50/150) × 15 mL = 5 mL.

43. **Answer = 200 mg.** Solve using Clark's rule: (60/150) × 500 mg = 200 mg.

44. **Answer = 16.5 mg.** Solve using Clark's rule. First convert kilograms to pounds: 1 kg/2.2 lb = 15 kg/X lb, where X equals 33 lb. Substitute into the equation: (33/150) × 75 mg = 16.5 mg.

45. **Answer = 0.76.** Specific gravity (SG) = Weight of a substance/Weight of an equal volume of water, where 1 mL of water weighs 1 g. You have been given the weight (95 g) and volume of the substance (125 mL = 125 g). SG = 95/125 or 0.76.

46. **Answer = 76 mL.** Specific gravity = 1.05 and weight is 80 g. Substituting into the equation for specific gravity: 1.05 = 80/X, where X = 76 mL.

47. **Answer = 125 g.** Specific gravity is 1.25 and equal volume of liquid is 100 mL. Substituting into the equation for specific gravity: 1.25 = X/100, where X = 125 g.

48. **Answer = 0.8.** Weight of substance is 60 g and it occupies a volume of 75 mL. Substituting into the equation for specific gravity: SG = 60/75, where the SG = 0.8.

49. **Answer = 2.5 g.** 1 L = 1000 mL. Convert % to a decimal (%/100 or 0.25%/100 = 0.0025). Solve using the following equation: Final volume (FV) × % (expressed as a decimal) = Amount of active ingredient (AI). 1000 mL × 0.0025 = 2.5 g of silver nitrate. In this situation, because it is a solution (w/v), the AI will be expressed in grams.

50. **Answer = 22.7 g.** 1 lb = 454 g. Convert the % (5%) to a decimal (0.05). Solve using the following equation: FW × % (decimal) = Amount of AI (g) or 454 g × 0.05 = 22.7 g. The AI is expressed in grams because it is a w/w problem.

51. **Answer = 1.125 g.** Convert % (0.45%) to a decimal (0.0045). Solve using the following equation: FV × % (decimal) = Amount of AI (g) or 250 mL × 0.0045 = 1.125 g. The answer must be expressed in grams because it is a w/v problem.

52. **Answer = 5 g.** 1:200 is a ratio. 1 L = 1000 mL. Convert ratio (1:200) to a fraction (1/200) and

express the answer as a decimal (0.05). This is a w/v problem and can be solved using the following: FV (1000 mL) × Percent as a decimal (0.005) = Amount of AI (5 g).

53. **Answer = 10,000 mcg.** Convert ratio (1:100) to a fraction (1/100) to a decimal (0.01). In this problem, the FV (1.0 mL) × % as a decimal (0.01) = 0.01 g. One is asked to answer the problem in micrograms, which can be converted by (0.01 g)(1000 mg/1 g)(1000 mcg/1 mg) = 10,000 mcg.

54. **Answer = 4.88%.** This is a dilution problem and can be solved using the following equation: Initial strength (IS) × Initial weight (IW) = Final strength (FS) × Final weight (FW). IS = 5%, IW = 120 g, FS (unknown), FW = 123 g. (5%)(120 g) = (X%)(123 g), where X = 4.88%.

55. **Answer = 60 tablets.** 8 oz of ointment is approximately 240 g. The problem can be solved using the following equation: FW × % (decimal) = Amount of AI (g) or 240 g × 0.15 = 36 g or 3600 mg (36 g × 1000 mg/g) of active ingredient. To calculate the number of tablets needed, divide the total amount of AI by the weight of one tablet, which is 36,000 mg/600 mg/tablet = 60 tablets.

56. **Answer = 30 mL.** This is a dilution problem and can be solved using (IS)(IV) = (FS)(FV), where IS (3%), IV (unknown), FS (1:200), and FV (6 oz). One needs to make sure that both the strengths and volumes are in common terms. Convert the ratio (1:200) to a fraction (1/200) to a decimal (0.005) to a percent (0.005 × 100 = 0.5%). Next, convert ounces (6 oz) to milliliters: (6 oz)(30 mL/oz) = 180 mL. Substitute into the following equation: (IS)(IV) = (FS)(FV) or (IV)(3%) = (0.5%)(180 mL), where IV is 30 mL.

57. **Answer = 64%.** This is a dilution problem and can be solved using the following: (IS)(IV) = (FS)(FV), where IS = unknown, IV = 2 oz, FS = 4%, and FV = 32 oz (4 bottles × 8 oz/bottle). (IS)(2 oz) = (4%)(32 oz), where IS = 64%.

58. **Answer = 6.67 mL.** This is a dilution problem and can be solved using (IS)(IV) = (FS)(FV), where IS = 75%, IV = unknown, FS = 4%, and FV = 125 mL: (75%)(IV) = (4%)(125 mL), where IV = 6.67 mL.

59. **Answer = 2.5%.** 1 L = 1000 mL. This is a dilution problem, where IS = 25%, IV = 100 mL, FS = unknown, and FV = 1000 mL: (25%)(100 mL) = (FS)(1000 mL), where FV = 2.5%.

60. **Answer = 76.8 mL.** This is a dilution problem, where IS = 75%, IV = unknown, FS = 72%, and FV = 80 mL: (75%)(IV) = (72%)(80 mL), where IV = 76.8 mL.

61. **Answer = 476 mL.** 1 gallon = 3840 mL. This is a dilution problem, where IS = 10%, IV = unknown, FS = 1.24%, and FV = 3840 mL: (10%)(IV) = (1.24%)(3840 mL), where IV = 476 mL.

62. **Answer = 51 g.** One ounce (wt) is approximately 30 g. This is a dilution problem, where IS = 10%, IW = 120 g (4 oz × 30 g/oz), FS = 7%, and FW = unknown: (10%)(120 g) = (75%)(FW) where FW = 171 g. The problem is asking for the amount of diluent to be added. FW − IW = Amount of diluents, or 171 g − 120 g = 51 g of diluent.

63. **Answer = 10 mL.** This is a dilution problem where the concentrations are expressed as ratios, but it can be solved in the same way. IS = 1:20, IV = unknown, FS = 1:100, and FV = 50 mL: (1:20)(IV) = (1:100)(50 mL), where IV = 10 mL.

64. **Answer = 91.94 mL.** This is a dilution problem using ratios as concentrations. IS = 1:6, IV = unknown, FS = 1:8, and FV = 125 mL: (1:6)(IV) = (1:8)(125 mL), where IV = 91.94 mL.

65. **Answer = 33 mL.** This is a dilution problem using ratios as concentrations. IS = 1:2, IV = unknown, FS = 1:3, and FV = 50 mL: (1:2)(IV) = (1:3)(50 mL), where IV = 33 mL.

66. **Answer = 25 mL.** 2 L = 2000 mL (2 L × 1000 mL/L). This is a dilution problem using ratios as concentrations. IS = 1:50, IV = unknown, FS = 1:4000, and FV = 2000 mL, where IV = 25 mL.

67. **Answer = 750 mL.** This is a dilution problem using ratios as concentrations. IS = 1:2000, IV = 500 mL, FS = 1:5000, and FV = unknown: (1:2000)(500 mL) = (1:5000)(FS), where FS = 1250 mL. The problem is asking for the amount of diluent to be added and can be calculated by subtracting the initial volume from the final volume. 1250 mL − 500 mL = 750 mL of diluent.

68. **Answer = 2400 mL.** 1 quart = 960 mL. This is a dilution problem asking for the amount of diluent (water) to be added in preparing this compound. IS = 70%, IV = 960 mL, FS = 20%, and FV = unknown: (70%)(960 mL) = (20%)(FV), where FV = 3360 mL. FV − IV = amount of diluent to be added or 3360 mL − 960 mL = 2400 mL.

69. **Answer = 1 mL.** This is a dilution problem using concentration expressed as milligrams per milliliter but can be solved the same way. IS = 5 mg/mL, IV = unknown, FS = 0.5 mg/mL, and FV = 10 mL: (5 mg/mL)(IV) = (0.5 mg/mL)(10 mL), where IV = 1 mL.

70. **Answer = 3.75 mL of cefazolin; 11.25 mL of diluent.** This is a dilution problem that can be solved using the following formula: (IS)(IV) =

(FS)(FV), where the IS = 1 g/5 mL or (1000 mg/5 mL), IV is unknown, the FS is 50 mg/mL, and the FV is 15 mL. (1000 mg/5 mL)(IV) = (50 mg/mL)(15 mL), where the IV = 3.75 of cefazolin. The problem asks for the amount of diluent that is needed and can be solved using (FV) − (IV) = Amount of diluent: (15 mL) − (3.75 mL) = 11.25 mL of diluent.

71. **Answer = 3 mL of vitamin B_{12} and 27 mL of diluent.** This is a dilution problem that can be solved using the following formula: (IS)(IV) = (FS)(FV), where the IS = 1 mg/mL or 1000 mcg/mL, IV is unknown, FS = 100 mcg/mL, and FV = 30 mL: (1000 mcg/mL)(IV) = (100 mcg/mL)(30 mL), where IV = 3 mL. The amount of diluent = FV − IV or 30 mL − 3 mL = 27 mL.

72. **Answer = 30 mL.** This is a dilution problem where concentrations are expressed as a concentration and a percentage. The concentrations need to be expressed in the same terms. Convert the ratio (1:4) to a percent (25%). This is a dilution problem that can be solved using the following formula: (IS)(IV) = (FS)(FV), where IS = 30%, IV is unknown, FS = 25%, and FV = 36 mL: (30%)(IV) = (25%)(36 mL), where IV = 30 mL.

73. **Answer = 0.35 mL.** This is a dilution where concentrations are expressed as both percentages and in grams per milliliter—therefore the concentrations must be expressed in the same terms; 28% means that that 28 g are in 100 mL of solution or 0.28 g/mL. IS = 42 g/mL, IV is unknown, FS = 0.28 g/mL, and FV = 52 mL: (42 g/mL)(IV) = (0.28 g/mL)(52 mL), where X = 0.35 mL.

74. **Answer = 1 mL.** This is a dilution problem with concentrations expressed as both percentages and a ratio. Convert 1:100,000 to a percent (0.001%); IS = 0.5%, IV is unknown, FS = 1/100,000, and FV = 500 mL: (0.5%)(IV) = (0.001%)(500 mL), where IV = 1 mL.

75. **Answer = 0.96 mL.** This is a dilution problem with strengths being expressed as both percentages and in milligrams per liter. w/v% is the number of grams per 100 mL of solution. Convert 100 mg/1000 mL to a percent, which is 0.01%.

76. **Answer = 379 mL.** This is a dilution problem with concentrations expressed in percentages. IS = 95%, IV is unknown, FS = 75%, and the FV is 1 pint (480 mL): (95%) × (IV) = (75%) × (480 mL), where X = 379 mL.

77. **Answer = 95%—5:9; 50%—4:9.** This is an alligation problem. Draw a tic-tac-toe table, placing the highest concentration (95%) in the upper left corner, the desired concentration (75%) in the middle, and the lowest concentration (50%) in the bottom left corner. Subtract the concentrations in a diagonal manner and place the number opposite the remaining concentration. 95% − 75% = 20 parts of 50%. 75% − 50% = 25 parts of 95%. Total all of the parts (45); 95% will require 25/45 (5:9) and 50% will require 20/45 (4:9).

78. **Answer = 7.5%—55.6 mL; 1:2000—64.4 mL.** This is an alligation problem. Convert 1:2000 to a percent (0.5%). Draw a tic-tac-toe table, placing the highest concentration (7.5%) in the upper left corner, the desired concentration (3.5%) in the middle, and the lowest concentration in the bottom left corner (0.5%). Subtract the concentrations in a diagonal manner and place the number opposite the remaining concentration. Calculate the proportions of each needed and multiply by the quantity to be prepared. 7.5%: (3 parts/7 parts) × 120 mL = 55.6 mL; 0.5%: (4 parts/7 parts) × 120 mL = 64.4 mL.

79. **Answer = 2.5%—109 mL; 0.9%—391 mL.** This is an alligation problem. Draw a tic-tac-toe table, placing the highest concentration (2.5) in the upper left corner, the desired concentration (1.25) in the middle, and the lowest concentration (0.9%) in the bottom left corner. Subtract the concentrations in a diagonal manner and place the number opposite the remaining concentration. Calculate the proportions of each needed and multiply by the quantity to be prepared. 2.5%: (0.4 parts/1.65 parts) × 500 mL = 109 mL; 0.9%: (1.25 parts/1.65 parts) × 500 mL = 391 mL.

80. **Answer = 20%—250 mL; 10%—750 mL.** This is an alligation problem. Draw a tic-tac-toe table, placing the highest concentration (20%) in the upper left corner, the desired concentration (12.5%) in the middle, and the lowest concentration (10%) in the bottom left corner. Subtract the concentrations in a diagonal manner and place the number opposite the remaining concentration. Calculate the proportions of each needed and multiply by the quantity to be prepared (1 L = 1000 mL). 20%: (2.5 parts/10 parts) × 1000 mL = 250 mL; 10%: (7.5 parts/10 parts) × 1000 mL = 750 mL.

81. **Answer = 5%—1.5 parts; 1%—2.5 parts.** This is an alligation problem. Draw a tic-tac-toe table, placing the highest concentration (5%) in the upper left corner, the desired concentration (2.5%) in the middle, and the lowest concentration (1%) in the bottom left corner. Subtract the concentrations in a diagonal manner and place the number opposite the remaining concentration. Calculate the proportions of each needed. 5%: 1.5:4 and 1%: 2.5:4.

82. **Answer = 20%—112.5 mL; SWFI—187.5 mL.** This is an alligation problem using IV solutions. Draw a tic-tac-toe table, placing the highest concentration (20%) in the upper left corner, the desired concentration (7.5%) in the middle, and the lowest concentration (0%) in the bottom left corner. Subtract the concentrations in a diagonal manner and place the number opposite the remaining concentration. SWFI is sterile water for injection and has a concentration of 0%, and D20W means 20% dextrose in water. Calculate the proportions of each needed and multiply by the quantity to be prepared. 20%: (7.5 parts/20 parts) × 300 mL = 112.5 mL; SWFI: (12.5 parts/20 parts) × 300 mL = 187.5 mL.

83. **Answer = 20% and 5%—250 mL; 20%—125 mL, 10%—375 mL.** This problem can be prepared using two different combinations (20% and 5%; 20% and 10%) to prepare 500 mL of D12.5. In both situations one must have a concentration above the desired concentration and one concentration below the desired concentration. Draw a tic-tac-toe table, placing the highest concentration (20%) in the upper left corner, the desired concentration (12.5%) in the middle, and the lowest concentration (5%) in the bottom left corner. Subtract the concentrations in a diagonal manner and place the number opposite the remaining concentration. Subtract the concentrations in a diagonal manner and place the number opposite the remaining concentration. Calculate the proportions of each needed and multiply by the quantity to be prepared. 20%: (7.5 parts/15 parts) × 500 mL = 250 mL; 5%: (7.5 parts/15 parts) × 500 mL. Draw a tic-tac-toe table, placing the highest concentration (20%) in the upper left corner, the desired concentration (12.5%) in the middle, and the lowest concentration (10%) in the bottom left corner. Subtract the concentrations in a diagonal manner and place the number opposite the remaining concentration. Subtract the concentrations in a diagonal manner and place the number opposite the remaining concentration. Calculate the proportions of each needed and multiply by the quantity to be prepared. 20%: (2.5 parts/10 parts) × 500 mL = 125 mL; 10%: (7.5 parts/10 parts) × 500 mL = 375 mL.

84. **Answer = 120 g.** This is an alligation problem to prepare an ointment. Draw a tic-tac-toe table, placing the highest concentration (2.5%) in the upper left corner, the desired concentration (1%) in the middle, and the lowest concentration (0.25%) in the bottom left corner. Subtract the

concentrations in a diagonal manner and place the number opposite the remaining concentration. Calculate the proportions of each needed. Set up a proportion to calculate the total weight of the preparation by using the 240 g of 0.25% ointment: 1.5 parts/2.25 parts = 240 g/X, where X = 360 g. To calculate the amount of 2.5% needed, subtract the amount of the 0.25% from the total weight of the compound: 360 g (total weight) – 240 g (weight of 0.25%) = 120 g (weight of 2.5%).

85. **Answer = 600 mL.** This problem can be solved by multiplying the rate (25 mL/hr) by the amount of time (24 hr): (25 mL/hr) × (24 hr) = 600 mL.

86. **Answer = 12.5 mL/hr.** Rate = volume/time (hr), or 1000 mL/8 hr = 125 mL/hr.

87. **Answer = a. 41 mL/hr.** Rate = volume/time, or 1000 mL/24 hr = 41 hr. A number less than a whole is rounded down in flow rates. **b. 10 gtt/min.** The problem can be solved by the following formula: Rate × Drop factor × Conversion factor = gtt/min: (41 mL/hr) × (15 gtt/mL) × (1 hr/60 min) = 10 gtt/min.

88. **Answer = 0500 hr on the next day.** Calculate the amount of time the IV will last (Time = Volume/Time) or 1500 mL/75 mL/hr = 20 hr. The first bag was hung at 0900 hours and will last 20 hours: 0900 hr + 2000 hr – 2400 hr/day = 0500 hr on the next day.

89. **Answer = 62.5 mL/hr.** Rate = Volume/Time, or 250 mL/4 hr = 62.5 mL/hr. **62.5 mg/hr.** Amount of drug/Time. 250 mg/4 hr = 62.5 mg/hr.

90. **Answer = 420 mL.** Volume = Rate × Time or 120 mL/hr × 3½ hr = 420 mL.

91. **Answer = 31 gtt/min.** Solve by using: Rate × Drop factor × Conversion factor = gtt/min: (1000 mL/8 hr) × (15 gtt/mL) × (1 hr/60 min) = 31 gtt/min.

92. **Answer = 80 mL/hr.** Solve by using: Rate = (gtt/min)/(Drop factor) × (Conversion factor): (20 gtt/min)/(15 gtt/mL) × (1 hr/60 min) = 80 mL/hr.

93. **Answer = 5 mL/min.** Calculate the amount of time 0.1 g (100 mg) would be infused into the body if the patient is receiving 1 mg/min by using a proportion: 1 mg/min = 100 mg/X min, which is 100 min. 100 mg is contained in 500 mL, which will take 100 min to infuse. The flow rate = Volume (500 mL)/Time (100 minutes) = 5 mL/min.

94. **Answer = 3.82 mL.** Convert the patient's weight from pounds to kilograms (280 lb × 1 kg/2.2 lb = 127.27 kg). Calculate the dose needed: (127.27 kg) × (150 units/kg) = 19,095 units. Solve

using a proportion: 5000 units/mL = 19,095 units/X mL, where X = 3.82 mL.

95. **Answer = 16 gtt/min.** Calculate the rate: (100 mL/1.5 hr) = 66 mL/hr. Calculate drops per minute by multiplying the rate by the drop factor by the conversion factor: (66 mL/hr) × (15 gtt/mL) × (1 hr/60 min) = 16 gtt/min.

96. **Answer = 25 gtt/min.** Calculate the rate (150 mL/2 hr = 75 mL/hr). Calculate drops per minute by multiplying the rate by the drop factor by the conversion factor: (75 mL/hr) × (20 gtt/mL) × (1 hr/60 min) = 25 gtt/min.

97. **Answer = 12 gtt/min.** Calculate drops per minute by multiplying the rate by the drop factor by the conversion factor: (50 mL/hr) × (15 gtt/mL) × (1 hr/60 min) = 12 gtt/min.

98. **Answer = 62 gtt/min.** Rate = 125 mL/hr; drop factor (DF) = 30 gtt/ mL and 1 hour/60 min (conversion factor [CF]). Solve using the following formula: Rate × DF × CF = gtt/min: (125 mL/hr) × (30 gtt/mL) × (1 hr/60 min) = 62 gtt/min. Remember drops per minute are always rounded downward when one has a fraction of a drop.

99. **Answer = $3,377,865.** Overhead is the sum of all the expenses a business experiences. In this problem, because there are two pharmacists, multiply the pharmacist salary by 2 and the pharmacy technician's salary by 3 to calculate the total salaries. Add up all of the expenses to obtain the overhead.

100. **Answer = $8.00.** Gross profit can be calculated by subtracting the cost, which in this case is the same as the average wholesale price (AWP) or from the retail price: $67.99 – $59.99 = $8.00.

101. **Answer = $4.00.** *Markup* is another term for gross profit. In this problem the markup is equal to retail price (13.99) – Cost (9.99), which is $4.00.

102. **Answer = 30%.** Markup rate is the markup dollars divided by the cost times 100. Calculate the markup: Retail price ($25.99) – Cost ($19.99) = $6.00. Divide the markup dollars ($6.00) by the cost ($19.99) and multiply by 100: ($6.00/$19.99) × 100 = 30%.

103. **Answer = $8.75.** Net profit is the retail price ($112.99) minus the cost of product or the actual acquisition cost ($99.99) minus any expenses ($4.25) associated with the product: ($112.99 – $9.99) – $4.25 = $8.75.

104. **Answer = $94.68.** Add the cost of the test strips ($67.50) to the overhead costs ($3.50) to obtain the total cost ($67.50 + $3.50 = $71.00). To calculate the selling price, add the total cost and net profit together to obtain the selling price: $71.00 + $23.68 = $94.68.

105. **Answer = $1911.** The pharmacy will receive a 2% discount off the total bill if the bill is paid in full within 30 days. $1,950.00 – (0.02)(1950.00) = $1911.00.

106. **Answer = 11.76.** Inventory turns can be calculated by dividing total sales by the inventory value or the average inventory value. Sales (3,000,000)/inventory ($255,000) = 11.76 inventory turns.

107. **Answer = 10.95.** The average inventory can be calculated by adding the initial inventory ($225,000) and the final inventory ($250,000) and dividing the sum ($475,000) by 2, resulting in an average inventory of $237,500. Divide total sales ($2,600,000) by average inventory ($237,500) = 10.95 inventory turns.

108. **Answer = a. 8.33 mg/capsule.** You have been given a formula that will yield 24 capsules. Divide the amount of hydrocodone bitartrate (0.2 g) by the number of capsules one is to prepare: 0.2 g/24 capsules = 0.00833 g/capsule. Convert 0.00833 g to milligrams by multiplying 0.0833 g × 1000 mg/g = 8.33 mg/capsule. **b. 430 mg per capsule.** Add up the total weight of all of the ingredients (10.4 g) and divide by 24 capsules. Each capsule will weigh 0.43 g. Convert grams to milligrams: 0.43 g × 1000 mg/g = 430 mg. **c. 75 mg.** 0.6 g of caffeine/24 capsules = 0.025 g of caffeine/capsule. Convert grams to milligrams. 0.025 g × 1000 mg/1 g = 25 mg. The directions state that the patient is to take one capsule three times per day. 25 mg of caffeine/capsule × 3 capsules = 75 mg.

109. **Answer = 10 1-g Carafate tablets.** Calculate the amount of Carafate needed for the compound; this can be done through the use of a proportion: 400 mg/5 mL = X mg/125 mL, where 10,000 mg of Carafate is the entire quantity. One can calculate the number of grams needed by using a proportion. 1 g/1000 mg = X g/10,000 mg, where X = 10 1-g tablets of Carafate.

110. **Answer = 43.2 g of iodine; 51.84 g of sodium iodide.** You have been asked to prepare 12 dozen 15-mL bottles, which is equal to (12)(12 bottles/1 dozen bottles)(15 mL) = 2160 mL of solution. The formula will make 1000 mL of solution. Calculate the amount needed of each ingredient by using the following formula: [Total quantity needed of compound (TQN)/ Quantity required for original formula (QRF)] × Amount of ingredient in original formula: (2160 mL/1000 mL) × 20 g of iodide = 43.2 g of iodide and (2160 mL/1000 mL) × 24 g of sodium iodide = 51.84 g of sodium iodide.

111. **Answer = Benzoyl benzoate**   **30 mL**
    Triethanolamine   **0.6 mL**
    Oleic acid   **2.4 mL**
    Purified water to make 500 mL   **120 mL**
This problem needs a smaller quantity to be made than is called for in the original formula. Use the following formula: (TQN/QRF) × Amount of each ingredient. (120 mL/500 mL) × 125 mL = 30 mL of benzoate; (120 mL/500 mL) × 2.5 mL = 0.6 mL of triethanolamine; (125 mL/500 mL) × 10 mL = 2.4 mL of oleic acid.

112. **Answer = Dextromethorphan**   **5760 mg**
    (5.76 g)
    Guaifenesin   **76,800 mg**
    (76.8 g)
    Flavored syrup to make 5.0 mL   **3840 mL**
This problem is enlarged from the original formula and can be calculated using the following formula: (TQN/QRF) × Amount of each ingredient. (3840 mL/5 mL) × 7.5 mg = 5760 mg (5.76 g) of dextromethorphan; (3840 mL/5 mL) × 100 mg = 76,800 mg (76.8 g) of guaifenesin.

113. **Answer = Coal tar**   **9.08 g**
    Precipitated sulfur   **13.62 g**
    Salicylic acid   **4.54 g**
    Lidex ointment   **108.96 g**
    Aquabase   **317.80 g**
This formula is going to be enlarged. One pound is equal to 454 g. This problem is not qs (or brought) to a final weight; therefore one must add up all the ingredients to determine the weight in the original formula, which is 100 g. The following formula can be used: (TQN/QRF) × Amount of each ingredient. (454 g/100 g) × Amount of each ingredient × 2.0 g = 9.08 g of coal tar; (454 g/100 g) × 3.0 g = 13.62 g of precipitated sulfur; (454 g/100 g) × 1.0 g = 4.54 g of salicylic acid; (454 g/100 g) × 24 g = 108.96 g of Lidex ointment; and (454 g/100 g) × 70 g = 317.8 g of Aquabase.

114. **Answer = Estriol**   **5 g**
    Estrone   **0.625 g**
    Estradiol   **0.625 g**
    Polyethylene glycol 1450   **14,500.5 kg**
    Polyethylene glycol 3350   **33,500.5 kg**
This formula is being enlarged. the following formula can be used: (TQN/QRF) × Amount of each ingredient. (2500 capsules/100 capsules) × 200 mg = 5 g of estriol; (2500 capsules/100 capsules) × 25 mg = 0.625 g of estrone; (2500 capsules/100 capsules) × 25 mg of estradiol; (2500 capsules/100 capsules) × 20 g = 0.5 kg of PEG 1450; and (2500 capsules/100 capsules) × 20 g = 0.5 kg of PEG 3350.

CHAPTER 2 REVIEW ANSWERS

1. a—Group purchasing organizations (GPOs) negotiate the best possible prices for hospitals; they do not purchase the medications for a hospital. The purchasing department of the hospital makes the purchases.

2. b—Some patients may experience difficulty swallowing capsules, caplets, and tablets. Solid dosage forms are extremely convenient for self-medication and are easy to package and dispense. Solid oral dosage forms lack taste or smell, which can prevent a patient from taking a medication.

3. a—Capsules are contained in a gelatin shell; the size of the shell can vary based on the amount of medication it will contain.

4. d—Tablets are prepared by compressing; capsules may be prepared using the "punch method."

5. a—Effervescent salts release carbon dioxide when dissolved in water; plasters adhere to the skin; powders may be administered either externally or internally; a troche, also known as a *lozenge* or *pastille,* dissolves in the mouth.

6. b—Liquids are easier to swallow than solid oral dosage forms.

7. b—Elixirs are clear, sweetened, flavored hydroalcoholic liquids containing water and alcohol and may or may not be medicated. Aromatic waters are solutions of water containing oils, which have a fragrance and are volatile; a suspension is a dispersion with two phases that has solid particles dispersed in the liquid. A syrup contains sucrose (sugar).

8. a—An emulsion is a liquid dispersed in another. Emulsions can be either oil in water or water in oil. A gel is a dispersion with extremely fine particles and when mixed is a semisolid dosage form. A lotion is a topical dispersion that contains insoluble substances; an ointment is a semisolid topical dispersion.

9. a—The date of the repackaging does not need to appear on the label, but it does need to be entered into the repackaging log. A repackaged medication must contain the generic name of the medication, the manufacturer's name and lot number, and the expiration date after packaging. The repackaging date can be either 6 months from the date the medication is repackaged or one quarter of the manufacturer's time, whichever is less.

10. b—The expiration date after repackaging does not need to be on the label.

11. c—Either the drug manufacturer or the FDA can issue a medication recall. Medication recalls can be one of three types, depending on the severity of the situation.

12. b—A modified unit-dose system can be known as a *punch card, bingo card,* or *blister card.*

13. b—A prime vendor agreement occurs between a pharmacy and a wholesaler; the pharmacy agrees to purchase the majority (80% to 95%) of their products from the wholesaler. In return, the wholesaler agrees to provide the pharmacy with a range of services, which may include electronic order entry devices, bar-coded labels, emergency service, and competitive pricing.

14. c—Syrups contain sucrose (sugar).

15. b—Liniments are considered solutions rather than dispersions because the solute is dissolved in a solvent. Liniments may be either an alcoholic or an oleaginous solution.

16. b—Emulsions possess a solute dispersed through a dispersing vehicle. Emulsions can either be oil in water or water in oil.

17. c—A pastille is also known as a troche or lozenge and dissolves in the mouth.

18. a—A collodion contains pyroxylin (tiny particles of cellulose) and can be dissolved in either alcohol or ether.

19. a—Suspensions are considered dispersions and have two phases.

20. d—A paste is a dispersion similar to an ointment, but it contains more solid material.

21. d—The Pharmacy and Therapeutics Committee (P&T), composed of physicians, nurses, pharmacists, and hospital administrators, develops the formulary for an institution.

22. b—Six months is the maximum amount of time that can be assigned to a repackaged medication.

23. a—The subscription contains special instructions to the pharmacist; the signa indicates directions to be typed on the label; the inscription consists of the name, strength, and quantity of medication; and the Rx symbol means "recipe" or "take."

24. a—Hazardous drugs and chemicals require the purchaser to receive a Material Safety Data Sheet (MSDS) from the manufacturer, distributor, or importer.

25. b—Ophthalmic products must be isotonic, or else damage can occur to the eye.

26. d—The patient must sign the back of each prescription he or she is requesting be filled in an easy-open container. A verbal authorization does not meet the requirement.

27. b—The patient's ID number is not required for a prescription; however, medication orders filled in a hospital do require the patient ID number.

28. d—No form is required.

29. d—Security requirements do not affect the storage of a medication. Environmental factors include light, heat, and humidity.

30. c—A solution is not a dispersion.

31. c—Sublingual tablets are not delayed release but rather immediate release.

32. d—Pills, tablets, and suppositories are all solid dosage forms.

33. d—OSHA is responsible for hazardous waste and materials because these substances may cause injury to the employee.

34. a—Class I recalls may cause death to an individual.

35. b—Products considered hazardous materials by OSHA require the purchaser to receive an MSDS form.

CHAPTER 3 REVIEW ANSWERS

1. a—Glass mortars and pestles are used to mix liquids, Wedgwood is used for crystals, and porcelain is used for powders.

2. a—The Department of Transportation (DOT) is responsible for the transportation of hazardous materials.

3. b—High-efficiency particulate airflow (HEPA) filters need to be certified every 6 months unless they become wet.

4. c—Radioactive Yellow III has the highest concentration, Radioactive Yellow II has the second highest, and Radioactive White I has the lowest concentration. Radioactive Orange IV does not exist.

5. b—Laminar flow hoods need to be certified every 6 months.

6. d—The *USP-NF* consists of drug monographs and standards. *Approved Drug Products with Therapeutic Equivalence Evaluations* is what is known as the *Orange Book. Drug Facts and Comparisons* and the *PDR (Physicians' Desk Reference)* provide valuable information about drug products.

7. b—Class A balances must have a minimum sensitivity of 6 mg.

8. b—Rubber spatulas are used because corrosive materials may react with the steel.

9. a—70% Isopropyl alcohol is used to clean laminar flow hoods. Rubbing alcohol will leave a film on the top of a laminar flow hood.

10. c—The lumen is the opening of a needle. The bevel is the angled tip of the needle where the

lumen is found. The hilt of the needle attaches to the hub of the barrel of the syringe. The shaft is the length of the needle.

11. a—Laminar flow hoods should be a Class 100 area, where there are no more than 100 particles that are 0.5 micron or larger per cubic foot of air. The number indicates the number of particles 0.5 micron or larger per cubic foot of air.

12. c—Pipettes should be used to measure volumes less than 1.5 mL.

13. d—Disease management services are reimbursed through the submission of an HCFS 1500 form.

14. d—The seller is responsible for the product during transportation.

15. a—Institutional pharmacies process medication orders instead of prescriptions. Ambulatory pharmacies process prescriptions.

16. c—Professional samples are frowned on because they may create a bias in purchasing.

17. b—Class B balances can weigh between 650 mg and 120 g and can be used for compounding.

18. d—A laminar flow hood must be on a minimum of 30 minutes before it is used to prepare an admixture.

19. a—A Type A hood can be converted to a Type B3 hood. A Type A1 hood does not exist.

20. d—Pharmacy balances must be certified every year by the Department of Taxation.

21. c—Finished radiopharmaceuticals are stored in the packaging area; the breakdown room is used to store empty or used radiopharmaceuticals before they are returned and dismantled for reuse; the compounding area is the compounding or dispensing area; and the storage and disposal area is used to store radioactive waste.

22. b—Face to face is the most effective way to communicate; the least effective way of those mentioned is a memo.

23. d—TJC does not certify retail pharmacies.

24. a—All pharmacies must have a Class A balance.

25. c—The air velocity of a laminar flow hood is 90 linear feet per minute (±20%).

CHAPTER 4 PRACTICE EXAMINATIONS ANSWERS

PRACTICE EXAMINATION I ANSWERS

1. a—ACE inhibitors have a potassium-sparing effect, which, if taken with potassium-sparing diuretics, may result in hyperkalemia.

2. d—30 mL (1 oz) MOM (Milk of Magnesia) PO (by mouth) ac (before meals) hs (at bedtime) prn (as needed).

3. c—Use the following equation: (IS)(IV) = (FS)(FV), where IS is initial strength, or 25%; IV is the initial volume that is being calculated; FS is final strength, or 10%; and FV is final volume, which is 4 fl oz, or 120 mL. This calculation yields 48 mL. Subtract the initial volume (48 mL) from the final volume (120 mL), which will yield the amount of diluent (72 mL).

4. a—"Hyper" means greater than, "hypo" less than, and "iso" the same as.

5. b—An elixir is a mixture of alcohol and water.

6. c—Convert pounds to kilograms (180 lb × 1 kg/2.2 lb = 81.82 kg). Calculate daily dosage (81.82 kg × 1.75 mg/kg/day = 143 mg/day).

7. c—Nifedipine is a calcium channel blocker. Beta-blockers are easily identified by the nomenclature syllable of *-olol*.

8. b—Generic drugs are nonproprietary drugs.

9. c—The *hypo-* prefix means low, and the root word *kalemia* means potassium.

10. d—Amino acids, dextrose, and lipids are used in preparing a total nutrient admixture, which is a parenteral form of nutrition for patients with specific conditions. Proteins are not used in this preparation.

11. d—UTI is an acronym for urinary tract infection.

12. c—A copy of the Controlled Substances Act and the *United States Pharmacopeia—National Formulary* are required in all pharmacies by the state boards of pharmacy. All pharmacies must maintain a library for reference.

13. d—There are 480 mL in a pint solution, and a teaspoon dose is equal to 5 mL. 480 mL/5 mL/dose = 96 doses.

14. d—Plastic is less expensive than glass, the pliability of the bag requires less storage space, and the bags are transparent.

15. b—Food and Drug Administration.

16. b—Anticholinergics have a tendency to dry up all bodily secretions as a side effect.

17. d—Vitamin K is a warfarin antagonist. It will increase clotting factors II, VII, IX, and X.

18. d—Unit-dose labels require the name and strength of the medication, expiration date of the medication, manufacturer's name, and lot number.

19. c—The patient is taking two tablets twice per day for a total of four tablets per day. Forty tablets divided by four tablets per day will last 10 days.

20. c—1.5 mEq/1 mL = 30 mEq/X mL, where X = 20 mL.

21. c—According to the Controlled Substances Act of 1970, the maximum number of authorized refills for a Schedule III to V drug is five.

22. b—Days supply = Total quantity dispensed/ Quantity taken per day (40 capsules/4 capsules/day = 10-day supply.

23. b—There are 24 hours in a day; if the drug is taken every 6 hours, four doses will be taken in a day's time.

24. c—There are 480 mL in 1 pint.

25. c—*Nephro* is the Latin word root for kidney.

26. d—An individual taking Lasix as a diuretic may lose potassium and require a potassium supplement. Aldactone, Dyazide, and Dyrenium are potassium-sparing diuretics.

27. c—1 mg of protamine sulfate will neutralize 90 to 120 units of heparin.

28. c—Solve using proportions. 1 L = 1000 mL. 100,000 units/1000 mL = X units/50 mL, where X = 5000 units.

29. b—The abbreviation "od" is derived from the Latin term *oculo dextro*, which is translated as right eye.

30. d—One teaspoon is equal to 5 mL, and the patient is receiving four doses per day for 10 days: (5 mL/dose × 4 doses/day × 10 days = 200 mL).

31. b—The generic name for Lodine is etodolac.

32. a—An individual undergoing "dig toxicity" (digitalis toxicity) may experience the following: arrhythmias, nausea, and vomiting. They may see yellow-green halos around objects.

33. b—An individual must determine how long the bag will last (1000 units/hr = 20,000 units/ X hr). The bag will last 20 hr. The rate of infusion can be calculated by dividing 500 mL by 20 hr, resulting in 25 mL/hr. Then, use the following formula: Rate × Drop size × 1 hr/60 min = gtt/min. Therefore, using (25 mL/hr)(15 gtt/mL)(1 hr/60 min) will yield 6 gtt/min.

34. c—Medicare is a federal program for individuals older than 65 years; Medicaid is a federal program administered by the state for individuals (families) who meet specific income guidelines; Workers' Compensation is for individuals who are injured while working.

35. c—Using Clark's rule [Weight (lb)/150] × Adult dose will provide the child with the correct dose: [(70 lb)/150] × 250 mg = 116 mg.

36. b—*Derm* means skin, *cerebr* means brain, *cranio* means skull, and *dent* means tooth.

37. d—According to the FDA, an X rating indicates that the medication is contraindicated in pregnant women.

38. c—Rx means to take a given product of a given strength and quantity.

39. d—AWP and capitation + dispensing fee are both types of third-party reimbursement formulas; a copayment is a predetermined amount of money or a percentage of money that one is responsible for paying on every prescription. A deductible is a yearly, predetermined sum of money payable before the insurer will begin making payments to an individual or institution.

40. d—The Controlled Substances Act requires that a pharmacy perform a biennial inventory of all controlled substances stocked in a pharmacy. An exact count must be performed on Schedule II medications and an estimated count must be done on Schedule III to V medications. An institution may perform an inventory more frequently if required by either state law or organizational policy.

41. d—30 tablets are dispensed, but one tablet is being taken every other day; therefore it will last 60 days.

42. d—Tuberculosis most often affects the lungs because *Mycobacterium tuberculosis* prefers an area of high oxygen content.

43. c—Sulfasalazine does not require monitoring through blood work. Patients taking lithium, phenytoin, and warfarin need to have frequent blood samples tested to ensure they are receiving the appropriate dose of medication.

44. b—Meperidine is a Schedule II drug that must be stored in a safe per the Controlled Substances Act of 1970.

45. a—The Accutane Law of 2002 does not permit refills on prescriptions of Accutane. The prescription must be handwritten by the physician and dispensed within 7 days of being written.

46. a—Set up the following proportion: 25,000 units/500 mL = X units/1 mL, where X = 50 units.

47. a—*Otic* refers to the ear.

48. b—According to the Controlled Substances Act, an individual may purchase only one 4-oz bottle of an "exempt narcotic" every 48 hr.

49. d—Ibuprofen is available over the counter as Motrin and Nuprin; naproxen sodium is Aleve; and ranitidine is Zantac. Tramadol is the prescription product known as Ultram.

50. d—Insulin is administered subcutaneously above and below the waist, in the buttocks, and in the upper arms.

51. a—The smaller the number in the denominator, the larger the value of the number.

52. d—"qs ad" are directions to the pharmacist in compounding a prescription "to make up to" a given weight or volume of a substance.

53. d—Imipramine (Tofranil) is used to prevent bedwetting in small children.

54. d—A potential side effect of ibuprofen is stomach irritation. To reduce this possibility, food should be taken to act as a buffer against stomach irritation.

55. b—Itraconazole is the generic drug name for Sporanox, which is available only by prescription.

56. d—Melatonin has been shown to be effective in assisting individuals fall asleep, especially when traveling in different time zones.

57. a—Only registered pharmacists are allowed by law to counsel patients.

58. c—The Kefauver-Harris Amendment requires that all drugs be pure, safe, and effective as a result of the thalidomide incident.

59. b—Forceps are used to prevent oils from the hands from being deposited on the weight, which may alter the composition of the weight.

60. d—Answer A is incorrect because it stated that tsp was tablespoonful instead of teaspoon; qod is every other day instead of four times per day; and answer C states penicillin G, whereas the prescription indicates Pen G. There is a difference between penicillin and penicillin G.

61. a—*Cardio* is derived from the Greek term *kardia*, meaning heart.

62. c—DAW2 means that a physician approved the dispensing of a generic drug but the patient requested the brand name drug. DAW means that the physician approved the dispensing of a generic drug; DAW1 indicates that the physician wants the patient to receive the brand name drug only. DAW5 means that the pharmacy has designated this drug as their generic drug of choice.

63. b—Alligation should be used to solve the problem. When subtracting the desired concentration from the higher concentration and subtracting the lower concentration from the desired concentration, one sees that equal quantities of each strength will be used.

64. d—St. John's wort has been used in the treatment of depression.

65. b—Itraconazole is the antifungal agent known as Sporanox.

66. c—The *Physicians' Desk Reference* contains information from the package inserts of more than 4000 prescription drugs.

67. b—Using Young's rule [Age (years)/Age (years) + 12] × Adult dose, the child will need a dose of 21.4 mg.

68. c—The Controlled Substances Act of 1970 allows an individual age 18 years or older to purchase a 4-oz bottle of an exempt narcotic every 48 hours.

69. d—Sulfisoxazole is a sulfa antibiotic.

70. a—URI is an acronym for upper respiratory infection.

71. b—Class A balances are used in extemporaneous compounding, not in the preparation of intravenous preparations.

72. a—Pharmacokinetics is the study of the absorption, distribution, metabolism, and elimination of a drug from the body. Pharmacognosy is the study of natural products; pharmacology describes how a drug works on the body; and pharmacopeia is a listing of drugs.

73. b—100 units of insulin are found in 1 mL of liquid.

$$\frac{100 \text{ units} = 40 \text{ units}}{1 \text{ mL} \times X \text{ mL}}$$

Cross-multiplying and dividing yields 0.4 mL.

74. b—Tylenol 3 contains 325 mg of APAP and 30 mg ($\frac{1}{2}$ gr) of codeine.

75. d—Beakers and graduates are not precise enough to measure a small volume such as 1.5 mL. A measuring device cannot have a capacity greater than five times the amount of volume to be measured.

76. c—GMP stands for Good Manufacturing Practices, which are followed in compounding prescriptions. The DEA is responsible for the Controlled Substances Act; the FDA for ensuring that food and medications are pure, safe, and effective; and OBRA 90 discusses Drug Utilization Review and counseling patients.

77. a—Compliance is an act of adhering to particular directions. The ease of administration is a factor in a patient's compliance in taking a medication. Both first and second pass are components of pharmacokinetics.

78. c—Metformin is the generic name for Glucophage. The other drug names are glipizide (Glucotrol), glyburide (Micronase or DiaBeta), and pioglitazone (Actos).

79. a—Zithromax is the brand name for azithromycin; other drug names are as follows: Biaxin (clarithromycin), Minocin (minocycline), and Floxin (ofloxacin).

80. b—A side effect of antianxiety medications, antidepressants, and anticonvulsants is drowsiness.

81. d—Even though both lotions and suspensions are dispersions, lotions are dissolved particles, whereas suspensions contain solid particles.

82. d—0.4 g is the same as 400 mg.

83. d—"os" means "left eye," which is the only difference among all of the interpretations.

84. b—Narcotics have a tendency to sedate an individual (i.e., to cause central nervous system [CNS] depression). CNS stimulation would have the opposite effect.

85. b—Calculate the amount of active ingredient by multiplying the final volume by the percent of clindamycin expressed as a decimal (480 mL × 0.02 = 9.6 g). Convert 9.6 g to grams by multiplying 9.6 g × 1000 mg/g = 9600 mg. Divide the total weight of clindamycin by the weight of each capsule (9600 mg /150 mg per capsule = 64 capsules).

86. d—The problem can be solved using a proportion: 125 mg/5 mL = 500 mg/X mL, where X = 20 mL.

87. b—AWP + dispensing fee is a common method of reimbursing pharmacies for medications. Calculate the cost of 30 tablets (100 tablets/$120.00 = 30 tablets/X), where X is $36.00 and the AWP for this medication; $3.25 is added to the AWP ($36.00), yielding $39.25.

88. a—The problem can be solved using the following formula: (IS)(IV) = (FS)(FV), where IS = 65%, IV = 1200 mL, and FS = 45%, or (65%)(1200 mL)/(45%) = 1733 mL. The amount of diluent added is equal to FV − IV, which is 1733 mL − 1200 mL = 533 mL.

89. d—Use the following formula: Rate (mL/hr) × Drop factor (gtt/mL) × (1 hr/60 min) = gtt/min. Substitute the following: (500 mL/6 hr) × (15 gtt/mL) × (1 hr/60 min) = 20.83 gtt/min. 20.83 gtt/min is rounded down to 20.

90. c—The Controlled Substances Act requires that a partially filled Schedule II prescription be filled within 72 hr if the pharmacy did not have the entire quantity for the patient. If it is not filled within 72 hr, the remaining quantity will become void.

91. c—Parchment paper may be used if an ointment slab is not available. After use, the parchment paper is discarded.

92. d—Counseling is a judgmental task that only pharmacists are permitted to perform. Pharmacy technicians currently are allowed to perform only technical tasks.

93. c—Oral medications are the most commonly used because of the ease of administration.

94. d—Nitroglycerin should be taken sublingually because of the urgency of obtaining relief from an angina attack. Sublingual medications bypass the digestive tract and are rapidly absorbed into the bloodstream by being placed under the tongue, which has a large blood supply.

95. c—Any errors made on a Form 222 cannot be corrected. This form must be retained in the pharmacy for at least 2 years.

96. c—The basic formula for medication reimbursement is drug cost + dispensing fee. There are many variations of this formula taking into consideration AWP, AAC, MAC, and percentages.

97. d—D10W stands for 10% dextrose dissolved in water. w/f% is the number of grams dissolved in 100 mL of solution. Using the following proportion, one can solve the problem: (10 g/100 mL = X g/1000 mL), resulting in 100 g.

98. b—A Class II drug recall is one in which the probability exists that the use of the product will cause adverse health events that are temporary or medically reversible. A Class I drug recall shows that there is a reasonable probability that use of the product will cause or lead to serious adverse events or death; a Class III recall means that the drug will probably not cause an adverse health event.

99. c—Calculate the total number of doses required (2 tablets/dose × 2 doses/day × 25 days = 100 tablets). Calculate the cost of 100 tablets ($321.66/500 tablets = X/100 tablets, where X = $64.33). Look for the fee on the table that corresponds to an AWP of $64.33, which would be $10.00. AWP + fee ($64.33 + $10.00 = $74.33).

100. a—TJC stands for The Joint Commission. Pyxis, Robot-Rx, and SureMed are automated dispensing systems.

PRACTICE EXAMINATION II ANSWERS

1. d—An individual may experience a severe rash as a result of photosensitivity to the sun if the patient is taking tetracycline. A patient should take tetracycline 1 hour before or 2 hours after a meal, which will prevent food and the medication from binding together. Antibiotics should be taken until they are completed.

2. c—2.79 kg = 2790 g; and 5 pints × 2 cups/pint × 8 fl oz/pint × 30 mL/fl oz = 2400 mL. 1 mL of water weighs 1 g. Specific gravity = Weight of substance/Weight of an equal volume of water, or 2790 g/2400 g = 1.16.

3. c—50 mg/1 mL = 75 mg/X mL, where X = 1.5 mL.

4. d—Drug names are as follows: sulfamethoxazole-trimethoprim DS (Bactrim DS), amoxicillin-clavulanate (Augmentin), cephalexin (Keflex),

sulfamethoxazole-trimethoprim (Bactrim or Septra).

5. a—Oxycodone acetaminophen is the generic name for Percocet, which is a Schedule II drug under the Controlled Substances Act. Prescriptions for Schedule II drugs cannot be refilled. The physician must write a new prescription if the patient requires additional medication.

6. a—This is an alligation problem, where the 2.5% is the highest concentration, 0.25% is the lowest concentration, and 1% is the concentration of the final product. $2.5 - 1 = 1.5$ parts of the 0.25%; $1.0 - 0.25 = 0.75$ parts of 2.5%. The total number of parts is 2.25 $(0.75 + 1.5 = 2.25)$. Set up a proportion to calculate the total weight: 1.5 parts of 0.25%/2.25 total parts of compound = 240 g of 0.25%/total weight of compound, where the total weight is 360 g. Total weight of compound – weight of 0.25% = weight of 2.5% (360 g – 240 g = 120 g).

7. c—The maximum number of refills allowed for a Schedule III medication if approved by the prescriber is five refills within 6 months of the date the prescription was written.

8. a—Elixirs contain alcohol.

9. d—ii (Roman numeral for 2) gtt (drops) os (left eye) bid (twice per day).

10. d—D5W means 5% dextrose in water. 1 L = 1000 mL. %w/v is defined as the number of grams per 100 mL of solution. Can be solved using the following proportion: 5 g/100 mL = X g/1000 mL, where X = 50 g.

11. d—Premarin is conjugated estrogen, unlike the other three products, which are different dosage forms of estradiol.

12. d—Laminar airflow hoods are used to prepare sterile products. Extemporaneous compounds are not sterile products. A Class A balance, a compounding slab, graduated cylinders, spatulas, and a mortar and pestle are a few of the pieces of pharmacy equipment used in extemporaneous compounding.

13. d—Gram is the basic unit of weight in the metric system.

14. d—Syrup contain sucrose (sugar).

15. d—DUE is an acronym for Drug Utilization Evaluation, which is mandated under OBRA 90.

16. a—1 quart is equal to approximately 0.96 L, or 1 L.

17. a—The patient would take a maximum of two tablets per dose with a maximum of six doses per day. 60 tablets (2 tablets/dose) at 6 doses/day will last 5 days.

18. c—Cocaine is a Schedule II drug under the Controlled Substances Act of 1970. Cocaine does have a medical use in the United States, but it has a high potential for abuse.

19. d—*Hypo* means low, *gly* means sugar, and *emia* means blood. Low blood sugar.

20. c—"qid" (four times a day) indicates how many times per day a medication would be taken. The terms "ac and hs" tell the patient when during the day the medication is to be taken.

21. c—10 mg/mL is the same as 0.01 g/mL, which is equal to 1%. Solve using the following formula: (IS)(IV) = (FS)(FV), where (10%)(IV) = (1%)(120 mL) and IV = 12 mL.

22. b—This problem can be solved using alligation, where 20% is the highest concentration, 3% is the concentration to be prepared, and petrolatum has a concentration of 0%. For the 20%, subtract the 0% from the 3%, which will require three parts of 20%; for the 0%, subtract 3% from 20%, which will give 17 parts of 3%.

23. b—Solve using the following formula (IS)(IV) = (FS)(FV); (2%)(120 mL) = (FS)(480 mL), where the FS is 0.5%.

24. d—Solve using the following formula: (Rate)(Kit size)(1 hr/60 min)=gtt/min, where (100 mL/0.5 - hr)(10 gtt/mL)(1 hr/60 min) = 33 gtt/min.

25. a—PO means by mouth.

26. b—Solve using Clark's rule: [Weight (lb)/150] × Adult dose = Amount of medication patient should receive. Convert kilograms to pounds (8 kg × 2.2 lb/kg = 17.6 lb). Substitute the given information: 17.6/150 × 10 mL = 1.2 mL.

27. c—A dry, nonproductive cough may occur as a side effect for patients taking ACE inhibitors.

28. a—Atorvastatin is the generic name for Lipitor, which is used in the treatment of hyperlipidemia (high cholesterol).

29. a—A Class A balance is a piece of required equipment for all pharmacies. Class A balances have a sensitivity of 6 mg.

30. d—Young men receiving trazodone should be warned of experiencing priapism (a prolonged erection).

31. d—Venlafaxine is the generic name for Effexor and is an SSRI.

32. c—A synergistic effect is a joint action of drugs in which their combined effect is more intense or of longer duration than the sum of their individual effects.

33. b—Using Young's rule: Age of child in years/(Age of child in years + 12) × Adult dose will yield 3.3 mg.

34. a—The Controlled Substances Act of 1970 requires that a pharmacy submit a DEA Form 41

in triplicate before the destruction of any controlled substances.

35. b—Inventory consists of products or goods available for sale.

36. a—A proper size syringe should not contain more than twice the volume to be measured.

37. b—Calculate by using the following formula: Final volume × Strength (expressed as a decimal) = Amount of active ingredient (g); 5 mL × 0.15 = 0.75 g, or 750 mg.

38. c—Pills, tablets, and capsules should be counted in multiples of fives.

39. c—1 gr is equal to approximately 65 mg; therefore 2 gr would weigh 130 mg.

40. c—Room temperature is 15° to 30°C (59° to 86°F).

41. a—Disulfiram (Antabuse) is used to treat patients who abuse alcohol. Disulfiram stops the metabolism of alcohol at the aldehyde stage, which causes aldehyde to accumulate in the body. If alcohol is consumed, the patient becomes extremely sick. This sickness is characterized by symptoms of blurred vision, confusion, difficult breathing, intense throbbing in the head and neck, chest pain, nausea, severe headache, severe vomiting, thirst, and uneasiness.

42. b—Look at the bottom of the meniscus or the lowest point of the liquid when measuring a liquid.

43. b—There are two types of emulsions: oil in water or water in oil. Emulsions are dispersions, in which one liquid is dispersed in another immiscible liquid.

44. a—Atenolol is the generic name for Tenormin. Other drug names are as follows: metoprolol (Lopressor or Toprol XL), nadolol (Corgard), and propranolol (Inderal).

45. a—Outside air flows into the back of the horizontal airflow hood and through the hood's HEPA filter and out toward the opening, and the air is recirculated into the room. A vertical airflow hood is similar to the horizontal hood except that the air cannot be recirculated into the room. This air goes through two HEPA filters and is released into an open area or is vented to the outside.

46. d—Using the formula (IV)(IS) = (FV)(FS), where 5% is the initial strength, 1 pint (480 mL) is the initial volume, and 1 : 50 (2%) is the final strength, the final volume would be 1200 mL.

47. c—Salicylates have the tendency to irritate the stomach and affect blood platelets before an overdose occurs. Tinnitus is a ringing in the ears and is a symptom of salicylate overdosage.

48. c—The following are the approved DAW codes used in pharmacy: DAW0, Generic allowed by physician; DAW1, Brand name required by physician; and DAW2, Generic allowed, but patient requested brand-name drug.

49. b—Military time begins at 12:01 AM and ends at midnight, which is 2400 hours. 0800 is the same as 8 AM.

50. c—GERD is an acronym for gastroesophageal reflux disease, which describes symptoms commonly referred to *heartburn*.

51. b—Norflex is a skeletal muscle relaxant.

52. a—*Osteo* is the word root for bone. The following word roots are for the other terms: cell *(cyte),* lymph *(lymph),* and muscle *(myo).*

53. b—Inderal can be used prophylactically for migraines; Imitrex, Midrin, and Stadol are used as abortive therapies for migraine headaches.

54. b—Clotrimazole is an antifungal agent.

55. a—An aseptic technique is the process of preparing sterile product to be injected into the body. Extemporaneous compounding, geometric dilution, and levigation are used in the production of nonsterile compounds.

56. c—Convert milligrams to grams (24 mg = 0.024 g) and solve the problem using proportions. $250.00/1 g = $X/0.024 g, where X = $6.00.

57. d—Calculate how long the bag will last [Volume/Rate or 1000 mL/(100 mL/hour)], which is 10 hr. Using military time, add 10 hr to 0800 hr to get 1800 hr.

58. c—Solve using the following formula: (IS)(IV) = (FS)(FV); (10%)(100 mL) = (0.9%)(X mL), where X = 1111 mL. To calculate the amount of diluent, subtract the initial volume from the final volume (1111 mL − 100 mL = 1011 mL of diluent).

59. b—An LCSW is a licensed clinical social worker, who works with individuals with affective disorders. LCSWs cannot prescribe medications.

60. d—Fexofenadine is available only as an oral preparation. The following are names for transdermal products: clonidine (Catapres TTS), estradiol (Estraderm or Climara), and fentanyl (Duragesic).

61. c—MedWatch is a program instituted by the FDA that involves the voluntary reporting of adverse health events and medical products.

62. c—The lumen is the opening in the needle by which medication is expelled from a syringe.

63. a—"Non rep" means do not repeat and is used to indicate that no additional refills are authorized.

64. b—All pharmacies dispensing controlled substances must register with the DEA by submitting a DEA Form 224.

65. c—Controlled-dose (CD), controlled-release (CR), and sustained-release (SR) products are time- or extended-release dosage forms. The abbreviation *ERF* does not exist in the practice of pharmacy.

66. b—DAW1 means the physician is requesting that the patient receive the brand-name drug.

67. a—Product names are as follows: atenolol (Tenormin), carisoprodol (Soma), nadolol (Corgard), and propranolol (Inderal).

68. b—Neither federal nor state law allows a patient to call a new prescription into the pharmacy. A patient may request a refill of a prescription by telephone.

69. c—Itraconazole (Sporanox) is an antifungal agent, which is taken by pulse dosing. Pulse dosing requires that the patient take one capsule daily for 1 week, skip 3 weeks, and resume. This form of dosing is effective therapeutically and is cost effective.

70. a—Policies are rules, procedures are involved with processes, protocol is concerned with appropriate behavior, and standards are expectations.

71. d—"i tab tid" means take one tablet three times per day. 30 tablets/3 tablets/day = 10 days' supply.

72. a—BS is an approved abbreviation meaning blood sugar.

73. c—Enalapril is the same as Vasotec. The generic name for Accupril is quinapril; Monopril is fosinopril; and Zestril is lisinopril.

74. b—"prn" means as needed for a particular condition.

75. a—Benztropine (Cogentin) is used to minimize the effects by responding to the excess muscle activity of antipsychotics.

76. c—Drug names are as follows: Zyprexa (olanzapine), Aricept (donepezil), Skelaxin (metaxalone), and Risperdal (risperidone).

77. d—Solve by calculating the amount of medication the patient is to receive daily: Weight of child × Dose × Frequency (30 kg × 10 mg/kg × 3 doses/day = 900 mg/day). To calculate the volume, solve using a proportion: 50 mg/mL = 900 mg/X mL, where X = 18 mL.

78. a—Tessalon Perles (benzonatate) is used as an antitussive because this agent anesthetizes the stretch receptors in the airway, lungs, and pleura but not the respiratory center.

79. b—A generic drug must contain the same active ingredients as the original brand-name drug; be identical in strength, dosage form, and route of administration; have the same use indications; meet the same batch requirements for identity, strength, purity, and quality; and yield similar blood absorption and urinary excretion curves for the active ingredient.

80. b—The generic name for Pepcid is famotidine.

81. a—A month is considered to have 30 days in it. Because the patient is taking the medication only every other day, the patient would be taking 15 tablets in 30 days.

82. d—Flow rate is a specific volume per unit of time (1000 mL/8 hr = 125 mL/hr).

83. c—The Pharmacy and Therapeutics Committee, composed of physicians, nurses, pharmacists, and administrators, determines the formulary based on the advantages and disadvantages of a medication and its cost effectiveness.

84. b—ii (2) caps (capsules) stat (immediately) then i (one) cap (capsule) q (every) hr (hour), max (maximum) 5 caps (5 capsules)/(per or in) 12 hr (hours).

85. a—According to the DEA and the Controlled Substances Act, medications placed in Schedule I have no medicinal use in the United States and have the highest potential for abuse.

86. c—*MAC* stands for maximum allowable cost and is used in reimbursement of multisource drugs by third-party insurance plans. Generic drugs are nonproprietary, whereas brand-name or trade drugs are proprietary drugs covered by a patent.

87. d—Olopatadine is the generic name for Patanol. Other drug names are as follows: brimonidine is Alphagan, ciprofloxacin is Ciloxan, and latanoprost is Xalatan.

88. c—DEA numbers are required only on the hard copy of a prescription for a controlled substance.

89. a—A unit dose is the amount of medication required for one dose. The order is for 40 mg. To solve for the volume desired, use 10 mg/mL = 40 mg/X mL or 4 mL.

90. c—One pair of gloves is worn underneath the cuffs of the protective clothing and the second pair of gloves goes over the top of the cuffs of the protective clothing.

91. a—MAOIs, SSRIs, and TCAs are used to treat depression. Antipsychotics are used to treat a different affective disorder.

92. b—NS is an abbreviation for normal saline (0.9%), which is one of the vehicles used in IV admixtures.

93. d—A corticosteroid ointment is more potent than a cream, gel, or lotion, assuming they are of the same concentration.

94. c—Lorazepam is a Schedule IV drug.

95. c—A combination of alcohol in any form or concentration may interact with metronidazole, causing extreme, unpleasant side effects from processes occurring in the liver.

96. d—Sublingual tablets are absorbed directly into the bloodstream by being placed under the tongue and therefore bypass the digestive system.

97. d—OBRA mandated that both a Drug Utilization Evaluation and an offer to counsel must be made to every patient. A Drug Utilization Evaluation is a technical task that a technician may perform, whereas counseling must be performed by a pharmacist.

98. c—Set the problem up as proportion using 3 mg/1 lb = X mg/60 lb, where X = 180 mg.

99. d—Regular insulin is the only type of insulin that may be added to an IV solution.

100. b—A nonproprietary drug is another name for a generic drug; a proprietary or trade name is another name for a brand-name drug; investigational drugs have not obtained FDA approval; and an OTC is an over-the-counter medication that does not need a prescription from a physician to be purchased.

PRACTICE EXAMINATION III ANSWERS

1. c—Postmarketing monitoring of medications is a tool for quality assurance to ensure medications are pure, safe, and effective. Adverse side effects are monitored, and any potential for harm is noted. If the medication may have detrimental effects on an individual, it may be pulled from the market by the manufacturer or the FDA. Recent examples include Rezulin, Redux, and Pondimin.

2. a—The abbreviation "hs" means at the hour of bed or hour of sleep.

3. c—According to the Controlled Substances Act of 1970, the maximum number of refills allowed by a physician is five refills within 6 months of the date of the prescription being written.

4. a—Colchicine is used in the treatment of gout and is not an NSAID.

5. d—Warfarin would be contraindicated with vitamin K therapy.

6. c—The abbreviation "os" means left eye.

7. a—A buccal tablet is placed between the gum and cheek. It is absorbed directly into the bloodstream and bypasses the digestive system.

8. a—A dosage schedule states exactly when a medication is to be administered to a patient, such as 8 AM or 4 PM.

9. d—Nitrofurantoin is better absorbed into the body if it is taken with food.

10. c—The suffix *-ectomy* means removal and is found in words such as tonsillectomy, vasectomy, and mastectomy.

11. b—Lorabid is a macrolide antibiotic.

12. b—To solve this problem, the following formula should be used: (IS)(IV) = (FS)(FV), and substitute the following: (50%)(120 mL) = (FS)(300 mL), where the final volume (FV) is calculated by adding 6 oz (180 mL) to the initial volume (IV) of 120 mL. The final strength (FS) is 20%.

13. b—Both horizontal and vertical laminar airflow hoods must be on for at least 30 minutes before being used in the preparation of aseptic products.

14. d—Hyperthyroidism—overproduction of the thyroid gland—may result in a goiter.

15. c—Noncompliance reports are a tool used to monitor savings and losses of a pharmacy when a Group Purchasing Organization (GPO) has negotiated specific prices for pharmaceutical products with a specific vendor.

16. c—A monograph is literature on a specific drug by the drug manufacturer that may include a description, indications, contraindications, adverse effects, and warnings. The *PDR* is an example of a collection of drug monographs.

17. c—*Drug Topics Red Book* is a good source of drug costs. Information found in the *Red Book* includes emergency information, clinical reference guides, practice management and professional development information, listings of pharmacy and health care organizations, drug reimbursement information, manufacturer and wholesaler information, product identification, Rx product listings, OTC and nondrug product listings, and complementary and herbal product referencing.

18. a—1 cubic centimeter (cc) = 1 milliliter (mL).

19. c—Ranitidine (Zantac) is not among the drugs to be excluded from using child-resistant containers under the Poison Control Act of 1970.

20. b—A patient would receive a maximum of six doses of (5 cc = 5 mL)/day for 5 days. The pharmacy would need to dispense 150 mL (5 fl oz) to fill the prescription.

21. a—Desyrel may cause a young male to experience priapism.

22. d—A biennial inventory is required of all controlled substances by the DEA every 2 years.

23. b—Amoxicillin is used prophylactically whenever a patient has a heart prosthesis, congenital heart disease, or mitral valve prolapse.

24. d—There are 30 mL to a fluid ounce. 240 mL/ 30 mL per fluid ounce = 8 oz.

25. a—Using the formula (IS)(IV) = (FS)(FV), where the initial strength (IS) is 30%, the final volume (FV) is 2.5 L (2500 mL), and the final strength (FS) is 5%; the initial volume (IV) will be 417 mL. The problem is asking for the amount of water (diluent) to be added. Use the equation Final volume − Initial volume = Amount of diluent to be added to get 2083 mL.

26. c—The patient is receiving 10 mg per dose and will receive three doses in 1 day. 3 doses × 10 mg/dose will equal 30 mg.

27. b—MAOIs inhibit the activity of enzymes that break down catecholamine; therefore the buildup of transmitters occurs at the synapse. Because of this buildup, MAOIs must be washed out of the system before treatment with another antidepressant is begun.

28. c—Joint

29. b—Ease of administration is an advantage of an oral dosage form. There are no special skills required to administer this form.

30. c—Convert 154 lb to kilograms (154 lb/2.2 lb per kg = 70 kg). Calculate the amount of drug the patient will receive per day (12 mg/kg/day × 70 kg = 840 mg). Multiply the amount per day times 5 days (840 mg/day × 5 days = 4200 mg). Convert milligrams to grams (4200 mg/1000 mg per gram = 4.2 g).

31. a—Young's rule calculates a dose based on a child's age and uses the following formula: [Age (years)/[Age (years) + 12] × Adult dose; [10/(10 + 12)] × 30 mg = 13 mg.

32. d—Online adjudication (electronic) is the method most commonly used to submit payments to insurance carriers. In certain situations a hard copy of the claim form (Universal Claim Form) may be required to be submitted for payment.

33. d—Pharmacy technicians are not permitted to counsel patients.

34. c—2.4 g = 2400 mg (1 g = 1000 mg); therefore 600 mg/1 tablet = 2400 mg/4 tablets each day.

35. d—Antihistamines should not be used; beta-blockers may constrict the bronchi; and many patients are sensitive to aspirin and NSAIDs.

36. c—Solve using the following equation: Final volume × Strength (expressed as a decimal) = Amount of active ingredient (g); 600 mL × 1/5000 = 0.12 g; convert 0.12 g to milligrams (0.12 g × 1000 mg/1 g = 120 mg). Calculate the number of tablets to dispense by dividing the total dose/dose per tablet: 120 mg/30 mg per tablet = 4 tablets.

37. b—Lansoprazole (Prevacid) is not an OTC product.

38. d—NPO means that the patient is not to receive anything by mouth, which means no food, liquid, or medication to be taken orally.

39. d—Solve by using the following formula: Final volume × % (expressed as a decimal) = Amount of active ingredient. Final volume × 0.2 = 40 g, where the final volume will be 200 mL.

40. d—MS (morphine sulfate) IM (intramuscularly) q (every) 4 h (4 hr) prn (as needed) for pain. The verb "inject" was chosen because of the route of administration.

41. a—Acetaminophen should be taken because it does not thin the blood like aspirin, NSAIDs, or narcotic analgesics. A person could hemorrhage to death if his or her blood is too thin.

42. c—1 L = 1000 mL. Solve using the following formula: (IS)(IV) = (FS)(FV); (70%)(1000 mL) = (30%)(X mL), where X = 2333 mL. To calculate the amount of water to be added, subtract the initial volume (IV) from the final volume (FV) (2333 mL − 1000 mL = 1333 mL).

43. b—70% isopropyl alcohol is used to clean both horizontal and vertical laminar flow hoods.

44. d—This is an alligation problem. Draw a tic-tac-toe table and place the highest concentration (10%) in the upper left corner; the lowest concentration (1%) in the lower left corner; and the quantity to be prepared in the middle (45 g of 2%). Perform the following: 10 − 2 = 8 parts of the 1% solution and 2 − 1 = 1 part of the 10%. Add the parts together (8 + 1 = 9 parts); calculate the amounts of each by concentration (10%: 1/9 × 45 g = 5 g; 1%: 8/9 × 45 g = 40 g).

45. c—International Units are a form of measure to indicate activity of a biologic product. Vitamin B is measured in milligrams.

46. d—i (1) cap (capsule) qid (four times per day) ac (before meals) and hs (bedtime).

47. d—The number size is inversely proportionate to the amount it will contain; the smaller the number, the greater the capacity of the capsule.

48. a—Capitation is a form of reimbursement used by insurance companies. This form of reimbursement favors the insurance company when the cost of the prescriptions exceeds the capitation being paid.

49. d—All except answer D are required on a Controlled Substance Administration Record, which is used to document controlled substance use in a hospital or long-term care institution.

50. c—Ciprofloxacin (Cipro) is a quinolone antibiotic.

51. a—AAC means actual acquisition cost, which means the pharmacy is reimbursed for what it actually paid for the medication after receiving discounts from either the manufacturer or wholesaler.
52. b—A PCA is a patient-controlled analgesia device used to infuse analgesics into the patient.
53. c—Zestril is the brand name for lisinopril. Other drug names are enalapril (Vasotec), fosinopril (Monopril), and quinapril (Accupril).
54. b—A fentanyl patch or Duragesic is a transdermal patch that will provide the patient with continuous medication for 3 days (72 hr).
55. d—If tetracycline is taken after it has passed its expiration established by the manufacturer, the patient may die. If the other products are taken after they have expired, the effectiveness will not be guaranteed by the manufacturer and the patient may experience side effects.
56. a—The inscription is the name, strength, and quantity of the medication to be dispensed; Rx means to take a particular drug, the signa means "write on label" and is direction to the patient; and the subscription contains instructions to the pharmacist, for instance regarding refills, packaging, and generic substitution.
57. c—Procedures are a way to avoid errors in performing a specific task.
58. d—A medication is guaranteed by the manufacturer to be effective until the last day of the month.
59. b—Solve using Clark's rule: [Weight (lb)/150] × Adult dose; [40/150] × 25 mg = 6.66 mg.
60. b—Suppositories are inserted into body orifices such as the rectum, urethra, and vagina. PR is an abbreviation meaning *per rectum*.
61. c—The abbreviation tid means three times per day.
62. d—Pharmacy technicians perform technical tasks; responding to a potential contraindication is a judgment decision, which only pharmacists can perform.
63. c—The FDA is responsible for ensuring that all medications are pure, safe, and effective. If a product is adulterated or misbranded, the FDA may issue a product recall if the manufacturer does not voluntarily issue one.
64. d—NSAIDs are indicated for use as an analgesic, an antiinflammatory agent, and fever reducer.
65. b—1 kg is equal to 2.2 lb; therefore 4.4 lb is equal to 2 kg.
66. c—Class I recalls are associated with serious adverse health consequence or death; Class II recalls are associated with drugs that may cause temporary or medically reversible adverse health consequences; Class III recalls are associated with drugs not likely to cause an adverse health consequence.
67. a—The suffix *-osis* means abnormal condition and is found in words such as *nephrosis* and *halitosis.*
68. c—A used needle should be disposed in a red plastic sharps container to prevent an individual from being injured by the needle.
69. b—One teaspoon is equal to 5 mL. "tid" means three times per day. The patient will be receiving 1 tsp three times per day, or 15 mL. The total amount of medication to be dispensed is 75 mL. 75 mL/15 mL per day = 5 days.
70. b—The first five digits of an NDC identify the drug manufacturer, the next four digits indicate the drug product, and the last two digits refer to the packaging of the drug.
71. c—Specific gravity = Weight of a substance/Weight of an equal volume of water or 170/150 = 1.13.
72. a—Benzocaine is a topical local anesthetic.
73. b—Cascara sagrada is used as a laxative; American ginseng is used to provide energy for the body; goldenseal is used for the immune system; and melatonin is used to induce sleep.
74. d—This is an alligation problem. Set the problem up with 10% in the top left corner, 5% in the center, and 2% in the bottom left corner. Calculate the number of parts of each strength to be used: 10% requires 3 parts (5 − 2) and the 2% requires 5 parts (10 − 5). To calculate the quantities of each, multiply ratio of parts by the total quantity to be prepared (10%: 3 parts/8 parts × 25 g = 9.4 g; 2%: 5 parts/8 parts × 25 g = 15.6 g).
75. c—A liter is equal to 1000 mL. Solve with the following proportion: 1000 mL/8 hr = X mL/hr, where X = 125 mL.
76. b—Methylphenidate (Ritalin) is a Schedule II drug according to the Controlled Substances Act.
77. b—Guaifenesin is an expectorant, whereas the other three products are bronchodilators.
78. c—Nifedipine is generic name for both Procardia and Adalat, which are calcium channel blockers.
79. b—Solve using Clark's rule: [Weight (lb)/150] × Adult dose; (25/150) × 100 mg = 16.67 mg (17 mg).
80. a—A prefix occurs before the root word, which is followed by a suffix. Vowels combine the prefix, root word, and suffix together.

81. b—The Controlled Substances Act allows for one 4-oz bottle of an exempt narcotic to be purchased by an individual older than 18 years every 48 hr.

82. d—An adverse reaction may occur if alcohol is consumed in any strength or form; stomach irritation is less likely to occur if it is taken with food; because metronidazole is an antibiotic, metronidazole should be taken until completion to ensure the infection has been eradicated.

83. b—The maximum number of different Schedule II medications legally allowed on a Form 222 is 10, which is found in the Controlled Substances Act of 1970.

84. b—Ciprofloxacin (Cipro) should not be given because it will affect the formation of the tendons in the body and may result in temporary damage.

85. c—Diuretics have a tendency to remove potassium from the body: *hypo-* means low, *-kalemia* means potassium.

86. c—Solve using the following formula: Final volume × Strength (expressed as a decimal) = Amount of active ingredient (g); 1000 mL × 1/1000 = 1 g. Convert grams to milligrams (1 g × 1000 mg/g = 1000 mg). 10 gr = 650 mg. Next, calculate the number of tablets by dividing the total weight by the weight per tablet (1000 mg/650 mg per tablet = 1½ tablets).

87. d—The Occupational Safety and Health Administration (OSHA) has enacted regulations to protect the employee at work. Regulations involving blood-borne pathogens, ergonomics, and personal protective equipment have been enacted for the safety of employees.

88. c—Reye syndrome may develop if a child who has been exposed to the virus causing chickenpox takes aspirin. Tylenol is highly recommended for children instead of aspirin.

89. b—Pharmacy technicians may accept new and refill prescriptions from a patient, but they cannot accept a new prescription that is called in to the pharmacy from a physician's office.

90. b—Calan and Isoptin are brand names for verapamil.

91. d—The abbreviation qid means 4 times per day. 40 capsules/4 capsules per day would yield 10 days.

92. c—The abbreviation *ac* means before meals.

93. c—The root word *cardio* refers to the heart.

94. d—*Intra-* means within; *hypo-* means below; *iso-* means equal, and *inter-* means between.

95. b—Inflammation is an indication for the use of steroids rather than a side effect.

96. c—*Inunction* refers to the process of rubbing a substance into the skin. Inunction is used when applying creams, lotions, ointments, and pastes.

97. b—Normal saline is 0.9%; therefore 1/2 NS would be 0.9%/2, or 0.45%. Solve using the following equation: (IS)(IV) = (FS)(FV), substituting the values (0.9%)(250 mL) = (0.45%)(X mL), where X = 500 mL, which is the final volume. FV − IV = amount of water to be added. 500 mL − 250 mL = 250 mL of water.

98. a—The Durham-Humphrey Amendment of 1951 required that the federal legend "Federal law prohibits the dispensing of this medication without a prescription" appear on all prescription medication containers. Answer B is required by the Controlled Substances Act of 1970 to appear on all prescriptions of controlled substances; answer C is required on any OTC product that is not in a child-resistant package as a result of the Poison Control Act of 1970; and answer D is a warning required by the Food, Drug, and Cosmetic Act of 1938.

99. a—Decongestants may cause CNS stimulation, which may cause the heart to beat harder, thus pushing more blood through the circulatory system and resulting in increased blood pressure. Decongestants do not decrease blood pressure.

100. b—D5W means 5% dextrose dissolved in water.

PRACTICE EXAMINATION IV ANSWERS

1. b—Calculate the volume of medication required to deliver the prescribed amount of drug per hour: 1 g (1000 mg)/250 mL = 250 mg/ X mL, where X = 62.5 mL. To calculate the flow rate, solve using the following formula: Rate (mL/hr) × Drop size (drop/mL) × 1 hr/60 min = gtt/min (62.5 mL/hr)(10 gtt/mL)(1 hr/60 min) = 10 gtt/min.

2. a—Absorption is the process of taking the drug from the administration site to the bloodstream; distribution is the process of taking the medication to organs and tissues; metabolism transforms the medication in the liver; and elimination (excretion) is the process by which the drug is removed from the body.

3. a—Benazepril is the generic name for Lotensin.

4. b—One must work at least 6 inches inside the laminar airflow hood to use proper aseptic technique.

5. c—"Milli" is a prefix meaning 1/1000. There are 1000 mL in 1 L.

6. b—For patients who are allergic to penicillin, there is a 10% chance they will be allergic to a cephalosporin.

7. d—The half-life of a medication is the amount of time required to eliminate one half of the amount of the drug from the body. Half-life is a tool used to determine dosing frequency of a medication.

8. b—Convert 10 g to milligrams (10 g × 1000 mg/ g = 10,000 mg). Divide the total weight by the weight per dose (10,000 mg/500 mg per dose = 20 doses).

9. d—Tricyclic antidepressants such as amitriptyline may be used in the treatment of chronic pain.

10. b—Capsules have a gelatin shell as an outer covering, unlike the other products mentioned.

11. d—Tablets are a solid dosage form, whereas creams, ointments, and suspensions are dispersions.

12. b—The Durham-Humphrey Amendment is being violated if a prescription drug is dispensed without a valid prescription.

13. c—Diltiazem (Cardizem) is a calcium channel blocker. Atenolol and carvedilol are beta-blockers, and lisinopril is an ACE inhibitor.

14. c—AWP stands for average wholesale price and is a term used in determining costs and calculating profitability of a product.

15. d—Singulair is a montelukast. Advair is a combination of fluticasone and salmeterol; Allegra D is fexofenadine and pseudoephedrine; and Combivent is albuterol and ipratropium.

16. d—Glucosamine has been shown to be helpful in treating arthritis, whereas feverfew may be used for migraines, ginger as an antiemetic, and ginkgo for circulatory issues.

17. b—During the process of geometric dilution, an individual is combining more than one ingredient. One begins by using the most potent (normally the smallest quantity) first in the mortar, then an equal amount of the next most potent drug is added. This process continues until all quantities have been added and mixed. During geometric dilution, the total quantity of drug being prepared is approximately doubling with each ingredient added.

18. d—A specific disease state, such as angina, requires a prompt response, resulting in nitroglycerin being taken sublingually and bypassing the digestive system. Oral medications do not require specific skills of the patient, unlike injectable medications, for which specific skills are necessary. The rate of action may be affected by the amount of time in which a therapeutic response needs to occur. An example would be an intravenous (IV) injection; IV injections provide a quicker response because the medication is administered into the bloodstream and gets to the site of action much more quickly than does an oral or topical dose. The shape, color, or taste of a medication does not affect the route of administration. The shape, color, or taste may affect the patient's compliance in taking a medication.

19. c—The patient will be taking one capsule four times a day; therefore the prescription will last 10 days.

20. b—Comminution is the act of reducing a substance to small, fine particles; blending is the act of combining two substances; sifting is used to combine powders; and tumbling is accomplished by combining powders in a bag.

21. a—Acetaminophen. Acetylsalicylic acid (aspirin), ibuprofen (Motrin), and naproxen sodium (Aleve or Anaprox) have the potential to irritate or ulcerate the stomach.

22. c—Glyburide is the generic name for both Micronase and DiaBeta.

23. a—Alendronate is the generic name for Fosamax. The other medications' brand names are calcitonin-salmon (Miacalcin), etidronate (Didronel), and raloxifene (Evista).

24. a—According to the FDA classification system, AA shows that the medication meets bioequivalence requirements.

25. d—A dispersion is not dissolved in a vehicle, but rather distributed throughout it. Suppositories are solid dosage forms, whereas dispersions are a liquid dosage form. Emulsions and lotions are liquid dosage forms. An ointment is a type of emulsion.

26. c—Phenytoin is the generic name for Dilantin, an anticonvulsant. The other drug names are Divalproex (Depakote), gabapentin (Neurontin), and valproic acid (Depakene).

27. a—Butorphanol was upgraded from the prescription drug Stadol to a controlled substance in 1997.

28. c—Using the formula 9C = 5F − 160, substitute 98.6 for the F and the answer will be 37°C.

29. c—Corticosteroids, loop diuretics, and thiazide diuretics have an adverse effect on lipid profiles.

30. b—Glipizide is the generic name for Glucotrol.

31. c—Risperidone (Risperdal) is an antipsychotic used to relieve symptoms but not cure the disease.

32. a—One of the ingredients of a compound must be a legend drug.

33. c—Olanzapine is the generic name for Zyprexa, olopatadine is the generic for Patanol, nefazodone is Serzone, and trazodone is Desyrel.

34. c—One dose is equal to 1 tsp (5 mL), which is taken three times per day for 10 days. The pharmacy will need to dispense 150 mL to the patient.

35. d—Ultralente insulin has a duration of 18 to 20 hours. Regular insulin lasts 5 to 6 hours; NPH insulin lasts 10 to 16 hours; and Lente insulin has a duration of 12 to 18 hours.

36. b—Class A balances, which are used to measure solid ingredients in compounding in a pharmacy, must have a minimum sensitivity of 6 mg.

37. b—Coreg is the brand name for carvedilol.

38. d—Tablets are produced by compression, capsules may be made by using the "punch method," and suppositories are made by compression and molding.

39. c—Even though both Wellbutrin and Zyban contain the same ingredient, bupropion, Wellbutrin is indicated only for the treatment of depression.

40. b—The Controlled Substances Act of 1970 allows for a maximum of five refills for Schedules III to V drugs within 5 months of the date the prescription was written.

41. c—Glyburide is the generic for Micronase. The brand names for the other generics are Amaryl (glimepiride), Glucotrol (glipizide), and Actos (pioglitazone).

42. b—Ipecac is an emetic to induce vomiting, Emetrol is an antiemetic, PEG is used as a bowel evacuant, and simethicone is an antiflatulent.

43. d—Using a proportion, calculate the amount found in 4 fl oz (120 mL): 50 g/1000 mL = X g/120 mL, where X = 6 g.

44. c—A loading dose of a medication is a greater than normal dose of a medication, which enables the drug to obtain a therapeutic level in the body sooner than normal.

45. b—The abbreviation w/v shows the concentration of a solid dissolved in a liquid. It is the number of grams dissolved in 100 mL of liquid.

46. b—Antitussives are used in the treatment of a dry, nonproductive cough, whereas expectorants are used if a patient has mucus or phlegm.

47. c—HCTZ is an abbreviation for the diuretic hydrochlorothiazide.

48. c—To convert a ratio to a percent, write the ratio as a fraction, divide the numerator by the denominator, and multiply by 100. 1:20 is the same as 1/20. 1/20 = 0.05; 0.05 × 100 = 5.00%.

49. a—An auxiliary label provides additional information to the patient. Patient product inserts (PPIs) are required for products containing estrogens; patient profiles provide the pharmacist information about the patient, such as illness, both OTC and Rx medications being taken, drug allergies, and demographic and payment information; and a prescription label provides information to the patient containing the name, strength, and quantity of drug and directions for usage as prescribed by the physician.

50. a—Aspirin does not reduce the level of cholesterol in the body. Fibric acid derivatives and HMG-CoA reductase inhibitors are classifications of drugs used to treat hyperlipidemia. Metamucil has been shown to lower cholesterol in the body.

51. c—A printer is an output device.

52. d—Rickets is caused by a deficiency of vitamin D. Deficiency of vitamin A results in night blindness, of vitamin B_1 in beriberi, and of vitamin C in scurvy.

53. b—CSAR stands for Controlled Substance Administration Record. CSARs are used in hospitals and other institutional facilities to acknowledge the administration of a controlled substance to a patient. The administrator must sign his or her name and the time of administration.

54. c—The Poison Prevention Act of 1970 permits certain medications (e.g., nitroglycerin) not to be dispensed in a child-resistant container.

55. d—Regular insulin should be drawn up first if it is being mixed with NPH insulin. Regular insulin does mix with Lente insulin, and glargine does not mix with any insulin.

56. d—Lamivudine is the generic name for Epivir (3TC); ddI (didanosine) is the generic name for Videx.

57. c—Food aids in the absorption of nitrofurantoin in the body. Amoxicillin (penicillin) is best taken on an empty stomach; minocycline and tetracycline (both tetracyclines) work best if taken on an empty stomach and should not be taken within 1 hour of ingestion of all dairy products because of chelation.

58. c—Specific gravity is a ratio of the weight of a substance to the weight of an equal volume of water (SG = Weight of substance/Weight of an equal volume of water): SG = 6565 g/5000 g: SG = 1.31.

59. c—*Hepato* is the Latin root word meaning liver.

60. d—U&C means the charge is the usual and customary charge that a patient would pay if his or

her third-party payer were not involved in the transaction.

61. d—An individual who recommends a product to a patient is performing a judgmental duty, which only a pharmacist may do.

62. c—Using Young's rule—[Age (years)/Age (years) + 12] × Adult dose—will give the appropriate dose for the child. Five months is approximately 0.42 years: (0.42/0.42 + 12) × 200 mg = 6.67 mg.

63. c—Midrin is a combination product used to abort a migraine headache but is not a selective 5-HT receptor agonist. Imitrex, Maxalt, and Zomig are 5-HT receptor agonists.

64. c—Using the formula (IS)(IV) = (FS)(FV), the initial strength is 25%, the initial volume is 600 mL, and the final volume is 700 mL (the initial volume + the amount of diluent). Inserting these values in the equation yields a final strength of 21.4%.

65. a—The *Drug Topics Orange Book* provides USP and NF drug standards and dispensing requirements.

66. a—Bupropion is generic name for the antidepressant Wellbutrin and the smoking-cessation product Zyban.

67. b—Nurses administer medication to patients and therefore would document MARs. Physicians diagnose and prescribe, pharmacists dispense, and pharmacy technicians assist pharmacists in performing their duties.

68. b—The first letter may be either an A or B. The second letter is the first letter of the prescriber's last name. Next, the numbers in the first, third, and fifth positions are added. Then the numbers in the second, fourth, and sixth positions are added; multiply this sum by 2. Add both sums together, and the correct number should be the last number.

69. d—The fluffy precipitate indicates the precipitation of dextrose; the solution must be shaken to ensure that dextrose is thoroughly distributed throughout the bag.

70. a—The Controlled Substances Act of 1970 allows no refills for Schedule II medications.

71. c—All prescriptions containing estrogens require the pharmacy to provide the patient with a Patient Product Insert (PPI).

72. b—The Drug Listing Act of 1972 provided a unique numbering system for each product. This 11-digit number identifies the manufacturer, the product, and its package.

73. c—Isoniazid (INH) is used to treat tuberculosis. Albuterol, ipratropium, and salmeterol are used to treat asthma.

74. d—The smaller the number, the more the substance is diluted.

75. d—i (Roman numeral for 1); gtt (drop); ou (each eye); tid (three times per day); ud (as directed).

76. d—Glyburide, an oral hypoglycemic agent, is used in the treatment of diabetes.

77. c—iss is a Roman numeral indicating 1½ gr. 65 mg/gr × 1½ gr = 97.5 mg.

78. b—Imitrex is taken at the onset of a migraine headache.

79. d—*ung* is a Latin abbreviation meaning ointment. Ointments are a dosage form applied externally on the skin unless otherwise directed.

80. a—Overhead is the sum of all the expenses in a business. Examples of overhead in a pharmacy include all the salaries of the employees, cost of inventory, the expense-associated utilities, supplies, licenses, and computer hardware and software.

81. c—m/100 mL = 100 g/X, where X = 1000 mL or 1 L.

82. a—Oxycodone + APAP is the same as Percocet and Tylox. Under the Controlled Substances Act of 1970, these products have a extremely high potential for abuse but they have a medicinal use in the United States.

83. c—A potassium supplement is taken for a deficiency of potassium in the body. *Hypo-* means below, and *-kalemia* means potassium.

84. b—In compliance with the Accutane Prescribing Law of 2002, all Accutane prescriptions must be handwritten by the prescriber and filled within 7 days of being written with the approved yellow seal attached and no refills authorized.

85. b—Oxycodone with acetaminophen is a Schedule II drug; according to the Controlled Substances Act, Schedule II drugs must be kept in the pharmacy safe when not in use.

86. b—Calculate the number of units per hour (20 units/1 min = X units/60 min [1 hr], where X = 1200 units). Calculate the volume to be infused per hour (100,000 units/1000 mL = 1200 units/X mL, where X = 12 mL in 1 hr). Calculate the number of gtt/min by using the following formula: (mL/hr)(drop size)(1 hr/60 min) = gtt/min. (12 mL/hr)(60 gtt/mL)(1 hr/60 min) = 12 gtt/min.

87. d—A minidrip or microdrip system yields 60 drops/mL.

88. c—An 80/20 report, also known as a velocity report, shows a detailed summary of purchasing history. It lists products that reflect 80% of your purchasing dollars.

89. a—Doxycycline is the only tetracycline that can be taken with dairy products.
90. c—Procardia (nifedipine) is a calcium channel blocker.
91. d—Multiply the cost ($2.00) by the desired profit (0.3), which will yield a profit of $0.60. Adding the profit ($0.60) to the cost ($2.00) will result of a selling price of $2.60.
92. a—Electrolytes are substances necessary to carry out the electrical activity of nerves and muscles in the body. One milliequivalent is 1/1000 of an equivalent weight and is used to measure replacement of electrolytes in the body.
93. d—Use this formula: Final weight × Percent (express as a decimal) = Amount of active ingredient. Both the percent (20%) and the amount of active ingredient (10 g) are provided in the problem. Place this information in the equation: Final weight = Amount of active ingredient/ Percent (as a decimal); final weight = 10 g/0.2, or 50 g.
94. a—Hazardous drugs are prepared in a biologic safety hood, intravenous solutions in a horizontal flow hood, antineoplastics in a vertical flow hood, and various extemporaneous products on an ointment slab.
95. c—Scurvy is a deficiency of vitamin C; deficiency of vitamin A results in night blindness; of B_1 in beriberi; and of vitamin D in rickets.
96. a—The Controlled Substances Act requires that all prescriptions for controlled substances have the physician's DEA number on them.
97. d—Lunesta is indicated for sleep.
98. d—240 mL of the prescription is to be prepared. The patient is to receive four doses of 5 mL daily or a total of 20 mL. To calculate the amount of Tussin to be taken daily, solve using a proportion (30 mL of Tussin/240 mL of total solution = X mL of Tussin/20 mL of total solution, where X = 2.5 mL of Tussin). Calculate the amount of guaifenesin (100 mg of guaifenesin/5 mL of Tussin solution = X mg of guaifenesin/2.5 mL, where X = 50 mg).
99. b—The abbreviation "pr" means per rectum.
100. d—A TPN solution must be isotonic to the blood or else the blood cells will either expand or collapse in the blood vessel. A hypotonic solution will cause the blood cells to collapse, whereas a hypertonic solution will cause the cells to expand.

PRACTICE EXAMINATION V ANSWERS

1. d—Rhinitis means a runny nose.
2. a—A small-volume parenteral contains 100 mL or less of solution.
3. b—Inhibition is the process whereby an agent can slow or block enzyme activity, which impairs the metabolism of drugs and as a result may increase their concentration. Additive effects are the combined effects of two drugs. Potentiation is an effect that increases or prolongs the action of another drug; the total effect is greater than the sum of the effects of each drug taken alone. Synergism is the joint action of drugs in which their combined effect is more intense or longer in duration than the sum of their individual effects.
4. c—Solve using the following formula: Final volume × % strength (expressed as a decimal) will yield the amount of active ingredient in grams: 250 mL × 0.25 = 62.5 g.
5. b—Elixirs, spirits, and syrups contain either alcohol or sugar; diabetics should not receive either of them; emulsions do not contain alcohol or sugar.
6. b—A flutter is a type of arrhythmia in which the patient's heart is beating 200 to 350 times per minute.
7. c—Sulfasalazine may cause photosensitivity in an individual if he or she is exposed to direct sunlight; one should drink plenty of water to prevent crystals from developing in the kidneys. Sulfasalazine has the tendency to change the color of urine from a yellow to an orange-brown color.
8. c—Solve by using the following formula: (Initial volume)(Initial strength) = (Final volume)(Final strength): (300 mL)(50%) = (300 mL + 200 mL = 500 mL)(Final strength), where the final strength is 30%. 30% means that there are 30 g in 100 mL. To calculate the number of grams in 500 mL, a proportion is used: 30 g/100 mL = X g/500 mL, where X = 150 g.
9. c—This is an alligation problem requiring an individual to make a 40% dextrose solution from both 60% and 10% dextrose solution. Place the 60% in the upper left corner, the 40% in the middle, and the 10% in the lower left corner. 60% − 40% = 20 parts of the 10% solution. 40% − 10%= 30 parts of the 60% solution. The total number of parts is equal to 50 parts. To calculate the required quantities of each solution, use a proportion. 30 parts of 60% solution/50 parts of 40 solution = X mL of 60% solution/ 1000 mL of 40% solution, where X = 600 mL of 60%. 20 parts of 10% solution/50 parts of the 40% solution = X mL of 10% solution/1000 mL of 40% solution, where X = 400 mL of the 10% solution.
10. a—The gauze swab will protect the finger from being cut by fine pieces of glass.

11. b—Inventory turnover rate is calculated by dividing the total sales by the average inventory value. $2,750,000/[($225,000 + $250,000)/2] = 11.58 turns.

12. c—1 pint = 480 mL. Solve by using a proportion: 2 mg/1 mL = X mg/480 mL, where X = 960 mg. Convert milligrams to grams (960 mg × 1 g/1000 mg = 0.96 g).

13. c—The Catapres TTS patch is changed weekly.

14. c—Percocet is oxycodone + acetaminophen. The other drug names are Tylenol C Codeine (acetaminophen + codeine), Vicodin and Lortab (hydrocodone + acetaminophen), and Darvocet N (propoxyphene + acetaminophen).

15. a—Convert pounds to kilograms (44 lb × 1 kg/2.2 lb = 20 kg). Next, calculate amount the patient is to receive each day (4 mg/kg × 20 kg = 80 mg/day). Next, calculate the volume to be given to the patient (30 mg/5 mL = 80 mg/X mL, where X = 13.3 mL).

16. d—OSHA stands for the Occupational Safety and Health Administration, which is concerned with employee safety; HIPAA stands for the Health Insurance Portability and Accountability Act, which is concerned with patient confidentiality; TJC is the Joint Commission, which is responsible for establishing standards for hospitals, nursing homes, and long-term care facilities and ensuring that the standards are maintained; OBRA is the Omnibus Budget Reconciliation Act, requiring drug utilization review and that an offer to counsel is to be made to every customer.

17. b—Elixirs are a clear, sweetened, flavored hydroalcoholic solution containing both water and ethanol; collodions are a liquid dosage form for topical application with pyroxylin dissolved in alcohol and ether; suspensions are a dispersion in which small particles of a solid are distributed throughout a liquid; syrup is an aqueous solution thickened with sugar.

18. b—The abbreviation "ou" means each eye.

19. c—Convert grams to milligrams (2 g × 1000 mg/g = 2000 mg). Set up a proportion: 2000 mg/30 mL = X mg/5 mL, where X = 333 mg.

20. d—Hyperalimentation and total parenteral nutrition are synonymous terms that describe the process of feeding patients who are unable to eat solids and liquids.

21. d—Latanoprost (Xalatan) must be refrigerated after opening.

22. b—Drugs names are Irbesartan (Avapro), candesartan (Atacand), losartan (Cozaar), and valsartan (Diovan).

23. a—Air flows in only one direction in a laminar flow hood, away from the hood in a horizontal flow hood and upward in a vertical flow hood.

24. b—During phase II, a final review is done on the ingredients of the agent in question. The public is able to give feedback. All data are taken into account. In phase I, advisors evaluate the agent in question to determine whether it is safe and effective when taken by the consumer or patient. During phase III, all the final evidence is presented and all aspects of the agent are exhausted, and the final monograph is published.

25. d—Drug names are Glucophage (metformin), Amaryl (glimepiride), glipizide (Glucotrol), and Micronase (glyburide).

26. d—As a patient ages, his or her ability to hear properly is reduced; the patient may begin to develop multiple disease states; as a result of multiple disease states, the patient is required to take multiple medications.

27. d—Vasotec is available as both an oral and intravenous dosage form.

28. d—Griseofulvin may cause photosensitivity in an individual, resulting in a severe sunburn or rash. Because it is a suspension, it should be shaken to prevent precipitation and needs to be stored at room temperature.

29. d—Tegretol is available as a chewable tablet, an oral tablet, and a suspension. As a transdermal dosage form, Catapres is known as Catapres TTS, a patch that needs to be changed weekly; Duragesic is a Schedule II medication that provides fentanyl as a narcotic analgesic and lasts for 3 days; and nitroglycerin is known as Nitro-Dur or Nitrodisc.

30. d—Prednisone is the generic name for Deltasone. The other drug names are lithium (Eskalith), methylprednisolone (Medrol), and prednisolone (Pediapred).

31. a—The sale of an "exempt narcotic" requires that an individual be at least 18 years of age and a resident of the community and that no more than one 4-oz bottle be sold in the original manufacturer's bottle every 48 hr. The patient must complete the exempt narcotic log (record), which includes the date of the purchase and his or her name and address. The pharmacist must see that the name, quantity of the product, and the selling price of the product are entered in the "exempt narcotic book." The pharmacist must sign his or her name in the book as the seller of the "exempt narcotic."

32. d—Etoposide must be prepared in a biologic safety cabinet because it is a plant alkaloid used in the treatment of cancer.

33. a—Bupropion (Wellbutrin or Zyban) is not an MAOI. MAOIs include phenelzine (Nardil), selegiline (Eldepryl), and tranylcypromine (Parnate).

34. d—Convert grams to milligrams (1.2 g × 1000 mg/g = 1200 mg). Use a proportion to calculate the volume to be infused (50 mg/1 mL = 1200 mg/X mL, where X = 24 mL).

35. c—Evista is used to treat osteoporosis.

36. c—The master formula sheet, also known as a pharmacy compounding log, indicates the amount of each ingredient used, the procedures used in the preparation, and the labeling instructions.

37. c—The prefix *hepato-* means liver.

38. a—At bedtime (hs), if needed (prn).

39. b—ASHP stands for American Society of Health-System Pharmacists.

40. b—A type II (cytolytic) reaction occurs because of the reactions of circulating antibodies of immunoglobulin (Ig) G, IgM, or IgA class with an antigen associated with a cell membrane. Type I (anaphylactic) reactions are produced when the antigen has stimulated the production of the antibody, which then becomes fixed to basophils and mast cells in the tissues. A type III (toxin-precipitin) reaction occurs when the precipitin complex is removed from the bloodstream by the reticuloendothelial cells in the spleen. A type IV (cell-mediated hypersensitivity) reaction depends on the presence of T-cell lymphocytes that combine with the antigen.

41. b—A list price is a synonym for suggested retail price. Discounted price, net price, and sale price reflect a reduction in price.

42. c—"Readily retrievable" means able to be provided to a third party, such as the DEA or representatives from a particular state board of pharmacy, within 72 hours.

43. d—Beta-2 agonists, cromolyn, and corticosteroids are treatments for asthma.

44. d—The state board of pharmacy will investigate all reported claims of medication error and will consider appropriate sanctions against all providers. The state board of pharmacy is concerned with the practice of pharmacy in a particular state, which includes the behavior of pharmacists. The DEA is concerned with adherence to the Controlled Substances Act; the FDA's priorities are to ensure that food and medications are pure, safe, and effective; MedWatch is concerned with adverse effects of medications.

45. b—H_2 antagonists do not have an interaction with phenobarbital. Beta-blockers, TCAs (tricyclic antidepressants), and warfarin have a negative drug interaction with phenobarbital.

46. a—The abbreviation "prn" means as needed for a particular indication. It also may refer to unlimited refills for a specific period as determined by either federal or state laws, whichever are the more stringent.

47. a—An emulsion may be either oil-in-water or water-in-oil.

48. d—A person's age affects the physical condition of his or her organs. A person's disease state can influence other organ systems, such as the liver and kidney, and whether a medication may be contraindicated with a specific disease. An individual's gender can affect how a medication is absorbed, distributed, metabolized, or excreted from the body.

49. d—The Controlled Substances Act allows for certain controlled substances to be purchased without a prescription under specific conditions. These substances are Schedule V drugs. The medications involve products containing specific amounts of codeine and paregoric. To purchase a container, the individual must be at least 18 years of age, the product must be packaged in the manufacturer's original container (4-oz bottle), the exempt narcotic log must be signed, the drug must be sold by a pharmacist, and the patient may purchase only one 4-oz bottle in 48 hours.

50. c—An anaphylactic reaction is an extremely serious allergic reaction that may be fatal. A person undergoing an anaphylactic reaction will experience tracheal constriction and difficulty breathing.

51. d—Taking fluoxetine, oral contraceptives, or theophylline with phenytoin will result in a drug interaction.

52. b—Nosocomial infections are hospital-derived infections.

53. d—Computers do all these activities.

54. d—A red C stamped on a prescription indicates that the medication is a controlled substance. All filled controlled substance prescriptions must be stamped with a red, 1-inch C.

55. a—Drug names are Capoten (captopril), Coreg (carvedilol), Catapres (clonidine), and Plavix (clopidogrel).

56. d—Glaucoma is a chronic disorder characterized by abnormally high internal eye pressure that destroys the optic nerve and can cause partial to complete blindness.

57. c—Fexofenadine (Allegra) requires a prescription. Chlorpheniramine (Chlor-Trimeton), diphenhydramine (Benadryl), and loratadine (Claritin) are all antihistamines available OTC.

58. d—Antihypertensives do not exhibit a drug-drug interaction with oral contraceptives. Antibiotics, anticonvulsants, and antifungal agents will reduce the effectiveness of oral contraceptives.

59. d—Type 2 diabetes can be controlled through behavior modification, which will result in a reduction of body weight. Type 1 diabetes requires insulin injections because of the body's inability to produce insulin; gestational diabetes will normally be reversed after pregnancy. Secondary diabetes is caused by various medications.

60. a—A "crash cart" is synonymous with a Code Blue cart. A Code Blue is announced whenever a patient develops a serious condition that may result in death. Serious situations involving the heart or the lungs are the more common causes for calling a Code Blue.

61. a—MAR stands for Medication Administration Record.

62. c—I-9s must be completed for all new employees in accordance with federal law. An employee must provide specific identification to prove his or her identity. Failure to provide documentation will result in not being hired. A business can face extremely high fines for not maintaining properly completed I-9s.

63. d—Prescriptions are medication orders written by a physician to be obtained through a community or mail-order pharmacy.

64. b—A modified unit dose is a drug distribution system that combines unit-dose medications blister-packaged onto a multiple-dose card instead of being placed into a box. Such packages are referred to as *punch cards, bingo cards,* or *blister cards,* and one card may contain 30, 60, or 90 units.

65. b—A HEPA filter is a high-efficiency particulate air filter found in a laminar flow hood to remove contaminants.

66. d—SMZ-TMP DS is the generic for either Bactrim DS or Septra DS, which are sulfa drugs used to treat urinary tract infections.

67. d—Celebrex is an NSAID, whose mechanism of action is by a COX-2 inhibitor.

68. b—Drug names are Prevacid (lansoprazole), Nexium (esomeprazole), Prilosec (omeprazole), and Protonix (pantoprazole).

69. d—Troches, lozenges, and pastilles are solid dosage forms that are administered buccally.

70. b—FDCA 1938 is the Food, Drug, and Cosmetic Act of 1938, which clearly defined adulteration and misbranding. Preparing prescriptions under unsanitary conditions is an example of adulteration.

71. b—Azactam (aztreonam) is a cephalosporin.

72. c—*Drug Topics Orange Book.*

73. b—25% means that there are 25 g in 100 mL of solution. Solve using a proportion: 25 g/100 mL = X g/200 mL, where X = 50 g. To calculate the kcal, solve using the following proportion: 1 g/3.4 kcal = 50 g/ X kcal, where X = 170 kcal.

74. c—Insurance companies prefer that generic medications be dispensed because of the potential savings to both the insurance company and the patient.

75. b—A bevel is the slanted part of the needle, the hub is the place of attachment of a needle, and the lumen is the opening of the needle. Coring refers to the fragments of a vial that contaminate a parenteral solution.

76. a—Drug names are Ativan (lorazepam), Dalmane (flurazepam), Klonopin (clonazepam), and Valium (diazepam).

77. c—The subscription on a prescription consists of directions to a pharmacist and may include compounding, packaging, labeling, and refill instructions and information about the use of generic medication.

78. c—The gauge of a needle is inversely proportional to the diameter of the needle.

79. c—A deductible is an amount an individual must pay before the insurance company begins to make a payment; coinsurance means that two parties are responsible for the payment; copayment means the insured party must pay a given amount of money each time before the insurance company begins to pay; and maximum allowable cost is the most the insurance company will pay for a generic medication.

80. b—i is the Roman numeral for one; gtt means drop; "ou" means each eye; and "bid" means twice per day. Instill one drop in each eye twice per day.

81. c—Januvia is used to treat type 2 diabetes. The other drugs and treatments are as follows: Estraderm (hormone replacement), Isordil (angina), and Nexium (GERD).

82. d—Zyrtec is available as an over-the-counter product.

83. d—Schedules II, III, and IV are monitored through prescription monitoring programs.

84. c—The abbreviation "dtd" is from a Latin expression meaning "give of such doses."

85. c—A microgram is the smallest unit of weight of the answers. Going from smallest to largest, they are microgram, milligram, gram, kilogram.

86. c—Zithromax is a macrolide antibiotic.
87. c—IV (intravenous). The other routes of administration are IA (intraarterial), IM (intramuscular), and SL (sublingual or under the tongue).
88. c—Cordarone is used to treat arrhythmias.
89. d—Spironolactone (Aldactone) is a potassium-sparing diuretic.
90. c—NPI stands for National Provider Identifier.
91. a—The gram is the basic unit of measurement for weight in the metric system.
92. a—Insulin is measured in USP units.
93. b—Carbamazepine (Tegretol) is used to prevent convulsions.
94. b—Anabolic steroids are classified as Schedule III medications.
95. c—A 1:25 ratio is converted to a percentage by dividing the first number of the ratio by the second number and multiplying the answer by 100.
96. a—Diphenoxylate (Lomotil) is a prescription medication used to treat diarrhea.
97. d—Nitroglycerin does not need to be placed in a child-resistant container per the Poison Control Act of 1970.
98. d—Vicoprofen is a controlled substance.
99. c—Premarin is not a transdermal estrogen product; it is taken orally.
100. d—Prescriptions for drugs in Schedules III, IV, and V may be faxed to a pharmacy from a physician's office.

PRACTICE EXAMINATION VI ANSWERS

1. d—Medicare Part D reimburses a pharmacy for prescriptions for Medicare recipients.
2. c—A patient taking milk with tetracycline experiences a drug-food interaction. Milk chelates (binds) with tetracycline, resulting in a loss of effectiveness of the medication. Adverse effects are undesirable effects of a medication; a synergistic effect occurs when the sum of the effects of two drugs is greater than their effects if taken separately.
3. c—1800 hours is the same as 6 PM. Military time begins at midnight, and each hour of the day corresponds to a specific time. Military time does not reset at noon. Military time does not consider AM or PM.
4. c—A "code blue" is a system to communicate to hospital staff that a patient is experiencing a life-threatening situation, such as cessation of his or her heartbeat or breathing. A code blue allows the hospital staff to respond with appropriate emergency procedures.
5. b—H$_2$ receptor agonists would aggravate a gastrointestinal problem rather than cure it or alleviate the symptoms.
6. c—Chewing benzonatate (Tessalon Perles) would result in the patient having excessive salivation.
7. d—Zidovudine is the generic name for Retrovir.
8. a—A pharmacy is to prepare a "stat order" as quickly as possible, within 5 to 15 minutes of receiving the order.
9. a—Body surface area is the most accurate method because it considers both the height and weight of the patient.
10. d—Solving the problem using the formula 9C = 5F − 160 will yield an answer of 50° F.
11. c—This problem can be solved by using a proportion. 4.4 mEq/1 mL = 45 mEq/X mL, where X = 10.2 mL.
12. b—A deficiency in vitamin B$_1$ causes beriberi; deficiency in vitamin A results in night blindness, dry corneas, and inability of the epithelial cells to shed; vitamin C deficiency causes scurvy; and vitamin D deficiency causes rickets.
13. c—A subscriber is the policyholder. A beneficiary is the individual who may receive a cash payout on the death of the subscriber; the dependent is an individual covered under an insurance plan. The patient may be either a subscriber or a dependent on an insurance plan.
14. b—Side effects of anticholinergic drugs include drying up of body fluids, which may cause a dry mouth, difficulty urinating or defecating, and inability to perspire and may cause the eye lens to become dry.
15. b—Convert the patient's weight in pounds to kilograms (13.2 lb × 1 kg/2.2 lb = 6 kg). Multiply the patient's weight in kilograms by the dose (6 kg × 25 mg/kg = 150 mg).
16. c—Multiply the percentage (expressed as a decimal) of talc by the total weight (120 g × 0.02 = 2.4 g or 2400 mg).
17. b—One of the first things to be done in lowering hypertension is to modify the person's lifestyle, which includes reducing sodium intake, eliminating excess calories from the diet, increasing physical activity levels, and reducing alcohol and nicotine consumption. Increasing the amount of sleep an individual receives has no effect on reducing hypertension.
18. a—Hydrochlorothiazide is one of the ingredients found in all the following medications: Diovan HCT, Dyazide, Hyzaar, and Zestoretic. Diovan HCT is valsartan and hydrochlorothiazide; Dyazide is triamterene and hydrochlo-

rothiazide; Hyzaar is losartan and hydrochlorothiazide; and Zestoretic is lisinopril and hydrochlorothiazide.

19. d—Protamine sulfate is used to counteract an overdose of heparin.
20. d—To convert a ratio to a percent, divide the first number by the second number and then multiply the answer by 100.
21. a—Medical record numbers are used only for patients in a hospital.
22. c—MDI is an abbreviation for metered-dose inhaler.
23. c—A solvent is the vehicle that contains the dissolved drug. A solute is the drug that is dissolved into the solvent; a solution contains both the solvent and solute; a syrup is an example of a solvent.
24. a—An arrhythmia is an abnormal heartbeat. Bradycardia, flutter, and tachycardia are examples of various arrhythmias.
25. c—%w/w is defined as the number of grams of a solute dissolved in 100 g. 30 g = 1 oz. Using a proportion of 1 g/100 g = X g/30 g, X = 0.3 g.
26. d—Each state has a board of pharmacy that is responsible for determining the licensing requirements of pharmacists in that state. The state board of pharmacy can suspend or revoke the license of a pharmacist in that particular state. The board of pharmacy is responsible for the practice of pharmacy in a state, which includes pharmacy technicians.
27. b—The prefix *fibro-* means muscle; *-algia* means pain.
28. a—120 mg is the minimum weighable amount on a Class A or Class III balance.
29. a—Capsules can be prepared using the "punch method."
30. c—Material Safety Data Sheets are required by OSHA and must be provided by the manufacturer, importer, or distributor of a hazardous chemical in the workplace. They must be in English and must contain the following information: chemical and common names; if a mixture, the chemical and common names of the ingredients; physical and chemical characteristics; physical hazards; health hazards; route of entry into the body; OSHA permissible exposure limit; precautions for safe handling and use; procedures for cleanup of spills; emergency and first-aid procedures; date of preparation of MSDS or date of latest revision; and the name, address, and telephone number of the manufacturer, importer, or distributor.
31. c—Most liquid antibiotics, including amoxicillin, must be stored in a refrigerator after they are reconstituted. Reconstituted antibiotics are good for 10 days after reconstitution.
32. a—Can be solved by using the following formula: Cost + [(Markup rate)(Cost)] = Retail price. $4.50 + [(0.30)(4.50)] = $5.85.
33. a—Drug names are as follows: Depakote (divalproex), Neurontin (gabapentin), Mysoline (primidone), and Depakene (valproic acid).
34. b—Color of ingredient does not need to be noted on the Master Formula Sheet.
35. b—*oculo* means eye, and *ultro* means each.
36. c—Laminar flow hoods used in the preparation of IV admixtures are a critical component of aseptic technique. The class of the HEPA filter used determines the number of particles allowed per given area.
37. a—A closed formulary is a limited list of medications that may be used in filling prescriptions in an institution or allowed by a managed care third party; an open formulary allows any medication to be dispensed; and a restricted formulary is a hybrid of both an open and closed formulary system.
38. c—Variable copayment may be affected by the cost of the prescription or if the agent is considered a lifestyle drug. Variable copayments may occur if a patient requests the brand-name drug when the physician has given permission for a generic to be used. A fixed copayment means that a patient pays the same copayment regardless of the cost of the prescription; percentage copayment indicates that a patient will pay a given percentage on every prescription regardless of the cost.
39. d—The *Physicians' Desk Reference* is a compilation of monographs submitted by the manufacturers and is published yearly.
40. b—The word root *osteo-* refers to bone.
41. a—

$$\frac{1\,gr}{60\,mg} = \frac{\frac{1}{4}gr}{X\,mg}$$

Cross-multiplying and dividing will yield X = 15 mg.

$$\frac{15\,mg}{1\,tablet} = \frac{15\,mg}{X\,tablet}$$

X = 1 tablet.
42. a—This is a proportion problem. 25,000 units/500 mL = X units/1 mL, where X = 50 mL.
43. b—One liter contains 1000 mL and 2 teaspoons is equal to 10 mL: 1000 mL/10 mL per dose will yield 100 doses.

44. c—An advantage of parenteral medication is that it is injected directly into the patient and the patient does not need to be conscious.

45. b—The Justice Department set up the Drug Enforcement Agency (DEA) to enforce the Controlled Substances Act of 1970.

46. a—An emulsion is a dispersion in which one liquid is dispersed into another immiscible liquid. Emulsions can be either water-in-oil or oil-in-water. Emulsions contain a third phase, which is an emulsifying agent used to prevent the emulsions from separating.

47. a—Presently, only pharmacists are allowed to accept new prescriptions being telephoned into a pharmacy from a physician's office, according to federal law.

48. d—The subscription consists of instructions to the pharmacist. These instructions may include the following information: compounding, packaging, labeling, and refill information and whether a generic drug is permitted to be dispensed.

49. d—Medications can be degraded by light, temperature, and moisture. Amber containers are used to block ultraviolet rays from breaking the medication down.

50. a—Amino acids, dextrose, and lipids are used to prepare a total nutrient admixture.

51. a—The Americans with Disabilities Act prohibits discrimination against an individual with a physical, mental, or emotional disability. The employer must make a reasonable accommodation for the employee. If the disability does not interfere with the individual's ability to perform a particular task, he or she must be considered for employment.

52. c—Doxycycline is in the tetracycline family of antibiotics.

53. a—IV is an approved pharmacy abbreviation for intravenous.

54. c—Pharmacies purchase their medications either directly from the manufacturer or from a secondary vendor such as a wholesaler. Chain pharmacy warehouses are a secondary vendor for a particular chain; GPOs negotiate prices for hospitals.

55. d—The Pharmacy and Therapeutics Committee, which is composed of physicians, pharmacists, nurses, and administrative personnel, develops the formulary for a hospital.

56. b—Methyldopa (Aldomet) is the only approved antihypertensive agent for pregnant women.

57. c—The abbreviation "qsad" means a sufficient quantity to make.

58. d—*USP-NF* stands for *United States Pharmacopeia—National Formulary.*

59. a—Group Purchasing Organizations (GPOs) negotiate prices for hospitals. They do not make the actual purchase of medications for hospitals.

60. c—The Federal Controlled Substances Act requires that all pharmacy records be maintained for a minimum of 2 years.

61. a—The hypothalamus regulates the body, and its goal is to maintain homeostasis within the body.

62. d—Pulse dosing of antifungal agents such as Sporanox has been found to be as effective as taking the medication daily and is cheaper for the patient.

63. b—The Pure Drug Act introduced the terms "adulteration" and "misbranding," but the Food, Drug, and Cosmetic Act of 1938 clearly defined these terms. Adulteration deals with the condition of the product, whereas misbranding is a function of the labeling aspect of the product.

64. a—The word part *-pril* is found in the nomenclature of ACE inhibitors.

65. b—Penicillin does not cause drowsiness; it should not be taken with juices or soft drinks because the acid in the beverages may break down the drug. It is best if penicillin is taken on an empty stomach for reasons related to absorption. Water is the best vehicle for taking medication.

66. c—The problem can be solved using the following formula: Final volume × Strength (expressed as a decimal) = Amount of active ingredient (g) or 100 mL × 1/10,000 = 0.01 g.

67. b—The patient would be receiving 500 mg daily instead of 250 mg per daily, which is twice the amount prescribed by the physician.

68. d—Multiply 500 g by 5% (500 g × 0.05 = 25 g).

69. c—The term 3% net means that a purchaser can reduce a purchase by 3% if he or she pays within a stated period (30 days in this case). Multiply $500.00 by 0.03 = $15.00 (amount of discount). Invoice – Discount = Amount to be remitted; $500.00 – $15.00 = $485.00.

70. c—A flow rate is a volume of liquid infused per period of time (hr). Calculate by dividing 1 L (1000 mL)/24 hr = 41.67 mL/hr. Flow rates are rounded downward instead of upward; therefore 41.67 mL/hr = 41 mL/hr.

71. d—The Controlled Substances Act states that controlled substance prescriptions and invoices containing controlled substances must be stamped with a red 1-inch C.

72. a—Glass mortars and pestles are best used for mixing liquids because of the smooth surface and because they will not stain as porcelain or Wedgwood will.

73. b—Selling price – Cost = Markup: $50.00 – $35.00 = $15.00. Markup/Cost × 100% = Markup rate ($15.00/$35.00) × 100% = 43%.

74. b—Calculate rate/hour and then divide by 60 min/hr (800 mL/12 hr = 66 mL/hr; 66 mL/hr/60 min/hr = 1.1 mL/min).

75. d—%w/v is defined as the number of grams/100 mL. Calculate using the following formula: Final volume × Percent (expressed as a decimal) = Amount of active ingredient; 500 mL × 0.1 = 50 g.

76. b—Solve using the following formula: Final volume × Fraction (expressed as a decimal) = Amount of active ingredient; 650 mL × 1/200 = 3.25 g. Convert grams to mg (3.25 g × 1000 mg/g = 3250 mg). 1 gr/65 mg = X gr/X mg, where X = 325 mg. Next, calculate the number of tablets needed by using the following proportion: 325 mg/1 tablet = 3250 mg/X tablets, where X = 10 tablets needed to prepare the solution.

77. c—%w/v is the number of grams/100 mL; 4 fl oz = 120 mL. Solve using a proportion: 5 g/100 mL = X g/120 mL, where X = 6 g.

78. c—Calculate the rate (1000 mL/4 hr = 250 mL/hr). Next, solve using the following formula: (Rate)(Kit size)(1 hr/60 min) = gtt/min or (250 mL/hr)(10 gtt/mL)(1 hr/60 min) = 41 gtt/min.

79. b—Two tablespoons = 30 mL. Solve using the following formula: (IS)(IV) = (FS)(FV); (30 mL)(85%) = (10%)(FV), where FV = 255 mL. To calculate the number of 3 fl oz (90 mL) bottles, divide the final volume by the volume per bottle (255 mL/90 mL per bottle = 2 full 3 fl oz bottles prepared).

80. d—According to the United States Pharmacopoeia, Syrup USP contains sucrose (sugar) dissolved in water.

81. c—Prescriptions can be written for only a 30-day supply.

82 a—The generic for Omnicef is cefdinir. The brand names for the other generic choices are Claforan (cefotaxime), Rocephin (ceftriaxone), and Cefzil (cefprozil).

83. c—Lorabid is a carbacephem. Azactam is a monobactam; Invanz and Primaxin are carbapenems.

84. c—Ketek is a ketolide. Dynabac is a macrolide; Keflex and Velosef are cephalosporins.

85. d—Sustiva is a nonnucleoside transcriptase inhibitor.

86. c—Heparin is administered intravenously to dissolve blood clots.

87. b—Use a proportion: 500 mL/4 hr = X mL/1 hr, X = 125 mL.

88. a—The monoamine oxidase inhibitors may interact with cured cheeses and red wines containing tyramine.

89. d—Miacalcin is not a bisphosphonate used to treat osteoporosis.

90. a—-*dipine* is a suffix that may designate a drug as a calcium channel blocker, -*mycin* designates macrolides, -*olone* designates steroids, and -*pril* designates ACE inhibitors.

91. a—Many antihistamines may cause drowsiness as a side effect.

92. d—Quality assurance monitors, evaluates, and improves the quality of pharmacy services.

93. d—The patient's telephone number is not required on a prescription label.

94. d—One could take two tablets every 4 hours, which would total 12 tablets in a day.

95. c—"Patient not found" or "invalid ID number" indicates the patient is not enrolled in the prescription plan based on the information entered into the system. It is advisable to check that the bin number, group number, and patient ID number were entered correctly.

96. a—Etoposide should be prepared in a biologic safety cabinet.

97. a—This is an example of a situation that requires a judgment to be made by the pharmacist. Pharmacy technicians perform technical tasks, whereas pharmacists perform both technical and judgmental tasks.

98. d—Zofran is indicated for severe nausea and vomiting, often when a patient is undergoing chemotherapy.

99. d—USP <797> regulates the practice of pharmacy in which sterile products are compounded.

100. b—Ambien is used to induce sleep and should be taken at bedtime.

Index

Note: Page numbers followed by *f* or *t* indicate figures or tables, respectively.